EDITED BY JOHN M. McINNES

A Guide to Planning and Support for Individuals Who Are Deafblind

UNIVERSITY OF TORONTO PRESS
Toronto Buffalo London

© University of Toronto Press Incorporated 1999
Toronto Buffalo London
Printed in Canada

ISBN 0-8020-4242-2 (cloth)

Printed on acid-free paper

Canadian Cataloguing in Publication Data

Main entry under title:

A guide to planning and support for individuals who are deafblind

ISBN 0-8020-4242-2

1. Blind-deaf.   2. Blind-deaf (Services for).   I. McInnes, J.M. (John M.).

HV1597.G84 1999   362.4′1   C99-930065-2

University of Toronto Press acknowledges the financial assistance to its publishing
program of the Canada Council for the Arts and the Ontario Arts Council.

This book is dedicated to the memory of Margot McGrath-Harding, 7 June 1954 – 19 June 1998. Margot was an innovator and leader in the field of Intervenor training as well as in many other aspects of support for persons who are deafblind. Her leadership will be greatly missed.

Contents

Preface

The purpose of this book is to address the problems faced by parents, Intervenors, para-professionals, and professionals who work with infants, children, youth, and adults who are ***congenitally*** or early adventitiously deafblind. Conventional wisdom has divided people who are deafblind into four classes. Both the July 1995 (No. 16) issue of *Deafblind Education*, the journal of Deafblind International (formerly the International Association for the Education of Deafblind People), and the Deafblind Division of the Canadian National Institute for the Blind identify persons who are deafblind as one of the following four types:

- Type one: individuals who were blind and become deaf.
- Type two: individuals who were deaf and become blind.
- Type three: individuals who become deaf and blind as a result of accident or disease after basic language and concepts have been formed.
- Type four: other.

This book will focus on individuals identified as *type four*. They are the infants, children, youth, or adults who were born with or who acquired the disability of deafblindness at an early age. Types one, two, and three have well-established agencies with long histories of interacting with and supporting individuals when they become deafblind. These individuals face many challenges and adjustments, which can be devastating without appropriate support. Throughout this book it is never suggested these individuals need any less specialized support than those identified as belonging to type four.

The type-four individual, who has been identified as 'other,' faces some of the same challenges, but the foundation upon which they stand to meet these challenges is different from that of the members of the first three groups. They have not had the opportunity to develop the language, communication skills, or cognitive and conceptual base upon which to build an understanding of their world. In addition, many individuals who are congenitally or early adventitiously deafblind have additional physical or intellectual disabilities from the time of their birth.

It is for the 'others,' their parents, and the professionals who work with them that this book is written. Our hope is that, after reading this book, all who work with them will approach the infants, children, youth, and adults who are congenitally and early adventitiously deafblind with new hope, increased knowledge, and improved skills, which will lead to greater understanding and success.

The basic premise throughout this book is that deafblindness is a unique disability, which requires a unique approach for support and a unique system to deliver that support. In the first three chapters the focus is on the identification of, planning for, and intervention for individuals who are congenitally or early adventitiously deafblind, regardless of their age. The ways that development of the individual with deafblindness is affected in the areas of communication, cognitive development, social-emotional development, and social sexual development are examined in chapters 4–7. The challenges faced by the deafblind individual and his or her family are considered from a family's viewpoint in chapter 8, and a framework is established for the next four chapters. In chapters 9–12 planning and support for preschool infants, school-aged children, and adults are dealt with. In chapters 12–16 the focus is on developing a support organization, advocacy, and physiotherapy, and on Intervenor, teacher, and consultant training. In chapter 17 a summary of the important points and questions raised is presented while a specific point of view is added to the text. A doorway to find deafblind services in various countries and on the internet and thus to facilitate communication among both parents and professionals at both national and international levels is provided in chapter 18.

Examples are used to illustrate a point or enlarge upon a subject throughout the text. In all cases except where stated otherwise, although the stories are based upon fact, the individuals referred to represent a composite of a number of individuals and/or incidents rather than identifying a specific person or incident.

The book is organized to prevent a constant repetition of key factors, such as explanations of deafblindness, Personal Plans, intervention, Intervenors, and consultants. For example, in chapter 1, the reader will find references to all of the above, but detailed explanations and specific information will be found in other parts of the text. A limited glossary is included to explain terms unique to the field. Items included in the glossary are printed in ***bold italic type*** when they first occur. In addition, a detailed table of contents will allow the reader to find specific information.

Throughout the text the term 'Intervenor' is spelled with a capital 'I' and an 'or' ending. This convention does not signify special status but rather follows the precedent set by *Intervention*, the magazine of the Canadian Deafblind and Rubella Association, and also to draw the reader's attention to the fact that the terms 'Intervenor' and 'intervention' are not derived from the dictionary definition of 'intervener' and 'intervention.' The term 'Intervenor' was first used by Ms J.A. Treffry and the author in the early 1970s to identify a person working with an individual who was deafblind. The term 'intervention' was developed at the same time to encompass the techniques and methods used by the Intervenor.

I would like to thank all the authors who so readily agreed to contribute their expertise to the writing of this book. Without the broad base of knowledge that they represent, this book would have been impossible. Each chapter has been read by at least two, and usually three, reviewers, who have recognized expertise in the particular field covered by the chapter. I would like to thank these forty-plus individuals who took time from their professional responsibilities to read and critique various chapters of the manuscript to ensure its completeness, accuracy, and readability.

I must also thank my wife who supported me throughout the writing and editing and who unstintingly lent her expertise and knowledge to assist me in the completion of the manuscript. Finally, I wish to recognize Catherine Frost for her suggestions and meticulous editing and the staff of the University of Toronto Press for their guidance in the preparation of this manuscript.

JOHN M. McINNES, CONTRIBUTING EDITOR

Contributors

Gary Bridgett is a specialist teacher of the deafblind, has worked as an Intervenor, as a teacher, and as a deafblind resource consultant at the W. Ross Macdonald School in Brantford, Ontario.

Norman Brown was a teacher when his son Stephen was born deafblind in 1966 as a result of congenital rubella, and Norman has been a parent member of Sense (the National Deafblind and Rubella Association) since then. Joining the staff in 1984, Norman was for eight years the family liaison officer at Sense before returning to university for postgraduate studies in 1992. Norman has lectured and taught on courses concerning deafblindness in the United Kingdom and abroad for a number of years and is at present Sense's specialist adviser on congenital deafblindness and joint program coordinator of the University of Birmingham Distance Education Course on Multi-Sensory Impairment. Stephen died in 1987.

Susan Campbell holds certification as a specialist teacher of the deafblind and a specialist teacher of special education. She has held the positions of teacher, educational coordinator, acting program director, and program support teacher in the Deafblind Program at W. Ross Macdonald School in Brantford, Ontario, and is a summer school instructor for the University of Western Ontario, London.

Rodney Clark is chief executive officer of Sense, the National Deafblind and Rubella Association in the United Kingdom. He has led Sense as it has grown from a volunteer parents' self-help group to major service provider for deafblind children and adults; played an important role for many years in the international deafblind field as secretary/treasurer of Deafblind International (DbI), and is providing leadership as Sense is now also operating internationally. He has received the DbI Distinguished Service Award for his work on behalf of the deafblind.

Gini Cloke is the mother of Ian, who was born deafblind as a result of maternal rubella in 1962. Gini has been involved in Sense since the early 1960s, initially as a parent member; has served on various committees and working parties; was a member of Sense Council of Management for many years; has been chair of the Adult Services Committee since 1986, and is also an active member of the European Deafblind Network. Gini is currently employed by Sense as librarian and a family liaison officer, and also is involved in training and giving presentations about Sense and family issues.

Mark Demerling is a graduate of McMaster University and Mohawk College. He has worked in the Deafblind Program at the W. Ross Macdonald School since 1981 and is currently community liaison worker, supporting young adults who are deafblind, their families, service providers, and government agencies in developing and/or obtaining appropriate adult services.

Sheila Eisler obtained a diploma in physiotherapy from the United Birmingham Hospitals School of Physiotherapy in 1963 and worked in England, Scotland, and Germany before moving to Canada in 1980. The author has worked as a physiotherapist at the W. Ross Macdonald School since 1980, gaining extensive experience in the treatment of multiply handicapped deafblind individuals between five and twenty-one plus years of age. She has lectured to groups of visiting professionals and parents on numerous occasions.

Douglas L. Geenens is a board-certified child, adolescent, and adult psychiatrist. He has worked with deafblind children and families throughout the United States. He is a faculty member at the Menninger Clinic in Topeka, Kansas, and has a private practice in Overland Park, Kansas.

Sharon Barrey Grassick is the senior officer for client services and training with the WA Deaf-Blind Association, and part-time visiting teacher for deaf with the Education Department, providing support to students who are deafblind. Originally from New York State, Sharon came to Australia in 1980 as a recipient of a Rotary International Award for Teachers of the Handicapped to study as a research assistant at North Rocks Deaf and Blind Children's Centre. Sharon is secretary of the Australian DeafBlind Council and now lives in Perth with her husband, Iain, and their son, Rob.

Randy Klump for the past seven years has been the technical coordinator for DB-LINK – the National Information Clearinghouse on Children and Youth Who Are Deaf-Blind – and NTAC – the National Technical Assistance Consortium for Children and Young Adults Who Are Deaf-Blind. He has sixteen years' experience in the field of social services, including over nine years' working with children and families.

Linda Mamer holds an EdD and currently works for the British Columbia Provincial Outreach Program for Students with Deafblindness. She instructs in the George Brown College Program for Intervenors for Deafblind Persons; has taught at the W. Ross Macdonald School with students who were visually impaired and deafblind; and is the national president of the Canadian Deafblind and Rubella Association.

Malcolm Matthews is director of policy and national services for Sense. His responsibilities include Sense's policy over the delivery of services and campaigning work. He has worked for Sense since 1989 and contributes to Deafblind International through editing the journal *DbI Review*.

Janis McGlinchey holds certification as a mental retardation counsellor; has experience in the Deafblind Program at the W. Ross Macdonald School, since 1977, as an Intervenor, residence counsellor, and currently as the communication coordinator; is a member of the Canadian Deafblind and Rubella Association and a founding member of the Intervenor Organization of Ontario; is on the advisory committee of the Intervenor Program, George Brown College, and is part-time faculty at Fanshawe College, Simcoe, Ontario.

Margot McGrath-Harding had extensive experience in the field of deafblindness. She began working as an Intervenor in the Deafblind Unit at the W. Ross Macdonald School, worked with the deafblind community at the Canadian National Institute for the Blind in Ottawa, and for the past seven years was a professor and coordinator of the Intervenor for Deafblind Persons Program at George Brown College in Toronto. She was involved in many aspects of education as a founding member of the Brampton Education Network and as a parent volunteer in her sons' schools.

John M. McInnes is certified as a supervisory officer, a specialist teacher of the deafblind, and a school principal. He has been a teacher, a school principal, a teachers' college master, an assistant superintendent of the W. Ross Macdonald School, the program director of Resource Services for the Blind and Deafblind, the executive director of the Group Home for Deafblind Persons, and a consultant. He is a past chairperson of the IAEDB; and for his work with persons who are deafblind has received a Lifetime Membership Award in CDBRA, the Canadian Commemorative Medal, the Anne Sullivan Award, and the IAEDB Distinguished Service Award.

Tom Miller is currently an educational supervisor at the Perkins School for the Blind in Watertown, Massachusetts. He has worked in the field of deafblindness and blindness for the past twenty-five years. He continues to develop and implement social/sex education programs and to consult and lecture on this topic both nationally and internationally.

Carolyn Monaco has been involved in the field of deafblindness since 1978 as a community school Intervenor, residential school Intervenor, a counsellor, a provincial resource consultant for students who are deafblind with the Ministry of Education and Training (Ontario), and a college instructor in the Intervenor for Deafblind Persons Program at George Brown College. She is president of the Ontario chapter of CDBRA and a director on the national board of CDBRA.

Stanley Munroe is the parent of a deafblind adult, a founding member, former president, and currently consultant for special projects for the Canadian Deafblind and Rubella Association, a professional biologist and retired public servant, province of Ontario. He holds Bachelor of Arts and Master of Science degrees from the University of New Brunswick.

Inger Rødbroe is a teacher in special education and has been involved in services for congenitally deafblind people for eighteen years. She is the head of the Assessment Department at Aalborgskolen (a resource centre for deafblind children in Denmark). Staff development is one of her main responsibilities. She is a member of the European Working Group on Communication and Congenital Deafblindness and is a consultant on deafblindness in East Africa.

Lauren Smith has been an Intervenor, a program coordinator, and the executive director of the Group Home for Deaf Blind Persons (Brantford) Inc. and currently is working for the CNIB national office.

Jacques Souriau is a psychologist. He has been the director of a school for deafblind children in France (Poitiers) for twenty-four years. He is also the head of a consultant service for deafblind children. He belongs to the European Working Group on Communication and Congenital Deafblindness.

Connie Taylor-Southall holds certification as a specialist teacher of the deaf, a specialist teacher of the blind, and a specialist teacher of the deafblind; was in the educational field for twenty-five years; and is currently executive director for Independent Living Residences for the Deafblind in Ontario, which is a community-based program for young adults who are congenitally deafblind.

William Thompson holds certification in a variety of educational fields, including principal, specialist teacher of the deafblind, and specialist teacher of special education. He was a teacher of the deafblind and a consultant with Deafblind Resource Services. Currently he is principal as well as acting superintendent of Deafblind Resource Services at the W. Ross Macdonald School in Brantford, Ontario, and is summer school instructor for the University of Western Ontario, London.

Elizabeth Van Kimmenaede holds certification in a variety of educational fields, including principal, specialist teacher of the deafblind, specialist teacher of the deaf, and specialist teacher of special education. She was a teacher of the deafblind and is presently the principal of the Deafblind Program at the W. Ross Macdonald School in Brantford, Ontario.

Bryndis Viglundsdottir was born in Iceland and educated there and in the United States in liberal arts and teaching/special education. She has been teaching in Iceland and Boston (at the Perkins School for the Blind, Deafblind Department) since 1956 and has been head of the Icelandic College of Social Pedagogy since 1976. She retired in 1998. Her other activities include writing and membership in the Association of Icelandic Authors. She has written educational radio programs and numerous newspaper articles on a wide range of topics, including being handicapped, the needs and rights of handicapped people, living in the West Fjords, stories for children, and the American Indians. She has translated into Icelandic books for publication and for Icelandic Radio. She belongs to several professional Icelandic and International Organizations and is on the executive of Deafblind International. She was awarded the Icelandic Falcon Cross for work on improving the quality of life for Icelandic people with special needs by the president of Iceland.

A GUIDE TO PLANNING AND SUPPORT FOR
INDIVIDUALS WHO ARE DEAFBLIND

1

Deafblindness: A Unique Disability

JOHN M. McINNES

Deafblindness is a unique disability,
which requires a unique approach to support
and a unique system to deliver that support.

Introduction

In this chapter I shall review suspected causes of deafblindness; the problems of
identification; errors in identification; problems faced by the individuals with
deafblindness; problems related to the low incidence of the disability; the need
for appropriate planning; and additional considerations that must be taken into
account. I shall also present a Canadian approach to supporting congenital and
early adventitious deafblind individuals at various stages throughout their lives.
My purpose in the chapter is to lay the groundwork for the chapters that follow.

Background

As we move into the twenty-first century, the importance and uniqueness of
each individual has become paramount in our thinking. The emphasis is no
longer on the disability but on the individual who has a disability. Terminology
has also changed. It is no longer correct to use terms such as the handicapped,
the blind, the deaf, the physically handicapped, and the mentally retarded when
the subject is an individual with a disability. This emphasis on the individual
and his or her uniqueness is extremely important when individuals with deafblindness are being considered. Each will have a particular degree of auditory
loss, and visual loss which may have been present at birth or acquired singu-
larly or in combination at different times after birth. The cause of the disability
may be **prenatal viral insult**, prematurity, other congenital afflictions, either

prescribed or recreational drug use by the mother, childhood diseases singly or in combination, or accident. *The only feature common to individuals who are deafblind is that all have some significant degree of deprivation in the use of their **distance senses*** (McInnes and Treffry, 1997, 2).

Causes of Deafblindness

A review of various records and reports from the last twenty-five years shows that in the late 1960s and during the 1970s more than half of the population identified and served as deafblind had rubella or suspected rubella listed as the causal factor and approximately 50 percent of the infants and children had moderate to severe additional disabilities. During the 1980s the number of individuals who were identified as congenitally or early adventitiously deafblind and who were identified as having additional moderate to severe disabilities gradually increased to 65–75 per cent, and as we approach the twenty-first century, the number climbs to 80–95 per cent in some areas. Little will be accomplished here in listing the hundred or more prenatal and postnatal diseases and syndromes that have been documented in various publications and reports.

Perhaps the most worthwhile observation is that the most prevalent causes identified are 'unknown,' followed by prematurity, Usher's syndrome, CHARGE association, meningitis, and various other syndromes and diseases, such as Cytomegloviris and Angleman's syndrome, and that the frequency of any but the most prevalent varies greatly according to the particular geographical area. David Brown notes in his article 'Trends in the Population of Children with Multi-sensory Impairment: 'Within the population of children with multi-sensory impairment the increase in the incidence and severity of multiple disabilities means that every aspect of living and learning becomes more challenging, both for the children themselves and for the families and professionals involved with them ... The fragmentation of the population into many small sub-groups defined by causal agent means that it is now much more difficult to predict development and to decide on educational approaches than was the case when working with a population consisting of mostly children with congenital rubella syndrome: whilst individualisation of assessment and educational programming has always been important ... it is now absolutely essential' (1997, 13).

The most important point to emphasize is that even when additional disabilities are present, either alone or in clusters, a child's deafblindness means that an ever-increasing number of professionals and semi-professionals will have to cooperate, plan, and work together for the deafblind individual's well being. Despite the fact that the person who is deafblind had, and will continue to have, additional disabilities, it is absolutely essential that the support received recognizes and is based on the fact that they are deafblind.

These comments help to set the focus of this chapter and those that follow. They point to the necessity of developing an approach specific to each individual and of implementing it in a way that meets that one individual's needs. In chapters 9–12 the focus is on how such development and implementation occurs at various stages in the deafblind individual's life.

Problems of Identification

In the 1960s and 1970s the problem was to gain recognition and provide services for the disability of deafblindness. In many areas the problem remains the same today.

Who Should Be Treated as Deafblind?

When we suggest that an individual is congenitally or early adventitiously deafblind, we are often met with statements such as 'I know that Jimmy can see. When he comes into the room he comes directly to me,' or 'I know that Susan can hear. She may have an auditory disability and need hearing aids, but she knows when I say NO! She just doesn't pay attention.' When Jimmy enters the room, he does not need much vision to see a big moving blob, nor does Susan require acute hearing to identify a repeated explosive sound that means something like '*bad*' or '*don't do that*' or '*stop.*' A limited ability to use some **residual vision** and/or hearing does not indicate the infant, child, youth, or adult does not have to be supported as deafblind.

A Defining Question

The question is not whether an individual with deafblindness has some residual vision and/or hearing, regardless of age. The questions to be asked about individuals with suspected vision and hearing loss are, in most situations of everyday living: (a) Do they have sufficient vision to compensate for loss of hearing and thus function as hearing-impaired persons? (b) Do they have sufficient hearing to function as if they were visually impaired? (c) Do they have sufficient residual vision and hearing to function as if they have no significant disability? If the answer to a, b, or c is NO, then the individual who has both a vision and a hearing loss is deafblind regardless of any additional disabilities.

A Russian Viewpoint
A. Meshcheryakov in his book, *Awakening to Life*, addresses the problem. He points out, 'Deaf-blindness is (usually) defined as the loss of sight and hearing from birth or early infancy and dumbness resulting from lack of hearing'; he

continues, 'The definition is inadequate. The definition of deaf-blindness from the pedagogical point of view should supply an answer to the question. Who needs to be taught as deaf-blind?' (1979, 70).

U.S. Congress Recognizes Deafblindness

In spite of the fact that government bodies, such as the United States Congress, find that deafblindness is among the most severe of all forms of disabilities, and there is a great and continuing need for services and training to help individuals who are deafblind attain the highest possible level of development (U.S. Code), many of the problems identified on pages 8–15 occur, and they may prevent or delay an individual from receiving appropriate services.

A U.S. Approach

Victor Baldwin, in a presentation at the National Symposium on Children and Youth Who Are Deaf-Blind, states that under the 1990 federal definition, 'The term "Children with deafblindness" means children and youth having auditory and visual impairments, the combination of which creates such severe communication and other developmental and learning needs that they cannot be appropriately educated without special education and related services beyond those that would be provided solely for children with hearing impairments, visual impairments, or severe disabilities to address their educational needs due to these concurrent disabilities.' He continues, 'The new federal definition not only ruled out programs that are designed solely for students who are blind or solely for students who are deaf, but also programs that are designed solely for students with severe disabilities.' It appears that the latter condition was added for the same reasons the first two were included. There was a concern that students who are deafblind were being placed in programs where the instruction might not focus on the unique conditions created by the dual sensory loss (Baldwin 1992, 48).

A Scandinavian Definition of Deafblindness

A Scandinavian study affirmed that deafblindness is a unique disability and must be approached as such. The Nordic Council of Ministers, on the advice of the Nordic Committee on Disability,[1] representing Norway, Sweden, Denmark, Finland, the Faeroe Islands, the Aland Islands, Greenland, and Iceland, adopted a definition of deafblindness that has formed a focal point for study by various professional groups. The Nordic definition states:

A person is deafblind when he or she has a severe degree of combined visual and auditory impairment. Some people who are deaf-blind are totally deaf and blind, while others have residual hearing and residual vision. The severity of the combined visual and auditory impairment means people who are deaf-blind cannot automatically use services for people with visual impairments or with hearing disabilities.

Thus, deaf-blindness entails extreme difficulties with regard to education, training, working life, social life, cultural activities, and information. For those who are born deafblind or who become deafblind at an early age, the situation is complicated because they may have additional problems affecting their personality and behavior. Such complications further reduce their chances of exploiting any *residual vision or hearing*. Deaf-blindness must therefore be regarded as a separate disability that requires special methods of communication and special methods for coping with the functions of every day life.

Definition Follow-up

A group of leading Scandinavian ophthalmologists and audiologists held a working conference in Dronninglund in August 1986 to study the Nordic definition and, as a result of their deliberations, issued the following statement as a guide to members of the medical profession throughout Scandinavia (adapted from a translation).

1. Deafblindness is a separate disability. It is characterized by the following criteria:
   - Serious problems in relation to communication with the environment
   - Serious problems in relation to orientation in the environment
   - Serious problems in relation to the acquisition of information.
2. Deafblindness may occur separately or in combination with other disabilities.
3. Upon suspicion that a person is actually suffering from deafblindness, or that it might develop in a person, the following diagnostic procedures should be carried out.
   - Examination of the hearing and vision functions by specialists experienced in deafblindness
   - In addition to the medical examination, an assessment related to the three functional criteria mentioned in (1) above
   - This assessment should be made by staff with special training (in the area of deafblindness) having a medical, social, and pedagogic background and adequate extensive education.
4. When diagnosing, one will find persons that fulfil the three functional criteria of deafblindness, but when using the current medical methods, one cannot register impairments of sight and/or hearing. These persons are also to be considered as being deafblind.
5. As deafblindness is a separate disability, all persons who are deafblind,

regardless of where they live and regardless of age and eventual (possible) institutionalization, should have access to special *habilitation* and *rehabilitation* (special aids, special teaching, special housing conditions, etc.).

It is evident from the definitions used on both sides of the Atlantic that deafblindness is recognized as a unique disability. It is equally evident that this disability requires an approach that differs significantly from that used with individuals who are challenged by blindness, deafness, or who have other severe multiple disabilities. Unless the person can function as an individual either with visual impairment or with auditory impairment and for whom no extensive additional allowances or adjustments are required, he or she must be supported as a person who is deafblind.

Recognition of Deafblindness as a Single Disability

Perhaps the single most serious problem faced by individuals of all ages who are congenitally or early adventitiously deafblind is the failure of the 'system' to recognize deafblindness as a single handicap. The importance of this oversight cannot be overemphasized. The 1990 Conference of the International Association for the Education of Deafblind People (IAEDB, since renamed *Deafblind International*) unanimously passed a resolution to change the spelling of *deaf-blind* to *deafblind*. This simple gesture was intended to lay to rest both the concept that the disability is deafness plus blindness and approaches to amelioration on the basis of whether the student was more deaf or more blind. At the time of writing, this spelling has been widely adopted throughout the world.

Alternative Labels

There seems to be a reluctance, particularly on the part of some individuals with *acquired deafblindness*, to use the term deafblind. This reluctance appears to have diminished since the advent of the *Deafblind List* on the Internet. Labels such as visually and auditorily impaired, multiply sensory deprived, multi-sensory impaired, Deaf and Blind, Blind Deaf and deaf-blind still may be found in contemporary literature. Such differences in labelling can cause confusion in the minds of the general population. It has been the author's experience that the term 'deafblind' itself is often the source of a significant problem. The use of the term, particularly prior to its being written as one word, sometimes has caused administrators to try to meet the needs of deafblind individuals by gathering together a group of experts from various specialties because they did not realize the need to hire a specialist in the field of deafblindness. Experts from other fields, while competent in those fields, do not understand the effects of a combined vision and hearing loss on the usefulness of their traditional practices. The problems associated with this approach are discussed in the following section (the combining experts from other fields error).

Errors in Identification

A variety of errors, both intentional and inadvertent, are made when individuals are being identified or assigned to support programs. Such errors (approaches) include, but are not limited to, the following:

- most significant disability
- identification as intellectually challenged
- additional disabilities error
- premature infants identification question
- combining experts from other fields

Most Significant Disability Error

Administrators often try to rationalize the decision of not providing support designed specifically to meet the needs of individuals who are deafblind by pointing out that the individual has some usable vision and/or hearing. They then try to identify which of these two disabilities presents the most severe problem and use their conclusion as the basis for placement, programming, and support.

The 'most significant disability approach' may be necessary to treat a person medically, but dividing them into parts for educational and developmental support is a flawed approach. It is sometimes contended that this most significant disability is ameliorated, the other problems will be significantly reduced or eliminated, and as a result, the individual's needs will be met. The error lies in not realizing that deafblindness is not an additive group of conditions, but is rather a single disability that affects overall development, socialization, and communication.

Identification as Intellectually Challenged Error

Some individuals who are deafblind have suffered severe brain damage from prenatal insult, disease, or accident. They require a specialized type of care. It is important that intervention techniques form the basis for such care. Experience has shown, that many of these individuals who are identified as 'low function-ing' require, and can benefit from, a Personal Plan approach. There is no excuse for denying the benefits of planning and support to an individual with deaf-blindness because he or she is identified as intellectually challenged.

MP was a young adult who was deafblind. He had been identified as 'retarded' (the term then in use) and was institutionalized at an early for his own good and that of the family. When the institution was closed in the late 1980s, he was placed in a program for adults who were deafblind. After a very slow and difficult adjustment, he now lives in an apartment, which he shares with another deafblind person, and takes care of his personal space and possessions. He shares responsibility for the part of the apartment that they both use, as well as taking his turn in being responsible for shopping and meal preparation. All this was accomplished through careful planning backed by the support of trained Intervenors who understood the importance of communication and how to 'do with' rather than 'for' him in a responsive rather than a directive environment.

Through mediation between the individual and the environment, he or she can be helped to experience, accept, organize, and react to external stimuli. Where the potential exists, the learned use of residual vision and hearing can provide important sensory information. If these benefits are to be gained, how-ever, the use of such sensory input must be taught and rewarded (see chapter 5). Essential motor skills, concepts, an effective means of communication, life skills, mobility skills, and social skills can be developed. Many of the individu-als, initially identified as low functioning, whom we worked with as infants and children in the 1970s are now living in their own houses or apartments supported by Intervenors. They are participating in a variety of community organizations, pursuing a variety of occupations or volunteer activities, and continuing to exhibit an ever-increasing level of competence and independence.

We always ask ourselves the following questions when we review a file of an individual who is deafblind and find, as a result of the application of standard-ized tests, developmental scales, or other diagnostic techniques, that a label indicating intellectual deficit or low functioning has been applied:

1. Who did the diagnosis?
2. Were the instruments used normed on a deafblind population?
3. How did the diagnostician communicate with the infant, child, or youth?
4. How did the diagnostician know that the communication was understood?
5. How did the diagnostician motivate the individual to respond?
6. How much experience had the diagnostician and/or the individual interpret-ing the results in working with and evaluating infants, children, or youth who are deafblind?

7. What type of program, if any, had the infant, child, or youth been receiving?
8. How long had the infant, child, or youth been in the program?
9. Where did the evaluation take place?
10. Was it a formative or summitive type evaluation?
11. Was a parent allowed and encouraged to be present at, and participate in the evaluation procedure?
12. Were both the infant, child, or youth and the parent at ease?

Complete and satisfactory answers must be found to these questions before a label identifying the individual as other than deafblind is acceptable. Until that time no label other than suspected deafblind should form even a minor part of the basis for placement or program planning.

It is true that some individuals with deafblindness have diminished intellectual abilities. Unfortunately, this identification is often made all too readily by professionals who have no understanding of the disability resulting from deafblindness. The older the individual, the more likely it is that the label of 'severely developmental delayed' or 'intellectually challenged' may be applied. Of course, a person who is deafblind is going to develop differently from an individual with both sight and hearing. The individual with congenital or early adventitious deafblindness will also develop significantly differently from an individual with a visual disability or an individual with an auditory disability.

The inability to obtain sufficient non-distorted information from the environment should never be confused with the inability to process it. It is not unusual to find the problem of lack of information confused with the lack of the ability to process it. To illustrate this point we suggest that you get a piece of paper and attempt the following:

1. List twelve Inuit words for snow.
2. Give the location of your house to the nearest minute and second of longitude and latitude.
3. Describe a 'Calabogie.'
4. To the nearest half-degree, give the surface temperature of lava.
5. Explain in detail why the ink in your ballpoint pen does not run out.
6. Say 'Hello' in Japanese.
7. Give the population of the capital city of your country within 100 persons.
8. Describe the difference between a rotary engine and a fuel-cell engine when used to propel an automobile.
9. Tell me about your spider gears.
10. What were the names of your great-great-grandfathers' wives?

If you cannot do all of the above, does this prove that you are mentally challenged, or do you simply lack the information to be able to 'perform' to my expectations of you? Always question both the diagnosis and the degree of intellectual challenge being assumed. In most cases the deafblind individual's lack of ability to obtain sufficient non-distorted information from the environment will be a far more significant factor than his or her ability to manipulate, store it, and apply it.

Additional Disabilities Error

Two new and disturbing arguments have arisen concerning the identification and support for infants and very young children who are deafblind and who have additional severe disabilities. First, it is sometimes argued that if they are identified as deafblind they will require the allocation of large amounts of scarce financial resources, and thus they will be best served in the long run by being placed in and programmed for under an already existing label. When there is hesitation to identify such infants and young children as deafblind, several important factors are ignored or forgotten. If an infant has a combined vision and hearing loss, which would otherwise cause them to be identified as deafblind, their ability to communicate with and interact with their environment will be so impaired that, regardless of other disabilities, the possibility of physical, social, and intellectual development will be severely limited unless specialized approaches are incorporated into the total approach used. Even when a therapist is able to interact successfully with a younger deafblind client, the application and practice of the skills being developed will not take place unless the specialized techniques needed to encourage the use of these skills and to promote practice between therapy sessions are used. When these techniques are used, the expected outcomes of the therapy sessions will occur. Without them, the proper chair will simply get bigger or the limb or hand will gradually become less responsive.

Second, some administrators, particularly those whose sole responsibility is for infant and preschool services, see this situation as short term. The child will no longer be their problem when he or she turns four, five, or six years of age. Such an approach completely ignores the fact that the early years are some of the most important periods for growth and development. In chapter 4, 'Communication,' Rødbroe and Souriau demonstrate the necessity of immediate identification and specialized approaches in the development of communication. If the larger picture is considered, it will be recognized that without such specialized approaches such infants will grow into adults who have a severely limited degree of self-sufficiency and thus will require that society spend more money to care for and support them for the rest of their lives. Even where the most significant disability is identified as being of a physical or intellectual nature, deafblindness will affect what is being learned, how it is learned, and how the learning is applied. Trying to meet the needs of the person who is deafblind by placing him or her in a program designed to meet the needs of individuals with another disability will not work. The person with deafblindness must have an approach specifically designed to meet his/her needs.

Another rationale used to justify the most significant disability approach is that such special programs provide the specialized services of a particular staff member, such as a nurse, physiotherapist, or speech therapist, or that such classes have a low teacher-student ratio. A realistic analysis will show the individual with deafblindness will use the services of specialized staff, such as the physiotherapist, for a limited time each day, and these usually can be made available without the particular placement.

Where a low student to staff ratio exists in programs designed to ameliorate other disabilities, it is because the three, five, or ten students with the specific disability found in the class represent the largest number of children with this disability the teacher of the specialized program can support. To expect that teacher and other support staff also to become specialists in the area of deafblindness is unrealistic.

Deafblindness is a unique disability that requires a unique support system. Attempting to use an existing program designed to support individuals with other disabilities, rather than identifying them as deafblind and supporting them as such, is not only ineffective, it is inexcusable.

Premature Infants Identification Question

Infants who are very premature may appear to have both serious visual and serious hearing losses. Some professionals argue that because they have **cortical visual impairment** and/or **central hearing loss**, they may grow out of it. While it is recognized that they will initially require treatment as infants who are deafblind, the disagreement arises as to whether they should continue to be supported as persons who are deafblind if they begin to use their residual vision and hearing effectively in some circumstances. One school of thought favours dropping the client as soon as he or she appears to function under some circumstances as if he or she were not deafblind. Another school feels that the infant, child, or youth will continue to need support as a person who is deafblind on into adulthood. This second group argues that the need for a wider understanding of, and communication with, the environment will continue to be effected; the ability to communicate will continue to be reduced; and the deafblind individual will continue to be faced with long periods of isolation.

Dr Rosemary Davidson stated, at the 1996 Vancouver Conference on Deaf-blindness, during a session devoted to evaluation and service, that in her experience children and youth continued to need support as individuals who were deafblind in spite of the fact that in many situations they appeared to function as individuals who have either a visual or an auditory challenge. She pointed out that factors such as changes in lighting, background noise, and many other circumstances will severely affect their interaction with others and the environment. Therefore, despite some appearances to the contrary, they will continue to need to be supported as individuals who are deafblind, regardless of age.

In the author's experience, the identification and support of premature infants as deafblind becomes an individual matter relating to the functioning of each infant as he or she grows and develops. If *in most*, not merely some, situations, an individual appears to begin to function as visually impaired, auditorily impaired, or in some extreme cases as non-sensorily impaired, rather than as if deafblind, the level of support and the use of specialized techniques can be gradually withdrawn. The contact with the family and the individual by the specialist in deafblindness should be continued. Periodic visits should be made to observe the current level of functioning in home, community, and school settings. The specialist, *in consultation with the family*, should be ready to re-establish immediately an appropriate level of support at the first indication of difficulty. Costly delay may result if the specialist is required to refer to a administrator or a review board for permission to re-establish services. Periodic, ongoing contact should continue for several years after the last evidence of difficulty has disappeared.

For example, PC is a young person who was supported as deafblind when she was an infant. This support was withdrawn, and within six months she was referred back to the deafblind specialists because she had become so unmanageable that the official diagnosis by local preschool authorities was 'severely emotionally disturbed and mentally retarded.' This scenario of dropping of service, breakdown in functioning, and re-referral to deafblind services was repeated three times before she reached her sixth birthday and twice more before it was accepted that she would continue to require ongoing support as an individual with deafblindness. Each time she appeared to function as a child with a hearing disability, a local authority decided that the designation as deafblind was inappropriate and had the support withdrawn. In fairness to these local authorities, whenever PC received appropriate support she did indeed appear to function as if she would no longer need either intervention or a Personal Plan. Happily, PC is now being supported as a young adult with deafblindness. She shows no emotional problems. She constantly is challenging all about her with questions concerning computers, internet researches, email, how her government support payments are being used, and so on.

It must be emphasized that the appearance of the ability to function successfully under some circumstances does not indicate that the person is not functioning as an individual who is deafblind. A good Intervenor will identify the particular circumstances where such abilities are exhibited and help the person who is deafblind to utilize, expand, and improve on his or her ability to function successfully at this level. The Intervenor will also realize that communication and isolation are two ongoing problems that must be constantly addressed. It is important that the Intervenor use a variety of techniques to check if the person who is deafblind really understands what he or she appears to have seen or heard. Such checking will often show that the information the person is receiving from the environment is distorted or incomplete. When the person is not supported appropriately and misunderstands or misinterprets information, behaviours may develop that will cause identification as emotionally disturbed, severely developmentally delayed, or mentally challenged.

Combining Experts from Other Fields Error

As a child enters the school years, educational and social service administrators are often reluctant to identify him or her as deafblind, either because they do not wish formally to identify another category requiring service or because of the cost involved in the specialized services required by this unique population. This failure to identify a child as deafblind sometimes results in attempts to meet his or her needs by bringing together experts on visual disability and auditory disability. Most of these experts have little understanding of the problems presented by deafblindness. They are experts in fields such as the use of vision to compensate for the loss of hearing and the use of a combination of hearing and tactile input to compensate for the loss of vision. This is not to say that these practitioners cannot learn to work with individuals who are deafblind. Many of the most knowledgeable experts in deafblindness came to its study from one of these areas. Without specialized training in the field of deafblindness, however, such professionals are no better able to meet the needs of a person who is deafblind than any other person. Teams whose claim to expertise rests solely on the fact that they have representatives from such fields are not prepared to offer adequate programming, counselling, and support for the person who is deafblind or for their families.

Problems Faced by the Individual Who Is Deafblind

The problems faced by this population are complex. They may

- lack the ability to interact with their environment

- have difficulty in communicating with others
- face long periods of isolation
- have a distorted perception of their world and the expectations of both family and society at large
- lack the ability to understand the results of their actions
- lack the ability to anticipate future events
- be deprived of many of the most basic extrinsic motivations
- have additional medical problems
- be placed in, and fail, programs designed to ameliorate other disabilities
- be judged according to inappropriate standards
- have extreme difficulty in establishing and maintaining interpersonal relationships
- have significant problems in developing and using an effective personal learning style.

These are but a few of the more serious results of the loss of the effective use of the distance senses. Workers in the fields of deafness, blindness, mental challenges, and physical disabilities often fail to grasp the significance or the complexity of the problem and attempt to implement partial solutions or to modify existing programs to meet the needs of the deafblind individual. Following is a discussion of some of the more common problems.

Modelling

The individual who is deafblind often has a difficult time watching, understanding, and modelling behaviour after family members and others with whom he or she comes in contact. Even if there is some residual vision, it is a continuing challenge to get him or her to look at what someone is doing and to imitate it. This is one of the main reasons hand-over-hand techniques are so strongly advocated as an initial instructional intervention technique (see chapter 3). With the use of techniques appropriate to the child's specific degree of vision and hearing loss, the deafblind child can be taught to model his or her attempts and compare results with those of his or her peers during suitable activities. Learning appropriate social behaviour through modelling is a much more difficult task and will take a long time to develop.

Developing a Learning Style

The deafblind specialist must help the individual to develop a unique learning style that

- takes advantage of any residual vision and hearing
- promotes sensory integration
- encourages curiosity
- takes advantage of his or her strengths
- promotes the setting of realistic individual goals
- builds self-confidence
- allows the individual to ask for assistance appropriately while still feeling free to reject such assistance.

Incidental Learning

It is unlikely that individuals with deafblindness, regardless of age, will obtain and assimilate a large amount of information from the environment when they are not assisted to do so. When they attempt to do so without intervention, the information received is often incomplete or distorted. Because of the frustrations arising from attempts to gather such information without Intervenor support, many individuals who are deafblind find it is easier to withdraw into themselves rather than continue to attempt the impossible. It is often far more frustrating to receive bits and pieces of information that seem disconnected or meaningless than to withdraw.

Peers who are not visually and auditorily challenged, as they develop cognitively, will gain much of their knowledge of people, places, societal norms, and an ever increasing variety of things without consciously being aware of absorbing the information. Little such incidental learning will be available to individuals who are deafblind. Not only will they have to be introduced to almost all learning using appropriate specialized techniques, they will also require a carefully constructed plan that will compensate not only for '*how*' but also for '*what*' they learn. The things learned by peers in both formal and informal groups or incidentally through the process of living in a family and growing up in the community will not be acquired in the same quantity or in a non-distorted form even where the individual who is deafblind has some residual vision or hearing.

Communication

As Rødbroe and Souriau (chapter 4) point out, communication is much more than the ability to sign. It encompasses an understanding of the concepts attached to each sign, interaction between two or more people, and a grasp of what each person understands by the sign or gesture as well as how the concept is modified by both the environment and the context in which it is used. A good

Intervenor must know not only how to communicate in the medium used by the specific individual with whom he or she is intervening but also what is understood by the individual when the gesture, sign, or finger-spelled word is used.

People are often extremely rude to individuals with deafblindness. It is so convenient – and totally unacceptable – to talk to others without signing when you would not hold the same conversation in the presence of an individual who could see and hear. It is often surprising, even to those of us who frequently work hands-on with deafblind clients, when an individual for whom we are intervening, if we fail to include him or her in our conversation, asks whom we are talking to and about what. Persons who are deafblind should not have to guess or feel left out when two or more sighted individuals are talking in their presence.

When we communicate with others, we use more than words. When speaking to someone else in the presence of a deafblind person, you should communicate what you are saying in such a way that the individual who is deafblind will know and understand. If you do not wish him or her to know what you are saying, then do what you would do if another hearing person was in the room: excuse yourself, explaining that you wish to talk to – and, going to a private place, do so. As a general rule, unless you wish to convey that communication is unimportant, include the deafblind individual in every conversation taking place in his or her presence.

Without adequate means of communication, progress through the stages of cognitive development appropriate to his or her age will not take place. Minimal progress is not necessarily evidence of low potential but may be due to lack of the necessary communication tools needed to perceive accurately, and respond meaningfully, to the environment. Even when there is in a Personal Plan in place, the Intervenor must constantly keep in mind that every experience must be designed to promote the development of communication skills until an adequate base of language, experience, and understanding is established. Limited experience leads to limited understanding, limited understanding to limited functioning, and limited functioning to limited experience. An unbreakable cycle leading to learned helplessness is formed. Or, from another point of view, a self-fulfilling prophecy that will ensure that the individual will be identified as low functioning has been put in place.

The basic concept in planning for the person who is deafblind is *meaningful communication can be developed by meaningful interaction within a reactive environment.*

Motivation

Motivation for the individual with deafblindness differs in many ways from that experienced by his or her peers.

Anticipation

The lack or diminished amount of non-distorted visual and auditory input reduces the deafblind individual's ability to anticipate coming events from environmental cues. Mother's entry into the room does not signify comfort, food, or cuddling. The teacher's entry into the classroom does not signal time to go to work. A peer's or employer's appearance does not signal the need for a change in behaviour. The inability to anticipate what will happen next can make each experience a new, puzzling, and/or frightening one. As the infant becomes a child, then a youth, and finally an adult, the inability to perceive the environment accurately often prevents anticipation of the results of his or her actions or the actions and reactions of others. Individuals who are totally blind and profoundly deaf receive little or no information about the ever-changing environment that surrounds them. Individuals with some residual vision or hearing often must face two problems. First, much of the information they receive may be distorted and may lead to mistaken interpretation. Secondly, people in their environment, even those who know them quite well, often assume that they see, hear, and understand more than they do, and thus, they expect them to reply or act appropriately.

With the support of a trained Intervenor, the individual who is deafblind can gather a great deal of useful, non-distorted information from the environment. Even then, the enormity of the task makes it impossible to receive the amount of complex information we receive incidentally or by directed attention. It is this constant flow of information that influences our every action, our every decision, and our opinions of others and that lays a foundation on which we can anticipate coming events. The problem may appear to be lack of intelligence or indifference, when it is, in fact, only lack of information.

The ability to anticipate provides a strong motivational factor. It allows us to review possible courses of action, evaluate choices open to us, and prepare both physical and social responses. Without the ability to anticipate, we often do not have the opportunity to 'prepare' and our inborn 'fight or flight' response takes over. It would not be viewed as unusual or inappropriate to resist if you are grabbed by the shoulder or wrists in a dark hall or while crossing an unlit parking lot at night. Yet individuals who are deafblind are labelled as tactile defensive or uncooperative when they resist when their hands are grabbed with no clues provided that will allow them to anticipate what is going to happen. Their behaviour is judged to be inappropriate. In addition, the ability to anticipate favourable outcomes provides a strong motivation to try.

Curiosity
Curiosity is another important motivational factor. The individual who is visu-

ally challenged is encouraged to be curious through the use of sounds. The individual who is auditorily challenged is encouraged to be curious through the use of visual stimuli. Individuals who are deafblind are deprived of such extrinsic motivation to stimulate their curiosity. Their whole world exists within the area of their random reach, blurred or restricted vision, and/or distorted sound and primarily within themselves. As the infant becomes a child, then a youth, and eventually an adult, the habit of being curious and of exploring is not developed unless it is stimulated and rewarded in infancy and reinforced at all stages of development up to and including adulthood.

The problem often arises because it is much easier to have a 'good' deafblind infant or young child, who does not explore, break things, and do the things that form part of the life of their siblings at that age. It is much easier to have children, youth, and adults who 'don't poke their noses' into things and conversations that don't concern them. If they don't do so, it may indicate that something is very wrong, and every effort must be made to rekindle the spark of curiosity.

Imitation

The ability to learn by imitation is a strong motivational factor that is severely restricted in the deafblind population unless appropriate intervention is available. Social patterning and skill acquisition are affected by the inability to perceive accurately and imitate either the actions or the creations of others. It is from these perceptions that the knowledge, skills, and attitudes of the individual who is deafblind and his or her perception of self and understanding of the expectations of others will primarily be formed. Intervention is necessary to help the person who is deafblind to overcome these problems and form accurate perceptions that will allow the use of imitation as an effective means of learning.

Emotional Bond

Love and affection form another set of basic motivational factors. Because of physical problems, tactile sensitivity, and parental tensions, the infant who is deafblind often has difficulty forming an emotional bond with his parents, family members, and peers. This bonding is of the utmost importance to the development of the individual who is deafblind. The absence of other effective extrinsic motivational forces makes the establishment of this bond essential (see chapters 4 and 6 for further discussion).

A strong motivational bond will not lead to inappropriate dependence or to the formation of an inappropriate self-image by the person who is deafblind. We all form such bonds. The development of a strong motivational bond is a preferable alternative to withdrawal into the total isolation of hypo-activity or a hyperactive life that uses motion, rocking, self-mutilation, and destructive behaviour to shut out the world.

These are but a few of the many extrinsic motivational factors that are diminished or absent in the life of the individual who is deafblind when appropriate support is not available.

Self-Stimulation

Another problem often faced by the congenitally deafblind person of any age is the severely reduced amount of stimulation received from his or her world. This isolation often results in the individual's finding inappropriate, substitute methods of stimulation, which unfortunately are often encouraged and rewarded. A discussion of the causes of and problems faced by infants and children who are deafblind will be found in *Deaf-Blind Infants and Children* (McInnes and Treffry 1997) and in chapter 6 of this text. It is important to note here that such children often are less mobile, less adventuresome, and more passive than most of their peers. Regardless of their age, many individuals who are deafblind are prone to develop a variety of self-stimulation activities, such as continuous motion, seeking long periods on a whirligig, swinging, poking the eyes, waving fingers before the eyes, rocking, staring at lights, or ritualistically repeating specific activities.

JR was a three-year-old child who was deafblind. She spent hours circling around the room in a seemingly random manner and appearing to examine first one object, then another. She had a small amount of residual vision, but careful observation over a period of time showed motion was one activity that she could use to shut out the world. The examining of objects was approved of by the family because she never broke anything. Visitors marvelled at her actions. The activity kept her occupied for hours at a time. She had found a socially acceptable means of self-stimulation.

SL was a young man who was deafblind. He attended a community-based program for the intellectually challenged. He sat at a table putting ten things in each envelope until a dozen envelopes were filled. He then emptied each envelope into a box and started the routine again. This was simply a self-stimulation activity that was tolerated (in fact actually approved of) by the staff of the centre. When it was suggested that he could stuff envelopes that would actually be mailed the staff explained that this was impractical because someone would have to go and get the fliers and someone else would have to stamp them and see that they were mailed. Who better than SL with the support of an Intervenor!

Another type of self-stimulation that is often fostered, approved of, and rewarded is the use of age-inappropriate puzzles or toys. Unfortunately, it is not unusual to see adults who are deafblind left sitting at a table with a puzzle designed for a preschooler. They will continually complete the puzzle and then dump the pieces on the table to start again. This is not even busy work; it is approved self-stimulation, pure and simple. Promoting such self-stimulation should not be an option. Craft projects, care of personal space, and a large variety of adult activities are more productive and rewarding.

In all of the above examples and in the countless ones that every person working in the field has observed, what is missing is meaningful communication with and feedback from the environment during age-appropriate activities. Without proper support, such as that supplied by an Intervenor, any activity can degenerate from a new experience to a routine and, if not supported appropriately, into a self-stimulatory activity. Cleaning a table after meals is a necessary routine; continually cleaning a table to the exclusion of interaction with individuals in the environment is self-stimulation! It is not what is done but how and when an activity is done that makes it either appropriate or self-stimulation.

Discipline

A problem sometimes arises because there is a strong temptation for those working with an individual who is deafblind, regardless of his or her age, to move the person about and to discipline behaviour without any, or insufficient, communication. Discipline through physical manipulation is a trap into which many fall. An explanation often given is that he or she is being 'placed out of harm's way.' As the child becomes a youth, size and strength make previously tolerable behaviour dangerous to him or herself and others. A slight physical resistance becomes an unmanageable one. Easily controlled physical responses become major behaviour problems that make physical restraint necessary. As the infant grows, frustrations grow, and eventually this course of action-reaction becomes a perpetual cycle that is hard to break, a level of USUAL behaviour that is hard to deal with. It is important, when one is dealing with an infant, that time is taken to ensure that he or she understands and can anticipate WHAT is going to happen and WHY. The time taken to communicate effectively at the infant and child stages will pay dividends when he or she becomes a youth or adult. When time is not taken, particularly with a high-functioning infant or child, the foundations are being laid for severe behaviour problems in the later years.

Problems Due to the Low Incidence of Deafblindness

There are a number of major problems that may result from the low incidence of the disability. These include, but are not limited to, the following:

- No pool of community knowledge
- Need for intervention misunderstood
- Establishing self-fulfilling prophecies
- Need for an appropriate Personal Plan.

No Pool of Community Knowledge

In most communities there is no pool of knowledge about and understanding of the disability of deafblindness. Such information is available to the family of an individual who is blind, physically disabled, deaf, intellectually challenged, or challenged by a combination of disabilities. This lack of community understanding constantly erodes the underpinnings of the family and can affect the level of service made available to the individual with deafblindness.

Members of the community try to relate the problems of the infant, child, or youth to disabilities with which they are familiar. Where disabilities in addition to deafblindness exist, they are often seized upon as the basis for labelling, and thus for service.

Need for Intervention Misunderstood

The basic need of the individual who is deafblind for appropriate intervention is frequently misunderstood by professionals from other support groups and by administrators. They often see requests for Intervenor support as requests for parent relief, and while parents of deafblind children certainly do need parent relief, this is a completely different issue. Workers and administrators in community support programs may become impatient with the family of the person who is deafblind when the family appears to refuse to be satisfied with existing levels and types of community services. Among the responses often received by the family of a deafblind individual is the assertion that if all mentally challenged persons had one-to-one support, they also would make extraordinary progress. Examination of this contention quickly shows that there is a substantial difference between being able to receive sufficient information from the world through sight and hearing and the ability to process such information.

The misunderstanding of the need for and the use of intervention arises from many sources and manifests in many ways. For example, with most disabilities, success is measured in part by the reduction of dependence upon people for assistance, and conversely, an increased need for additional human support is indicative of a deterioration. *As individuals with deafblindness improve in their level of functioning and knowledge of the options open to them, MORE, not less, intervention is needed.* As the individual who is deafblind becomes more aware of the world about him or her and as his or her levels of intellectual and social functioning improve and, above all, the need for meaningful communication grow, the need for intervention increases. Extended periods with little or no meaningful stimulation will no longer be tolerated. Communication and meaningful activity will be demanded. The basic human needs for information, communication, and social interaction will cause an ever increasing level of stress if they are not met. Existing in the 'silent night' with brief, meaningful contact with others will no longer suffice as awareness of the world increases. When such support is denied, the family is only too aware of the development of emotional problems by deafblind individuals and of the lost opportunities for continued improvement towards supported independence that are missed. The concept that the higher the level of functioning the greater the need for human support (intervention) flies in the face of the conventional wisdom associated with most other disabilities.

Establishing Self-Fulfilling Prophecies

When the only understanding that community professionals have is based upon their knowledge of other disabilities, it is extremely easy to set up a self-fulfilling prophecy for the individual who is deafblind. If a deafblind person has been identified as low functioning and he or she is placed in a program for individuals who are intellectually challenged, deaf, emotionally disturbed, or blind, and is treated like any other person in the program, the result will be a very low-functioning and/or problem individual who eventually will be dropped from the program for 'lack of progress' or because of 'behaviour problems.' The initial assessment of their potential will seem to have been correct. It is not that teachers in such programs are incompetent. It is simply that their training and experience cause them to look for success indicators that mark progress for others and are not applicable to the individual who is deafblind.

CB is an example of such a case. When he was registered in preschool, he was placed in a program for the mentally challenged because of his developmental delay. That is, he was not performing as a person without disabilities would perform at the same age. From the records available, it would appear that no consideration was given to his visual and hearing loss, yet he was functioning as if he were severely visually impaired and profoundly deaf. Because he did not do the things that indicated progress in other children in the class, such as sitting quietly during 'circle time' or lining up, taking turns, exploring his environment, playing with others, and sharing, his behaviour was taken as 'proof' that he was indeed intellectually challenged.

To compound the problem, when his placement was questioned after he had been in school for some time, he was tested with two parts of a standardized battery of tests, one of which was used to test blind children and the other to test deaf children. It is obvious that the person who administered the test did not understand that this approach was inappropriate because

- the part tests had not been normed on a deafblind population
- the learning styles of students who were blind or deaf bore little or no relation to how CB learned
- the ability of the tester to communicate with CB was based upon techniques used with deaf students, not upon the adapted communication techniques employed with deafblind persons
- simply because others had used the same (mistaken) approach in the past, the psychologist assumed that this validated the use of such a testing procedure and the results.

In any case, the part tests were administered and the resulting 'score' was inevitable. It was 'proved' that the original diagnosis was correct. He was intellectually challenged and functioning at a twenty-two-month level. The professionals felt satisfied, but the parents knew that the results were ridiculous.

As far as the parents were concerned, CB certainly did many things that no two-year-old child did. He dressed himself, looked after all his self-care needs with minimum prompting, aided in shopping, food preparation, and other basic 'jobs' at home with intervention, enjoyed eating in local fast food restaurants, attended and took part in church services, could follow two- and three-step instructions, and had extensive receptive and a somewhat limited expressive manual communication vocabulary when the adapted communication he learned at home was used. At school he was taught language primarily from vocabulary lists, not in context, as Geenens, Souriau, and Rødbroe point out is essential for development of understanding and communication skills. The only thing that seemed to matter to the community professionals was that the prophecy be fulfilled.

Need for an Appropriate Personal Plan

Identifying an individual of any age as deafblind is only the first step. He or she will need ongoing formative evaluation, a Personal Plan, and appropriate support to carry out the activities necessary to provide opportunities to achieve the objectives identified in the program (see chapter 2). Unfortunately, without an appropriate Personal Plan and the support of trained Intervenors, individuals who are deafblind will exhibit many of the characteristics associated with the diagnosis of intellectually challenged or emotionally disturbed. Eventually, such individuals will fail when they are placed in programs designed to meet the needs of other groups. Even where the diagnosis has some validity, individuals will not be able to perform to their potential unless they are supported by the techniques and methods needed to support persons with deafblindness.

Students who are enrolled in a nursery school, preschool, elementary school, secondary school, or even college or university and who do not face the challenge of deafblindness do not confine their learning to three or four hours per day. Exposure to environmental stimuli takes place throughout their waking hours.

- They have opportunities for patterning their actions and behaviours after peers.
- They are constantly challenged to solve new problems by modifying previously acquired solutions.
- They frequently take part in two-way and social group communication.
- They are obtaining feedback concerning every attempt at mastering a skill.
- They are continually learning the concept of responsibility as it applies to both their age and the specific activity taking place at the moment.
- They are beginning to understand the expectations of parents, other family members, peers, and the public as they apply to them.
- They are continually finding out the consequences of each and every thing they do.

For the student who is deafblind to have anything approaching the same opportunities, a carefully written Personal Plan, not merely a school-based *Individual Educational Plan*, or *IEP*, must be developed. The environment must be peopled with individuals who are knowledgeable about his or her level of functioning and changing needs. It is only when the Personal Plan holistically incorporates individual, family, community, medical, and educational needs and activities that individuals who are deafblind will be able to develop to their potential. The older youth and adult who is deafblind should be encouraged to try new experiences and will do so if an emotional bond has been developed with the person providing the intervention. We seek the company of friends and often try new things because of who is asking us to do them. When we act for this reason, our relationships with our friends and loved ones are viewed as 'normal.' Such a relationship between an Intervenor and an individual who is deafblind is not only equally as appropriate, but essential. Simply having an Intervenor and a relationship, however, is not sufficient. There must be a Personal Plan and carefully chosen activities that provide opportunities to compensate for the disability of deafblindness.

A Canadian Approach

Introduction

Whether there is a 'Canadian Approach' probably depends more on where you are viewing the multitude of efforts across Canada to support individuals with deafblindness than on the identification of a clearly defined approach or set of rules. Two things are clear, however, to all who seek to identify and understand the 'Canadian Approach.' First, the Canadian philosophy is based on:

- the recognition of the uniqueness, needs, and personal worth of the individual
- the lack of a local pool of accurate community knowledge about deafblindness
- the demographics of the vast service areas
- the place of the individual who is deafblind and his or her family in all aspects of support and decision making
- the need for professionals with specific training in deafblindness
- the need for a Personal Plan that encompasses all aspects of support from the time of identification
- a consistency of approach by all parties from the time of identification onward
- the use of the process of intervention to support the individual with deafblindness.

Second, it is a philosophy that is not unique to Canada. It is true that certain specific aspects evolved in Canada and emphasis on particular techniques are more pronounced, but parts or all of this philosophy are being applied in many programs throughout the world. Even within Canada, the overall philosophy has been modified to meet the local needs as defined by service organizations, government, the background and training of the professionals involved, and financial considerations.

Identification

Every attempt must be made to identify the individual with deafblindness at the earliest possible age. Wherever possible, the identification should be made at birth or shortly thereafter. If a suspicion exists that an infant or child is deafblind, he or she should be treated as deafblind until it has definitely been shown that the identification is inappropriate. Under no circumstance should services be delayed until such identification is resolved.

The Individual

The Canadian philosophy stresses the uniqueness of the individual and his or her personal degree of both vision and hearing loss. Even where the individual has some degree of residual vision or hearing, he or she is considered deafblind if he or she has both a vision and a hearing loss and does not have sufficient hearing to compensate for the loss of vision and/or sufficient vision to compensate for the loss of hearing during activities of everyday living.

The individual who is deafblind has many unique challenges to overcome. Unless special provisions have been made, deafblindness significantly restricts all types of interaction with the environment, including, but not limited to, the ability to obtain sufficient non-distorted information, the ability to communicate with others, and how and what the individual with deafblindness learns.

Deafblindness may be accompanied by other challenging disabilities. Even where additional medical problems exist, the individual who has a significant vision and hearing loss must be identified as and supported as deafblind. Therapeutic and other programs must be incorporated into the overall support plan to assure the integration and the attainment of the objectives of such programs through appropriate methods of presentation, feedback, and reinforcement.

Some individuals are congenitally or early adventitiously deafblind; others are later adventitiously deafblind. While each group has many challenges in common, each has many significantly different challenges also. Individuals who are deafblind and their advocates in each group must work together to attain community and governmental support while at the same time recognizing both the common and different challenges faced by the other.

A Low-Incidence Disability

The fact that deafblindness is a low-incidence disability has three distinct outcomes that must be taken into account in developing a support system. First, there is usually no pool of community knowledge about deafblindness. Access to the professional knowledge base may vary according to the size of the population centre and geographical location. Often, realistic expectations concerning the person who is either congenitally or early adventitiously deafblind are non-existent among both the general population and community medical or educational professionals. As a result, doctors, therapists, educators, and community support workers may view the infant, child, youth, or adult with deafblindness on the basis of their experiences with other disabilities. Early-childhood educators, teachers (both generalists and specialists) and school administrative personnel may attempt to force the student with deafblindness into an existing program with or without some modification to it.

A mistake often made by professionals from other fields is failure to differentiate between the ability to gather non-distorted information from the environment and the ability to process such information. Such failure often causes the individual with deafblindness to be inappropriately labelled 'intellectually challenged' or seriously to overestimate the extent of his or her challenging condition.

The Family and the Individual

Another of the aspects that tends to set the Canadian philosophy apart is the emphasis on the place of the individual with deafblindness in his or her nuclear and extended family and the place of the family in helping to define the support system to be used. Because of the low incidence of the disability and the lack of community support, families often become desperate, particularly when they feel circumstances are denying their infant or child appropriate support or when community professionals see requests for such support as the family not 'pulling their weight.' It should be the role of agencies and professionals serving the deafblind community immediately to assist the family to advocate for an appropriate type and level of support and to ensure an adequate level and frequency of ongoing support, so families are not forced to turn to inappropriate sources. Where the deafblind individual is unable to accept some or all of the personal responsibility, the family or advocate must receive support in all aspects of decision making. Deafblind individuals and, where appropriate, their families must be given all the facts concerning the problem being addressed and must be encouraged to contact and be supported when they wish to initiate contact with other families of individuals who are deafblind.

The ultimate goal of teaching every skill, routine, or concept is for the person who is deafblind to decide who will offer what help and when. Until this level of functioning has been reached, the family, or the advocate in cases where the family is not available, should have the final say as to the goals of the Personal Plan, what community support will be utilized, and by whom the support will be given.

As soon as possible, the individual, or the family in cases where the individual with deafblindness has not acquired the necessary skills, should have the final say in hiring, training, evaluating performance of, and, if necessary, firing the individuals providing personal support. It is the responsibility of all support organizations and their representatives to provide the information and training necessary to enable the individual, the family, or the advocate to accept and fulfil this role.

A Personal Plan

The concept of the Personal Plan includes the aspirations of the individual with deafblindness, or, where this is not yet appropriate, the family. The Personal Plan will also include any educational or therapeutic program that has been developed. It will emphasize the development of the knowledge, skills, and attitudes necessary to enable the individual with deafblindness, regardless of age, to have an appropriate, effective, and contributing place in the family, school, and community. The development of the Personal Plan must be based upon ongoing formative evaluation focused on areas of present and future progress, not on a series of isolated summative evaluations focused on identifying what the infant, child, youth, or adult with deafblindness cannot do or identifying the place upon some scale that they appear to occupy.

Implementation of the plan will stress the effective use of educational, family and community resources. Above all, the individual or, when appropriate, the family or advocate should have the final say in all aspects of the development, implementation, and evaluation of their Personal Plan. The ownership of the Personal Plan lies with the individual with deafblindness, or, when appropriate, with his or her advocate, not with the professional.

The Personal Plan must stress what we in Canada call the 'Total Communication Approach.' (This concept differs from 'Total Communication' as used in the deaf community.) This approach stresses both receptive and expressive communication and requires that they be incorporated from the time a skill, routine, or concept is introduced, regardless of the age of the deafblind person. Communication must take place before any activity, during the activity, and after the activity has taken place. Such communication must give the individual with deafblindness an ability to anticipate what is going to happen, to know what is happening, and to receive feedback about how well the activity was performed.

The Personal Plan approach utilizes three types of intervention: General Intervention; Instructional Intervention, which encompasses the Presentation Sequence, the Interaction Sequence, and the Reaction Sequence; and Social Intervention.

The Personal Plan also emphasizes creating a reactive environment that gives the individual, regardless of age, appropriate control over what he or she does, when and for how long he or she will do it, how well it will be done, and with whom it will be done. In the implementation of the Personal Plan, when inappropriate behaviours are being targeted, behaviour substitution, not behaviour eradication, is emphasized, because denial of contact with the environment is counter-productive and may lead to withdrawal and other serious long-range behaviour problems when it is used with individuals with deafblindness and because aversive techniques often have severely negative and long-lasting effects.

Professionals

The Canadian Approach emphasizes the need for professionals with a high level of training and specialization in the area of deafblindness. This level of specialization may be arrived at in a number of ways, depending on the role of the specialist. The knowledge necessary to support the individual who is deafblind, his or her family, and community professionals, such as therapists, medical practitioners, social workers, and educators, will not be gained by assembling a committee of individuals with backgrounds in the amelioration of vision problems, hearing problems, developmental delay, behaviour modification, and so on. Deafblindness is a unique disability that requires specialized knowledge.

The role of the specialist is not to replace the community professional but rather directly and indirectly to support such professionals through education and involvement in the development of a Personal Plan. Professionals are not superior beings; they simply have more knowledge of a narrow field, and the application of this knowledge should be controlled on the basis of the wider interests of the infant, child, youth, or adult with deafblindness.

Intervention

'Intervenor' is a term attached to anyone providing appropriate support for an infant, child, youth, or adult with deafblindness. An Intervenor may be a parent, a sibling, a volunteer, or a trained professional. The level of expertise will vary from that acquired by an Intervenor working with one individual to that of a college graduate who is highly trained and knowledgeable in the needs of all individuals with either congenital or adventitious deafblindness and the techniques and methods used to support individuals with congenital or *acquired* deafblindness. Working with one deafblind individual does not, in itself, provide sufficient background to support another infant, child, youth, or adult with deafblindness.

'Intervention' is a term that describes the process of interaction between the individual with deafblindness and the Intervenor who is providing support. The specifics of the process that should be used at any one time are determined by the needs of the person who is deafblind, not by the skills of the Intervenor. The Canadian Approach recognizes that there are three distinct types of intervention: General Intervention; Instructional Intervention, and Social Intervention.

The ultimate goal of the Intervenor must be to facilitate all aspects of communication; to empower the individual with deafblindness, regardless of age, to ask for help appropriately; and to pass to the individual with deafblindness an appropriate degree of control through the use of a reactive rather than a directive environment.

Conclusion

The application of this Canadian Approach will be examined in greater depth throughout this book. The intent in this chapter is simply to outline briefly the basis upon which this philosophy is based. To encourage thought, several chapters have been written by individuals from other countries. Their work illustrates how the same approach is applied in different settings and gives insight into their philosophies and delivery systems.

Summary

1. A person who is deafblind has both a significant vision and a significant hearing loss and is not able to function in most situations of everyday living as either a person who is visually impaired or a person who is auditorily impaired.
2. Deafblindness is defined as not having sufficient vision to compensate for the loss of hearing and not having sufficient hearing to compensate for the loss of vision.
3. Deafblindness is a complex problem requiring specific approaches, techniques, methods, and programming designed to meet the needs of the infant, child, youth, or adult who is deafblind.
4. Among the identified causes of deafblindness prematurity is the most prevalent. A major concern is that more than 50 per cent of the cases are not identified as to specific cause.
5. Because of the low incidence of the disability, parents of deafblind infants and children face additional problems.
6. The Canadian Approach encompasses a broad approach with specific emphasis on the dignity of the person who is deafblind, communication, a reactive environment, and intervention, among other things.

NOTE

1 The Nordic Committee on Disability is an institution for Nordic congenitally disabled. The operation is subordinated to the Nordic Council of Ministers (i.e., the

governments of Denmark, Finland, Iceland, Norway and Sweden). Postal address: The Nordic Committee on Disability, P.O. Box 303, S-161 26 Bromma, Sweden.

REFERENCES

Baldwin, Victor (1992) *Proceedings of the National Symposium on Children and Youth Who Are Deaf-Blind*, Teaching Research, Western Oregon State College, 23 September
Brown, David (1997) 'Trends in the Population of Children with Multi-sensory Impairment,' *Talking Sense* 43(2). Published by Sense, the National Deafblind and Rubella Association, ed. Sarah Talbot-Williams
Conference on Deafblindness (1996) *Living and Learning, a Lifelong Adventure*. Vancouver. University of British Columbia, May
McInnes, J.M., and J.A. Treffry (1982, 1993, 1997) *Deaf-Blind Infants and Children: A Developmental Guide*. Toronto: University of Toronto Press
Meshcheryakov, A (1979) *Awakening to Life*. Moscow: Progress Publishers
United States Code, Title 29 – Labor, Chap. 21, 1901 Congressional Findings

2

Developing a Personal Plan

JOHN M. McINNES

Deafblindness is a unique disability,
which requires a unique approach to support
and a unique system to deliver that support.

Introduction

The second of the essential elements to support the individual with congenital deafblindness is the Personal Plan. In this chapter the following points will be covered:

- Discussion of why a Personal Plan is needed
- An overview of the process of writing the Personal Plan
- Identification and detailed suggestions for the development of the four mandatory and two optional sections of the Personal Plan
- Examination of the relationship between objectives and activities
- Identification and discussion of the need for a Reactive Environment in the implementation of the Personal Plan
- Consideration of both the need for parental involvement and support, intervention, and a community network as well as other factors that should be considered during the development and implementation of the Personal Plan.

The phrase '*of the individual who is deafblind and/or, where appropriate, his or her parents*' is used purposefully to stress that we must always work towards having the person who is deafblind make age-appropriate decisions or contributions. Unfortunately, in many cases such decisions are left in the hands of parents or professionals far too long, and the deafblind individual is not taught to make age-appropriate decisions, to understand the consequences of such decisions, or to accept responsibility for these consequences.

Background

The Personal Plan[1] concept was developed to meet the needs of the individual with deafblindness, regardless of age or level of functioning. The Personal Plan will differ markedly from an *Individualized Educational Plan* (*IEP*) or an *Individual Pupil Plan* (*IPP*). These approaches are designed to meet the educational needs of a student who is faced with intellectual, physical, or other challenges. The most important difference is that the Personal Plan is designed to cover twenty-four hours a day, 365 days a year, not simply the time the infant, child, or youth spends in school. Another important aspect of the Personal Plan is that it must be delivered in a Reactive Environment.

The Personal Plan compensates for the disability caused by a combined severe vision and hearing loss. It must be stressed, however, that *the deafblind individual will NOT live a more regimented life* than other members of his or her family, nor should anyone expect that parents or other family members will be involved in 'programming' (in the worst sense of the word) twenty-four hours a day.

The well-written plan will take into account and reflect the resources of time, energy, and finances of the family; the material, moral, and physical support and expertise available in the community; and the availability of ongoing consultative support. The implementation of the plan must be designed to fit within and accommodate the normal routines that the family, residential setting, and/or community have already established.

An initial plan for an infant may involve little more than support for the parents through sharing of information, demonstrations of techniques and methods to encourage communication between the parents and the baby, and helping the parents to identify and react to the infant's attempts at communication. Until the parents are comfortable with the consultant and the process, the plan may contain only an abbreviated history, a brief description of functioning, and a few key objectives. The greatest mistake any consultant can make is to develop a plan that so exhausts and discourages the family and/or community workers that the plan is ignored (see chapter 9).

Why a Personal Plan Is Needed

Experience has shown that there are several problems that arise when standard programming approaches are used with the deafblind individual. The most frequent problem takes place when he or she is placed in a preschool or educational program that has no provision made for the transfer of knowledge and skills to the home and community. In most non-residential school programs the individual will spend approximately the same number of days at home – approximately 182 – as he or she spends in school.

When the child attends a local community school, educators traditionally feel little or no responsibility for out-of-school hours except, perhaps, to assign homework. It is felt that the school has no responsibility for teaching parents how to teach skills such as reading or subtraction, let alone how to implement the broad-ranging developmental, social, and educational learning that is taking place in the home and community.

The program for a deafblind student must assume such responsibilities, and where the teacher in the community school does not have the expertise, then a support person with expertise in deafblindness must form part of the programming team. The family is also an essential part of this team, as is every professional and support person who works with the deafblind student in the home, school, and community. If the family is not involved in plan development and implementation, the child with deafblindness is doomed to spend half his or her life in an environment that features isolation, has communication deficits, and in which a set of different and often either too low or unrealistic expectations are held for him or her.

Simply sending home a comprehensive report card and a vocabulary list is not sufficient. Parents must be supported so that they can identify and work towards the achievement of realistic expectations. Such training will not be accomplished by one, or even several, weekend training sessions or by a short one- or two-week workshop. *Parental training and education must be evolutionary in nature* and implemented by continued close contact between the consultant for deafblindness and the family. (See chapter 16 for a detailed description of the consultant's role.)

The residential school staff or the consultant in deafblindness, as experts in deafblindness, have a responsibility to

- develop a Personal Plan for the student
- educate family members and individuals in the community who come into regular contact with the student
- educate other members of the staff of the school the student attends, including vice-principals, principals, and senior administrators.

This broad-ranging approach is necessary if appropriate priorities, appropriate staffing, and appropriate classroom and school-based decisions are to be made. The setting of such priorities and the making of such decisions are necessary to facilitate the implementation of the preschool or student's Personal Plan. The plan must identify and provide for the development and application of the knowledge, skills, and attitudes necessary for success in educational, family, and community settings. It is unlikely that an individual with deafblindness will make progress in all areas of development when family, educators, and/or community workers do not have an understanding of the *success indicators* specific to the infant, child, or youth with deafblindness and the skills necessary to provide support.

Another problem almost sure to arise when a comprehensive plan is not developed is that of *learned helplessness*. Expectations held by medical professionals, therapists, and family members often are based upon their knowledge of the effects of other disabilities and thus are inappropriate when applied to the deafblind child. In addition, such expectations may even conflict because different bases for assumptions are being employed. Individuals with deafblindness often are seen as severely developmentally delayed when developmental steps are expected in a specific order based upon studies of infants and children without or having other disabilities, such as deafness or blindness.

As a result of expectations and presumed delay based on 'normal' developmental patterns, inappropriate programming decisions are sometimes made. When the individual who is deafblind does not meet such expectations it is sometimes inappropriately assumed that little or no further progress can be expected in a particular area. Such a decision frequently leads to a change in focus from development to maintenance and thus to the encouragement of learned helplessness.

Older children, youth, and adults with deafblindness also may be left to function at the level of learned helplessness. Once they have acquired the basic life skills, such as putting on clothing and minimal eating skills, no more is expected of them. During the carrying out of age-appropriate activities, basic rules for working with individuals who are deafblind, such as the following, must not be ignored (see chapter 3).

- Every activity must stress communication.
- Individuals must be supported to do for themselves by teaching them to ask for assistance appropriately.
- Do with, but NEVER do for, when individuals are engaged in age-appropriate activities.
- Continually seek to expand deafblind individuals' knowledge of their world.

The specialist in deafblindness must explain the application of these basic rules as they apply to the activities engaged in by each child and according to his or her age and present level of functioning.

There is never any excuse to have children, youth, or adults engage in activities that are not age appropriate. Activities like sorting silverware from the dishwasher are age appropriate to teach classification, numeration, and so on. Using materials like puzzles and blocks designed for preschoolers are not age appropriate when the individual is an older child, youth, or adult. There is no excuse for having a deafblind adult do and redo a preschool puzzle 'because he likes it.' There are many adult activities that can provide greater rewards.

Another reason a Personal Plan is required is that the absence of the effective use of the two distance senses severely affects both intrinsic and extrinsic motivation. Some understanding of the significance of the disability may be gained by the following.

- *Explain* why a non-challenged infant or young child would stack blocks.
- Next, *explain* why an infant or young child with deafblindness would stack blocks!
- *Relate* these reasons as to why the deafblind infant or young child would stack blocks to learning skills such as sitting, standing, toilet training, walking, eating with a spoon, dressing him or herself, working at a job, keeping personal and shared space neat and clean, and behaving in an age-appropriate manner.

If appropriate, rewarding activities are not available, individuals with deafblindness may try to cope by withdrawing. They may adopt learned helplessness as a means of coping. They will simply stop trying to 'do for' themselves with or without assistance and may become tactilely defensive or present challenging behaviours when pressed to participate in an activity.

Some of the most frequently heard reasons for setting up a situation where an individual will develop learned helplessness are the following.

- It is easier to dress him rather than to expect him to do the buttons, zippers, and ...
- She is so small and has so many other problems that I can't expect ...
- I don't have time to ...
- He's deafblind and couldn't possibly learn to ...
- She's deafblind and has so many difficult problems to overcome that ...
- He is (fill in the reason you like) and can't be expected to make decisions about ...

The fact is that, with

- knowledgeable and trained family members, educators, and community professionals

- a comprehensive Personal Plan that identifies specific objectives and their accompanying success indicators
- appropriate intervention,

in most cases he or she CAN succeed!

There never can be any acceptable excuse for promoting learned helplessness. We continue to acquire new skills and gain knowledge throughout our lives. Until the youth or adult with deafblindness acquires the knowledge and skills necessary to make plans to live in an expanding, rather than a shrinking, confining world, we must ensure that his or her plans provide challenges, new and expanding concepts, and opportunities for growth.

The Personal Plan

The Basis of the Plan

A Personal Plan starts with a blank sheet. It will

- be based upon the infant, child, youth, or adult's present level of functioning, not on an existing program or scale
- cover all the waking hours
- incorporate physiotherapy, occupational therapy, educational program goals, recreational goals, social goals, and so on within its structure, rather than their existing as isolated, non-connected items or events
- be written by a professional who is a specialist in the development, education, and support of the individual who is deafblind
- incorporate input from the person who is deafblind and, as appropriate, from parents, medical and educational professionals, Intervenors, global family members, friends, and volunteers
- be based upon the framework described in the following pages or a similar comprehensive approach
- not be implemented until it is approved of and signed by the youth or adult who is deafblind or, where more appropriate, the parents or advocate of the deafblind individual
- be written and implemented within the capabilities and within the established routines of the family and within the resources of the community support services
- be the basis for all evaluation of the individual for whom the plan was developed.

The Purpose of Writing a Personal Plan

The purpose of writing any Personal Plan must be to aid the individual to

develop to his or her full, unique potential as a human being and as a participating member of his or her family and of society. In more practical and operational terms, the goal is to provide each individual who is deafblind with a
plan designed to fit his or her needs, interests, abilities, past performance, and
present level of functioning. The plan must be delivered at the rate, in the
depth, and by the methods best suited to the individual's learning style and the
available resources of the family, school, and community; and the individual
must be evaluated in terms of his or her improved level of functioning as
shown by the success indicators (objectives) identified in his or her Personal
Plan.

If the Personal plan is being developed by a youth or adult who is deafblind,
he or she should be encouraged to look for both 'new worlds to conquer' as well
as the improvement of existing skills and the broadening of personal concepts.
No professional working with an adult who is congenitally or early adventitiously deafblind should feel that the adult has reached some final plateau and
needs only to be maintained. Encouragement to make decisions, try new things,
meet new people, and visit new places should form a part of the implementation
of each plan regardless of the age or level of functioning of the individual for
whom the plan is being developed.

It is equally important that the adult who is congenitally or early adventitiously deafblind, his or her advocate, and concerned staff be involved in plan
development. When a plan is being developed, the developer must take into
account

- the aspirations, priorities, and goals of the individual, or, where more appropriate, those of the parents and/or advocate
- recommendations of Intervenors, family members, and community professionals
- present and future community resources available for support as the plan is
  being implemented
- the medical prognosis.

If the plan is not seen as worthwhile by the family, it will have little chance of
continuing success. One of the best ways for the professional to ensure that the
family will see the plan as worthwhile is to encourage their active participation
in plan development. Token consultation of parents, advocates, and/or staff is
not enough. In fact, it is insulting to the very people whom the developer must
rely on for a major part of its implementation.

Another purpose of the Personal Plan approach is to give the parents, family
members, Intervenors, therapists, educators, or any other professional or community worker an understanding of where their contribution fits into overall

development. The approach should ensure that no professional effort is made in isolation and that everyone involved in daily routines and special activities understands which skills should be introduced and practised.

While each Personal Plan is designed to meet the specific needs of one individual, it is recognized that there are elements that may be found in more than one person's plan. Just as an architect will use many of the same concepts, theories, materials, and techniques found in many buildings to design a building to meet a unique set of requirements, the developer writing a Personal Plan for a given individual will incorporate tested methods, modifying some approaches and developing new techniques and approaches to ameliorate this specific individual's needs.

Writing a Personal Plan

How does one start designing a Personal Plan? When faced with this task, both parents and professionals outside the field of deafblindness find this one of the hardest questions to answer. Tried and true approaches that have worked with others often seem less effective when used to develop a plan for the individual who is deafblind. A plan developed to meet the needs of one person who is deafblind cannot usually be directly applied to another. Application of a set of global *goals* and/or *objectives* or ones that were written for another individual is perhaps one of the most common reasons that a plan for a specific individual is inappropriate or fails. Sometimes planning attempts deteriorate into searches for an appropriate placement in some existing program designed to serve children with vision, hearing, or physical challenges. This approach is flawed and inappropriate.

The approach to programming outlined in this chapter provides a guide to the development and implementation of a Personal Plan. It is designed to provide a complete picture of the functioning of the individual who is deafblind, a set of clearly identified five-year goals, and attainable objectives that will provide a description of what will constitute success in the coming six or twelve months. A graphic overview is presented in figure 2.1.

A Basic Concept

One underlying concept that must be constantly kept in mind is that the infant, child, youth, or adult for whom the plan is written CANNOT FAIL. The developer may over- or underestimate the progress expected in a given area in the next six or twelve months for many reasons, such as illness of the individual, disruption of the family or residence, or simply because he or she lacked the information to make a more accurate judgment. It is extremely difficult to

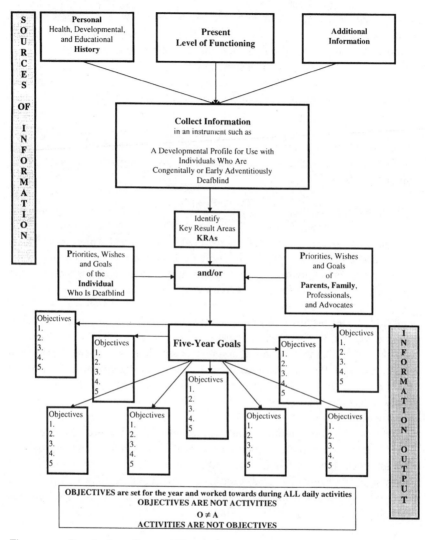

Figure 2.1   Developing a Personal Plan

predict how an individual who is deafblind will be functioning next year. Such a prediction must be attempted, however, because there is no educational or developmental program with appropriate, identified milestones in which he or she can be placed.

Plan Content

The Personal Plan consists of four mandatory and two optional sections. The required sections are:

1. Personal Health, Developmental, and Educational History
2. Present Level of Functioning
3. Five-Year Goals
4. Six- or Twelve-Month Objectives

The optional sections are:

5. Resources Required for Implementation
6. Implementation Schedule.

Part One: Personal History

The first step is to update or, in the case of a first plan, collect and record a detailed personal history. This detailed history will provide one-third of a platform upon which the Personal Plan will be developed. Without in-depth knowledge of the individual's history, it is impossible to interpret adequately the present level of functioning, to form a basis for the setting of five-year goals, or to gather the information necessary to write twelve-month objectives. The emphasis in this section on health, developmental, and educational history should be as follows:

• It acts as a safeguard against inappropriate judgments being made by people who do not have a long association with the individual who is deafblind. After it has been collected, the history should be summarized into a short readable form.
• It serves to prevent people working with individuals with deafblindness from requiring that they engage in activities that may, because of past or present medical or other problems, place them in jeopardy or that have been tried and found unsuitable for a variety of reasons.
• It assists in the identification of, for example, the late manifestations of Rubella in adults who are deafblind.

The personal history will be assembled from many sources, chief among which will be the family. We have found that use of *The Developmental Profile for Use with Persons Who Are Deafblind* (McInnes et al. 1994) or a similar instru-

ment, such as the *Callier-Azusa Scale* (1966), ensures that all important information will be collected systematically and organized in a useful manner prior
to summarizing.

The first response by many individuals when they read the suggested contents of Part 1, is that there is too much work required. In reality, once the initial
information is obtained and the section is written, the only work involved is
upgrading the existing section by adding any changes that have taken place or
any new information that has been obtained during the previous year (or six
months in the case of an infant's plan). The individual's history doesn't change,
but it becomes ever more vital that everyone working with him or her has an
accurate understanding of what went before if inappropriate conclusions are to
be avoided.

The personal history should include the following.

Health History

A complete health history, including, but not limited to

- a neonatal history
- a report on the condition of the infant at birth, including the **APGAR** score if
  available
- a description of neurological impairments and their significance
- audiological information, including a chronological history of hearing tests,
  their results, and an indication as to whether the examiner felt the tests were
  successful
- vision information, including a chronological history of tests, their results,
  and an indication as to whether the examiner felt the tests were successful
- a comprehensive functional inquiry
- a detailed chronological record of hospitalization, childhood diseases, and
  periods of convalescence.

Therapeutic History

A therapeutic treatment history, including, but not limited to

- a chronological list of treatments detailing the reasons the treatment was
  given, the reason the treatment was terminated (if not ongoing at present),
  and the name of the therapist
- a description of the treatment, emphasizing modifications made to compensate for the individual who is congenitally or early adventitiously deafblind

- a description of the provisions made for the application of the skills by the person and/or other follow-up activities between therapy sessions
- a description of how the therapist communicated with the individual and whether the communication was successful.

Developmental and Educational History

An educational and/or developmental program history, including, but not limited to

- a description of each program's content
- a description of the infant's, child's, or youth's level of participation in each aspect of the program
- the parents' evaluation of the significant gains made as a result of participation in the program
- the reason the program was terminated, if not ongoing at present, as given by both the program director and the parents.

Family History

A family history, including, but not limited to

- serious or prolonged illness of individual family members that had an effect on the infant's, child's or youth's, and in some cases the deafblind adult's program or support received from within the family
- problems in acquiring appropriate support and a description of which agencies provided useful support, when, and how often
- a family's estimate of its resources and the circumstances that may limit their use.

Accumulation and Wording of Material

The accumulation of this history will take patience and tact. The actual wording of the summary of this information that will be placed in the Personal Plan should be subject to the client's or, where appropriate, the parent's or advocate's approval.

While all of the above information is vital to the developer, the decision about whether it should be recorded or made available to anyone other than the developer is the prerogative of the family, the advocate, or the individual who is deafblind. On the other hand, it should be explained that the more complete the information available to the person providing intervention and support is, the better the intervention and support will be.

Part Two: The Present Level of Functioning

The purpose of part two is to give a complete description of the present level of functioning of the individual. The emphasis is upon how the individual functions in everyday situations. The description should be in plain language. For example, a description of an eighteen-month-old infant's use of residual vision might be as follows:

John recognizes familiar people at approximately four feet. He responds to signs and gestures presented at the midline approximately twelve inches away. He tracks objects occasionally, left to right and up and down and vice versa, with prompting. He examines objects using his right eye at approximately three inches and stops using his vision when presented with a loud auditory or strong tactile stimulus.

Note: The above would be only one aspect of a statement of John's present level of functioning. The areas of functioning that should be addressed in *all* Personal Plans include

Auditory Functioning	Leisure and Recreation Activities
Cognitive Functioning	Problem Solving
Communication Skills	Receptive Language
Expressive Language	Sensory Integration
Fine Motor Skills	Social and Emotional Development
Gross Motor Skills	Visual Functioning
Intervention Usage	

Other areas that may be addressed, depending on the age of the individual, include but are not limited to

Banking	Family Relationships
Budgeting	First Aid
Care of Personal Space	Food Preparation
Care of Possessions	Intervenor Evaluation
Dressing Skills; care of,	Intervenor Selection
buying, and choosing clothing	Intervenor Training
Eating/Dining Skills	Measurement

Money

Orientation and Mobility

Peer Relationships

Personal and General Safety

Personal Hygiene

Recognition of expectations of
   family, peers, and others

Recognition of Societal Norms

Sexual Functioning

Shopping

Time; telling and planning
   use of

Other information concerning overall functioning that any contributor may feel is important may be included, for example, acceptance of responsibility (a) for a child: putting away toys after use; (b) for a teenager: saving money for a trip.

The combination of an understanding of how the individual is currently functioning and of his health, developmental, and educational history accomplishes two important things. The plan developer now has two-thirds of the basis for developing twelve-month objectives. The Intervenor also has the information necessary to identify and use the most effective techniques and methods during routine activities.

Care should be exercised when an instrument that was not developed specifically for use with individuals who are deafblind is selected. Using scales or profiles designed for use with the general population or with individuals who have some other challenging condition is *not recommended* (see chapter 4). Many such instruments require the person to use vision and/or hearing to attain identified milestones. In addition, such instruments may focus on knowledge and skills that the person is expected to have learned incidentally or to have discovered and practised through non-directed interaction with the environment. It is highly unlikely that the infant, child, or youth who is deafblind will have an extensive collection of knowledge and skills developed in this way.

The following could be a report on the Present Level of Functioning of KN, a twelve-year-old girl who has a small amount of functional vision and hearing. She also has problems with ongoing ear infections. The health record shows suspected CHARGE Syndrome, although she does not present a classic case. Her family consists of a father, a mother, and a fifteen-year-old brother.

KN continues to have frequent occurrences of ear infections in both ears. She has two behind the ear aids but never has had a long enough period free of ear infection to have had them successfully introduced in such a way that they become an important part of her functioning. She will wear them for varying periods of time at the request of her Intervenor, but she soon removes them and places them back in the box.

KN appears to use her right eye to examine objects she holds at the right corner of her eye at a distance of six to eight inches and to use her left eye to read manual communication at a distance of approximately three feet. She does not appear to integrate visual information from both eyes or auditory input with visual input from either eye.

KN spontaneously uses approximately 400 receptive signs and over 250 expressive signs. On the rare occasions that she wears her aids, she responds to twelve spoken words correctly, but she has only one word, 'no,' that she uses expressively. Currently she is beginning to make a specific sound, 'Mae–e' to identify her key Intervenor (Anne Marie). She is beginning to differentiate among Braille cells when they are presented in a game format and appears ready to begin to learn to read Braille. Whether she will require Braille as a primary means of reading in the future will depend upon whether there is a continued deterioration in her eyesight. She recognizes approximately sixty symbolic representations when they are used in her calendar or for shopping, and she will copy large-print words from a model to her own paper.

KN follows two- and three-step directions, combines previously learned skills to solve new problems, and has preferences as to which Intervenor she will choose for a specific activity. She becomes frustrated with people who underestimate her abilities and/or who use a directive approach when working with her. When frustrated or annoyed, she prefers to go to her room and shut her door vigorously or, if away from home, to go directly to the car and avoid any communication. The periods usually last from five to fifteen minutes. At school, such actions are viewed as inappropriate and she is seen as ungrateful and uncooperative. These actions usually result in punishment, which consists of placement in a corner and removal of her Intervenor for periods of up to one hour. Such treatment often results in a repeat of the offending action, and a cycle is set up that usually lasts all day.

Academically, KN is on a grade-four class register. She is doing arithmetic at grade-three level, participates in group activities with two peers whom she has taught to sign, and takes great pride in making detailed, illustrated notes in history. Her Intervenor helps her to copy the notes from the blackboard by fingerspelling them to her letter by letter, after which KN signs the note back with the Intervenor's assistance. She spends approximately one-third of her time in the grade-four class; one-third doing activities in the school with the Intervenor that are specifically designed for her, such as her weekly therapy sessions, introduction to Braille, and so on; and one-third using community resources, such as shopping, other life skills, mobility, and swimming, which are not within the school curriculum.

The therapist (Ms T) reports that there continues to be a need for more extensive application of the range-of-motion exercises throughout everyday activities. She also reports that KN continues to be tactile defensive and non-cooperative. She has agreed to have Mother and the Intervenor attend the therapy sessions and to try the techniques suggested by the Intervenor and consultant from the Deafblind Regional Centre, who acts as a case manager, to overcome the tactile defensive responses and non-cooperation. As of this date, the therapist has had only two sessions since this new approach has been introduced, but she says that there seems to be some improvement and hopes it will continue.

Overall, the parents, the teacher, and the principal are pleased with the progress KN has made since her transfer to his present school from the J.C. Crawsley School for Community Living. The principal has indicated on several occasions that had KN attended her local school from kindergarten on and been supported by an Intervenor and consultant, in his opinion she would be functioning at an even higher level.

Socially, KN gets along very well in the schoolyard during recess and noon hour. She and her Intervenor are accepted by KN's peers, who often invite her to participate in their activities. At home, her social contacts and leisure activities are still very limited. In spite of the family's best intentions, she has long periods of inactivity and no friends outside family members. Her horseback riding was a success but was dropped after one month for financial reasons.

With her Intervenor, KN prepares simple meals for the family, orders meals appropriately in the local restaurant, and does the family grocery shopping on Saturdays. KN receives an allowance and banks a portion of it each week. She is starting to understand the concept of saving to make a 'big' purchase of something she wants in the future. Sometimes she does not receive a full allowance because, like many twelve-year-olds, she has to be reminded that she has a responsibility to keep her room neat and clean.

KN has excellent self-care skills and follows well-established daily and weekly routines. She brushes her teeth twice daily, showers and washes her hair daily, and usually remembers to clean the sink or bathtub after use.

KN has problems in accepting changes in plans. If a scheduled activity has to be cancelled because an Intervenor is ill or a family member has to change priorities, she becomes very upset and may be angry with the person involved. This anger sometimes lasts for two or more days.

The objective of assembling the information necessary to write the above description of KN's present level of functioning is to

- promote discussion among all concerned during its assembling and writing
- give an agreed-upon picture of the key areas of functioning
- identify key areas for plan development.

During the writing of KN's Present Level of Functioning it became obvious that several conflicting techniques were being used in areas such as discipline and particularly in communication. As a result of the consultation required to write this description, it was decided that changes had to be made. There is much value in the discussion required to decide what should be included in the description of the Present Level of Functioning when it is written by all those involved rather than written by one person and presented to others for approval.

Key Result Areas

The concept of Key Result Areas (KRAs) evolved from educational practices in North America. As curriculums became less regimented in the latter part of the twentieth century, educational professionals in North America and elsewhere began to place emphasis on developing specific measurable objectives to describe exactly which skills, knowledge, and attitudes a student would develop as a result of being involved in a particular curriculum. The more the development of curriculum was left to individual educational authorities, school staffs, and even individual teachers, the more the need to show clearly what was being accomplished was emphasized.

It became the norm to have the objectives for each curriculum written in terms that described observable and measurable behaviour. Individual Pupil Plans (IPPs) and Individual Educational Plans (IEPs) became the order of the day. Such plans, when developed, were often presented to parents for their approval. This practice informed the parents about what was being taught and shared the onus of ensuring that the pupil received an adequate education.

It soon became evident that it was impossible to describe everything the student would learn, and attempts to do so led to plans of unmanageable length. It also became evident that many teachers who had excellent teaching skills did not have sufficient training in curriculum development to independently design programs, and, in addition, many lacked the time to do so. Numerous solutions evolved, including, for example, duplicated lists of objectives produced by a board, school committees, or available commercially from which the teacher could choose. These approaches, of course, defeated much of the individualization that was being attempted, particularly with children who had been placed in 'special' classes.

The temptation always exists to fit the individual deafblind pupil into a predetermined program and, if the pupil does not make the expected progress, to identify the pupil, not the program, as having failed. In the previous two or three decades, pupils with deafblindness were often put in programs for individuals with other disabilities. Professionals and parents working with the student who was deafblind soon found neither the objectives developed to meet the needs of children with other disabilities nor the suggested sequencing of these objectives was suitable for their students. Often such programs did not address all areas of development or take into account the fact that what was taught could not be based upon assumed knowledge formed as a result of incidental learning. In addition, it was soon realized that without specific provision things taught would not be spontaneously or successfully applied in the out-of-school hours.

An appropriate plan for the individual who is deafblind must take into account the fact that development and practice take place throughout all waking hours, not only in the portion traditionally the responsibility of preschool programs, school-based programs, or adult workshops. The plan must integrate objectives arising out of the educational, medical, developmental, recreational, and life-skills areas, yet it must avoid the problem of having so many objectives that it looses its effectiveness. At the same time, the Personal Plan must identify and describe what actions will indicate success. To accomplish these requirements the concept evolved of identifying *key areas* in which specific results were desired or expected.

Before writing the objectives for a Personal Plan you must identify the specific areas that will be targeted. This identification will be based upon the deafblind individual's history, present level of functioning, and his or her aspirations, priorities, and personal goals, and, where applicable, those of his or her parents, extended family members, and/or advocate. The process found most successful for identifying Key Result Areas (KRAs) consists of the following six steps.

1. Review the past history and the previously written description of the level of functioning.
2. Add any new information to the History section.
3. Describe the individual's present level of functioning. In the process of describing the present level of functioning, review each of the behavioural objectives for the previous period and decide if it has been surpassed, accomplished, or not accomplished.
4. Record in point form the priorities, wishes, and personal goals of the individual who is deafblind and, where applicable, those of his or her parents, extended family members, and/or advocate.
5. Review the five-year goals written in the previous plan to ensure continued relevancy.
6. Identify the most important areas by consolidating the information assembled.

The areas that are identified as most important become the Key Result Areas and will form part of the basis for writing or revising existing five-year goals.

Part Three: Five-Year Goals

Before we discuss the writing of five-year goals as they apply to a deafblind individual, please write your answers to the following questions on a piece of paper:

1. You are going out in your car. How much money will you take with you?
2. What clothing will you take with you?
3. What provisions will you make for mail, care of your house, and emergencies?

Decide whether you are person A, B, C, or D. Turn to the end of the chapter to see how you made out. Were your answers to these questions appropriate? The point is that, unless you know where you are going, you may be completely off in your Personal Plans. Five-year goals set the direction, which in turn governs all aspects of the Personal Plan. This setting of five-year goals is necessary because the approach of 'plugging' the deafblind child into a program designed for others is unsuccessful, and very few will have the opportunity of having their deafblind infant or child attend a comprehensive total program designed specifically to meet his or her needs as a deafblind child.

One has only to look at the parents of an infant or child without disabilities to understand the need for long-term goals. The parents of a one-year-old non-challenged infant usually have a dream for their child. The parents, extended family members, friends, and society all have a set of expectations as to what their child will be like as a two-year-old or a six-year-old, and it is upon these expectations that the parents' dreams are based. Parents may even be able to say what they expect their child will be able to do as he or she completes the first year of school. In addition, there usually are a clearly identified set of mile-stones and options that are defined in part by their culture, in part by educational authorities, and in part by family traditions. Their infant or child will be judged against these criteria by family, friends, neighbours, and society at large.

The parents of a child who is deafblind usually do not know what to expect and often are too concerned with today to worry about what the future holds. Life often seems to go from one crisis to the next. Parents need encouragement to dream and the support of a professional with training and experience in working with individuals who are congenitally or early adventitiously deafblind if they are to form realistic expectations. There must be a replacement or modification of the societal norms and family traditions. The parents must be assisted to develop the confidence that can grow only from seeing their child move towards identified goals. Not every expectation will become reality, but realistic expectations will provide both hope and strength for everyday functioning.

Discussion and setting of five-year goals provide direction for both the plan developer and the individuals providing support. Without direction, it is next to impossible to identify objectives for the next twelve months or to see progress clearly. Unless goals are identified and shared, it is possible that those involved will have different and even conflicting priorities and may even be attempting to go in opposite directions. Both parents and professionals often choose to avoid writing such goals. Parents may be reluctant to look ahead; simply surviving the day or the week seems safer and all that can be coped with. As a consultant, the author has frequently taken more than two or three visits, over a period of time, to work with the parents until they were comfortable in identifying and articulating such goals. Even when they have begun to dream, it will take time to trust the world not to laugh at or ridicule the dream.

What Are Goals?

Goals are not objectives to be attained. Goals are the stars that guide us on our journey, while objectives are the specific landmarks that indicate our progress towards our goals. Because goals represent what we wish to accomplish eventually, we recommend the following framework within which to write them. We have found it easiest to start with a statement such as '*By June 200–* (a date five years in the future) *John* (now a two-year-old) *will* (enter information under the following headings).

Living Space Goals
a) Where will he be living? (At home, in a residential setting, etc.; have his own room, share a bedroom, etc.)
b) What personal responsibilities will he have? (For putting away toys, picking up clothing, etc.)
c) How much responsibility will he have within the family?

Example: *Living Space*

By June 200–, John will

a) be living with his family in Marytown

b) share a bedroom with his younger brother

c) put away his toys after use

d) take his share of responsibility for helping with family chores, such as setting and clearing the table, looking after his area in the garden, and helping to put the soiled clothing in the clothes basket

e) attend church summer camp and CDBRA, Ontario, camp with his Intervenor.

Specific Functioning Goals

Other areas in which specific goals will be identified may include some or all of the following as well as those areas that will be specifically relevant to the individual according to his or her age, and present and expected future level of functioning. The following questions can help to identify five-year goals.

Specific Functioning Goals

What areas of development, such as the use of functional vision and hearing, motor skills, communication, language development, and so forth, are likely to show long-term improvement?

Life Skills Goals

What will be expected in areas such as

a) care of self

b) care, purchase, use, and discarding of possessions

c) management of money

d) use of specific family resources

e) use of community resources

f) peer relations beyond family?

Education (Work, if Applicable) Goals

a) Where will schooling or work will take place?

b) What type of education or pre-vocational training, work-related skills, and social skills will be needed?

c) Will volunteering in the community be part of his or her future?

Leisure and Recreation Goals

a) What indoor individual activities will be pursued when on his or her own, or with intervention?

b) What indoor activities in which others will participate with him will he engage in?

c) What family activities will be participated in with other family members?
d) What outdoor recreational activities will be pursued on his or her own, or with intervention?
e) What outdoor recreational activities will be participated in with peers?

Intervention Goals
a) What amount of intervention will be needed?
b) What part will the individual who is deafblind play in deciding who the Intervenor will be for various activities?
c) What part will the deafblind individual play in hiring, training, scheduling, and/or evaluating the Intervenor?

Writing the Five-Year Goals

The first step in writing five-year goals is to have a series of discussions with the individual who is deafblind and/or the parents or the advocate, as appropriate, after all have agreed upon what should be written in Part Two, 'The Present Level of Functioning.' This step should be attempted even if the child or youth is placed in a residential program or an institutional setting.

As the five-year goals are developed, the discussion provides an opportunity to identify educational, developmental, and in some cases treatment options. Questions as to what is reasonable to expect and how development, interests, and activities will both parallel and differ from his non-challenged peers can be discussed in safety.

When all of the discussion is completed, the next step is for the developer to formulate a provisional set of goals. The professional consultant in deafblindness, community workers, and the parents should view this first attempt as a basis for further discussion and revision. The consultant should then revise the goals according to the consensus reached by the team. The final step is for the individual who is deafblind and/or the parents and any others directly involved, to approve the five-year goals.

The initial set of five-fear goals will rarely be formulated in one or two weeks and certainly not in one meeting. The individual and/or parents and others need time to think about what has been discussed and what will be discussed at the next meeting concerning the future.

As time passes and trust develops between the parents and the developer, goal setting will become part of a systematic process for developing a Personal Plan. There is no excuse for five-year goals being developed and approved solely by professionals on the basis of their perception of the individual's and/or the family's needs. The goals, like the person about whom the expectations are being formed, are part of a family and its expectations. They provide the direction, and the professionals will identify the means of getting there when they write the twelve-month objectives.

Part Four: Twelve-Month Objectives

The Personal Plan will contain behavioural objectives in each of the areas identified in the five-year goals. These goals usually should involve some aspect of the following:

- Communication and language development
- Social and emotional development
- Gross and fine motor development
- Cognitive conceptual development
- Perceptual development
- Educational (subject related) progress
- Leisure and Recreation
- Life skills development.

Within each of the above areas actions that demonstrate expected progress should be described in behavioural terms.

These plan areas will remain relatively constant during the period of birth to twelve years of age, regardless of the specific age of the individual, his or her level of functioning, or the presence of additional disabilities. As the age increases, areas may need to be added or removed. Within the subsections of Part Four, twelve-month objectives expectations will change. For example, within the plan area of gross and fine motor development, sitting will become walking, then running and climbing, and gradually will evolve into specific pursuits, such as swimming, bowling, woodworking, typing, skiing, and other individual leisure and recreational activities. Progress within an activity can be shown as the individual progresses from doing the activity occasionally, with assistance, through several stages until he or she is doing the same activity frequently, or when required, with appropriate intervention.

In the teenage years and as the individual progresses towards and into adulthood, the behavioural objectives identified for each will become increasingly influenced by the individual's and family's preferences, the individual's lifestyle, and academic, recreational, and employment-related expectations. The individual's peers, who are not challenged by the disability of deafblindness, will acquire many of the more advanced skills of adult living through incidental learning, but the youth who is deafblind will obtain little or no non-distorted information in this manner. The plan must begin to focus on the specific skills he or she will need to live as an adult as soon as level of functioning permits. *Information, skills, and attitudes must be identified and taught, they will not be 'caught.'*

Writing Behavioural Objectives

The following are guidelines that we have found helpful when writing objectives for a Personal Plan. These guidelines are based upon the author's experience and should be modified to accommodate individual tastes.

General
a) When the infant is less than two years old, the behavioural objectives usually will be designed to identify the progress expected in the next six months. Behavioural objectives written for individuals who are two or older usually reflect the progress expected in the next twelve months.
b) Behavioural objectives MUST describe actions of the individual that will demonstrate the progress that is anticipated. Behavioural objectives for therapeutic or educational parts of the Personal Plan may focus partly on areas needing remediation, but, in general, educational and developmental objectives should focus on areas of strength.
c) Each goal may result in identification of a number of specific areas about which objectives will be written.
d) As a general rule, not less than five or more than ten behavioural objectives should be written in any one identified area.
e) As the individual gets older and attains a higher level of functioning, these general rules will not apply in areas such as motor development or leisure and recreation, where subareas, such as swimming, camping, running, and so on, each may have three–five behavioural objectives identified for the next twelve months.
f) Each behavioural objective will describe WHO will do WHAT, WHEN, and HOW WELL. These behavioural objectives will be the success indicators looked for by everyone involved with the implementation of the Personal Plan as signs of progress.

WHO
To identify WHO without needless repetition, the list of behavioural objectives in each area should begin with the general statement, such as

By June 200–, John will (a date representing twelve months in the future)

a) run down hill without assistance, upon request
b) demonstrate his enjoyment of vigorous physical activity by ...

WHAT

The What part of the behavioural objective describes exactly *what you expect to see the individual do*. In the above example anyone observing John will be able to state whether he could *run down hill*. If the WHAT identifies some knowledge that John will gain or a particular attitude identified as desirable for him to form, then the WHAT will state at least three observable actions identified as signifying that the objective has been accomplished. For example, if it has been identified as an objective that John should have a basic understanding of the computer, then you will have to identify a number of things that you expect him to be able to do to DEMONSTRATE the desired knowledge.

Example: *Computer Skills*

By 30 June 200–, John will

Demonstrate a basic understanding of the computer by

a) turning on the computer and printer upon request and without assistance.
b) when directed, opening Windows 98 and Microsoft Word 7.0, Excel 5.1, or Corel Draw 6 without assistance
c) locate, load, work on, and save a file in Microsoft Word and Excel frequently, without assistance
d) occasionally print a copy of work in progress, without assistance
e) set up and dismantle a computer and printer, connecting cables correctly, with intervention.

You may disagree that being able to do the five tasks listed above demonstrates a basic understanding of the computer and wish to substitute alternative ones. The point is that when John's Personal Plan is being written, everyone involved will work on it until they agree on the activities that will demonstrate his understanding of the computer.

The same technique is used when you identify social attitudes that you wish John to develop. There is no excuse for failing to state the key concepts or the key attitudes you wish him to develop. Bloom (1971) points out that writing behavioural objectives that describe desirable outcomes in the *Affective* (feelings) *domain* and *Cognitive* (knowledge and understanding) *domain* is no more difficult than writing objectives in the *Psychomotor* (skills) domain. Identify the behaviours that will DEMONSTRATE that the individual who is deafblind knows or feels what you are trying to promote.

Example: *Social Attitudes*

By 31 December 200–, George will demonstrate his liking for swimming by

a) frequently requesting that swimming be included in his weekly calendar without prompting
b) frequently assembling his towel, swim trunks, soap, and swimming cap without prompting
c) frequently changing into his swimming trunks at the pool without prompting
d) occasionally requesting swimming as an activity for Jim (his sighted friend) and himself.

How Well
The HOW WELL describes the conditions or limitations that are present. Terms such as *without spilling, with assistance, without assistance, with prompting, without prompting,* and *with intervention* can be used, provided the exact meaning of each term has been agreed beforehand by all parties. The author has used the following terms for many years and has found that they provide descriptions everyone can understand.

TERM	DESCRIPTION
with assistance	Requires hand-over-hand guidance. The mode used by the Intervenor primarily during the AWARENESS stage of Instructional Intervention.
without assistance	Does not require continuous hand-over-hand interaction throughout the activity but does require some verbal or physical direction. Corresponds with the beginning of the ACQUISITION stage.
with prompting	Demonstrates an understanding of the process and has the necessary motor skills but requires a non-directed prompt from time to time to complete the activity. Corresponds to the APPLICATION stage.
without prompting	Has the understanding and skill necessary to complete the activities and solve problems arising naturally from the activity but does not yet seek intervention appropriately when required. Corresponds to the more

advanced level of the APPLICATION STAGE and continues into the TRANSFER and GENERALIZA-TION STAGES.

with intervention   Knowledge, attitudes, and skills have been integrated and will be used as the basis for further learning. *The person who is deafblind understands the desired outcome and asks for intervention when his multi-sensory deprivation makes it necessary.* The highest level of functioning occurs when the person who is deafblind, not the Intervenor, decides when intervention is required and asks for it appropriately.

occasionally   More than twice in the period agreed upon (usually three to four weeks); often signifies that the area is ready for development.

frequently   More than 50 per cent of the time during the period agreed upon. *Note*: If the individual performs the task more than 50 per cent of the time but not as often as you like, you have a problem with MOTIVATION, not knowledge, skill, or attitude development.

The following examples may help to clarify the desired type of behavioural objectives.

Example: *Gross Motor Skills*

By 31 March 200–, George will
1. be happy when swimming.
Not a well-written objective. How will you know he is happy? A more appropriate example is given in the previous section under 'Social Attitudes.'
2. not self-abuse more than five times during a forty-minute swimming period.
Adequate, if everyone agreed upon what 'self-abuse' means when the Personal Plan was being written. It is negative, however, and the author would rather stress what Frank *will* do, that is, frequently refrain from 'picking at his arm' and return to the activity being engaged in at the time, when prompted.
3. put on and tie his boots without prompting each time he gets ready to go outside. Adequate, but if he fails to tie his boots on one occasion, he fails to attain the objective. It would be better to state as an objective, frequently put on and tie his boots without prompting, when preparing to go outside.
4. improve his eating habits. Unacceptable: 'Improve' compared with what? It would be preferable to specify desired behaviours:

a) frequently eat his meals without throwing food.
b) frequently drink his beverages without spilling.
c) frequently keep his hands out of non-fingerfood, without prompting.
d) occasionally recognize the difference between fingerfood and non-fingerfood, with prompting.

5. frequently prepare lunches consisting of soup and a sandwich or a hot dog and dry potato chips with intervention. Good. Describes WHO (George) will do WHAT (prepare lunches) WHEN (frequently: i.e., more than 50 per cent of the time), and HOW WELL (with intervention).

Part Five: Resources Required for Implementation (Optional)

If a new plan is being established or an existing plan modified, it is usually wise and sometimes necessary to identify all associated costs and so forth and to indicate where the financial and other resources will come from. For instance, the costs of intervention may be met from many sources, including government agencies, service clubs, and volunteers, and the family's contribution should always be recognized. Additional expenses also may arise in the areas of transportation, community program registrations, meals away from home, and so on. The author's experience has been that if these expenses are not identified before additional support is requested, it will be much more difficult to add them later.

Part Six: Implementation Schedule (Optional)

If a new plan is being introduced or additional community programs or services are being incorporated into the existing Personal Plan, dates and information as to who will provide the plan, monitor results, and be the liaison with the developer and the family should be included. In addition, a schedule of quarterly reviews of the Personal Plan giving dates, times, locations, and naming the people involved also should be included.

Implementing The Personal Plan

The careful development of a Personal Plan will not, in itself, ensure that the plan will be implemented successfully and that the appropriate techniques and methods will be utilized. The well-written Personal Plan is much like a personal travel guide obtained from one of the automobile associations. You have a vehicle (the Personal Plan) in which to travel, a personal road map directing you towards your destination (five-year-goals) and specific landmarks (behavioural objectives) that will indicate that you are making progress. All of these advantages, however, do not guarantee success. Your vehicle may break down or you may drive poorly and end up in a ditch. In the final analysis, the successful partnership consisting of the individual with deafblindness, family members and/or advocate, the community professionals, and the Intervenors will determine whether a Personal Plan will be successful or not.

There are two additional essential elements in the implementation of the Personal Plan: the actions of the Intervenor and the environment in which the daily activities will take place.

The Actions of the Intervenor

The concept of intervention and the actions of the Intervenor are described in detail in chapter 3. When the Intervenor is implementing a Personal Plan, there is an overriding philosophy that should guide his or her actions. The Intervenor must constantly remember that

Personal Plan behavioural objectives are NOT daily activities.

$$O \neq A,$$

that is, OBJECTIVES are not the same as ACTIVITIES.

Each activity will provide the opportunity to work on many objectives. The implementation of the Personal Plan MUST emphasize the use of ongoing personal and family routine activities to provide the opportunity to work on the knowledge, skills, and attitudes that have been identified. All activities, from getting up in the morning to getting dressed to go outside, from eating breakfast to making a snack, from learning to keep an activity box to making choices concerning the coming week's activities, present opportunities for working on expressive and receptive communication, attitudes, and a variety of cognitive and motor skills. For the infant, interactive play with the intervenor provides the same opportunities for development that the child's non-challenged peers get from interacting with others and with things in their world. For the deafblind youth or adult, a shopping trip provides endless opportunities for growth and development. This should not be interpreted as indicating that all activities should be used primarily for Instructional Intervention. Providing support through the use of General Intervention or Social Intervention is equally important (see chapter 3).

The success of the activity-based plan is dependent upon the use of clearly identified objectives. Little, if anything, in the development of the individual who is deafblind can be left to incidental or accidental learning.

Creating a Reactive Environment

The success of the Personal Plan approach depends, in part, on the involvement of the individual in a Reactive Environment. The Reactive Environment will not simply emerge or happen because you have identified goals, written specific objectives, and planned appropriate activities. You must motivate the individual who is deafblind, regardless of age, to participate in activities, be curious, reach beyond him or herself, and gain satisfaction from contacts with the world. In addition, someone must be there to receive attempts at communication and respond appropriately. This is hard, demanding work. A Reactive Environment is one that responds to the individual. For example, one of the earliest and loudest and ongoing forms of communication can be a temper tantrum or obvious anger. When this expression happens, analyse the situation and communicate that you understand the cause. You don't necessarily let the individual have his or her way, but you should communicate understanding.

Frances, a twenty-eight-year-old, profoundly deaf, totally blind, and physically handicapped woman who had spent her early years in an institutional setting either in bed or in a wheelchair, now lives with two deafblind companions in the community and has progressed to the stage of going to a restaurant to eat. On one occasion, Frances had a soft drink and fries. She decided she wanted another drink and signed 'drink please.' When told 'no,' she asked again three times and then in frustration swept the table contents onto the floor. Each time, the Intervenor explained that they had enough money for only one drink, and when the unacceptable behaviour took place, she firmly removed Frances from the restaurant. At this stage, objectives being worked on included several focusing on money and budgeting; buying a second drink or allowing others to buy one would have been inappropriate. Currently, Frances is successfully budgeting her pension; she herself could now decide on and buy a second drink.

As the Intervenor noted in her anecdotal record: 'It was quite a scene. Several people offered to buy her another drink.' All offers were politely refused. After they had returned home and Frances had calmed down, the incident provided the basis for several good dialogues. The next time Frances went to the restaurant she was reminded about one drink before they left home and again as they entered the restaurant. After several visits, no further problems arose. In Frances's case the problem was solved after a few visits. Unfortunately, the norm is to make many visits before the problem is solved. Incidentally, it has been found that the restaurant should be selected with care and, in the beginning, off-peak hours, when there are few other customers, are usually the best times to introduce visits.

Meaningful communication with the environment requires understanding of the environment. Take time to ensure that the individual who is deafblind has been able to explore his or her surroundings and to gain an understanding of them before activities are begun. Don't assume he or she knows what is there or what you expect of him or her. If you want to gain insight into the problem, blindfold yourself and, allowing no auditory input to take place, try the following.

1. Complete some simple tasks.
2. Next, communicate what you want to do tomorrow to a friend who does not know sign.
3. Then, ask her without speaking, where she got her shoes and what she wishes to eat next Sunday for supper.

The frustration you feel at not being able to find something that you think is in a particular place, being unable to seek assistance, or communicate simple ideas will assume new dimensions.

The Reactive Environment is not created for a few minutes or hours of each day. It is a total approach to rearing, working with, implementing a Personal Plan, and supporting the person who is deafblind. Communication, understanding, and subsequent development should not be stopped and started indiscriminately. We continually identify, explore, solve problems, and acquire new knowledge. We must provide suitable opportunities for the individual who is deafblind to have the same type and number of experiences regardless of his or her age. Never say, 'She is too young, too disabled, too —.'

Find a way to make it meaningful. During the Application Stage of an activity (see chapter 3), be sure that the individual who is deafblind has experiences that provide him or her with an opportunity to identify common problems and to solve them successfully. You will see indications when enough of an activity has taken place for the time being. Look for this message and respect it. You can always go back later if more experience or practice is needed.

Structure situations to ensure successful attempts in most cases. Be sure the individual understands when he or she has been successful and why. The Reactive Environment must also be structured to encourage and reward the use of residual vision and hearing. The individual who refuses to wear his hearing aids or glasses is not receiving sufficient benefit from them during daily routines and special activities to make them worthwhile. This is YOUR problem, not his or her problem.

The Reactive Environment must provide for basic needs, including security, love, and affection. A necessary component of 'security' is the feeling that one has the ability to control one's world. To control it effectively, the infant, child, youth, or adult who is deafblind must both perceive reality and be able to anticipate future interactions and their probable results. To be effective, the implementation of the Personal Plan must be designed to allow the individual to do both.

A Reactive Environment is not the same as a Permissive Environment. It is an environment designed to encourage the same control over interaction with the world enjoyed by peers who are not challenged by the disability of deafblindness. Most non-challenged infants, children, and youth are allowed to protest and present arguments in a courteous manner against rules, regulations, and arbitrary decisions of parents, family members, peers, and others many times each day. The arguments are not always successful, but they are allowed to take place. In a healthy family atmosphere children will be included in family planning, at a level appropriate to their ages, and allowed to voice their opinions, objections, or support for proposals.

Older youths and adults have an even greater degree of freedom in the actions they may take to 'live their own lives.' A challenging condition, such as deafblindness, should never be used as an excuse to take away this fundamental right. When severe disabilities enter the picture, there must be a conscious and purposeful effort to ensure opportunities for the exercise of options available to peers who are not faced with the same level of challenging disabilities. In many cases this stripping of human dignity is accomplished by doing nothing, doing for rather than with, or by creating a directive environment where all important decisions are made without real consultation with the child, youth, or adult. Sometimes, in the implementation of a Personal Plan, it is thought to be enough if the individual makes a limited choice. He or she is permitted to choose juice or milk but may not choose to say 'No, I want to skip lunch,' or choose to go to McDonald's.

It takes hard work to create a Reactive Environment. It takes real, concentrated, conscious effort, beginning with the infant and never ending, to include the individual who is deafblind in age-appropriate decisions. It is easy to use the excuse that he or she is too low functioning, doesn't have the experience necessary, or doesn't have the skills required to make the decision or carry out the actions arising from the decision. The real reason is often that it requires of others too much effort and time. The creation of a Reactive Environment is sacrificed to expediency through a rush to accomplish nothing worthwhile and to get nowhere important.

Decisions, Choices, and Responsibility

The Reactive Environment we are proposing is NOT an environment without rules, regulations, responsibilities, or tasks. A Reactive Environment is one in which each individual is treated with respect by others, listened to by others, and encouraged to communicate his or her ideas, and become a contributing member of the family or peer group. It must be stressed that in a Reactive Environment, for every opportunity to make a choice, to decide on a course of action, or to solve a problem, there is a consequence and a responsibility for that consequence.

Non-deafblind individuals learn that responsibilities accompany their actions and decisions in many ways. For infants, children, youth, and adults who are deafblind, the meaning of responsibility and consequences must be taught, because such concepts will not be acquired incidentally. During the implementation of the Personal Plan, it will take careful structuring and infinite patience to provide appropriate opportunities to develop understanding of the concept of responsibility for one's actions. The individual's environment will dictate the opportunities, but it does not have to dictate the results.

For example, CL decided, after finishing school, that she wanted to live at home with her parents, have a job, and participate in community recreational activities. Through a long slow process she has learned to operate within the family's budget when purchasing food and housekeeping necessities. She is now learning to anticipate other monthly bills and to establish a system to ensure that each is paid on time. Her parents have done an outstanding job of teaching her both the routines of daily living and the responsibility for seeing that these routines are carried out.

BP is a young man who is deafblind and lives in his own apartment within a setting designed to provide appropriate intervention and support. He has taken many years to understand group and community expectations and the necessity to conform to societal rules. He has progressed from the attitude that 'This is my apartment and my life and I will not do anything I do not want to' to volunteering to assist others by Brailling various catalogues used in the public library to make them useful for people who are blind.

Creating a Reactive Environment is not something that is done when the person who is deafblind becomes old enough. It begins when the infant is encouraged to indicate that he or she wants '*more*' or the activity is '*finished.*'

Example: Completing the Calendar

A child, totally blind and profoundly deaf and in a wheelchair, interacts with his Intervenor while creating a calendar for the following week:

Intervenor: Prompting the child to pick up a tactile card that indicates swimming symbols, signs (using adapted sign language) and says, *'When will you go swimming?'*

Child: Finding the symbol that indicates Tuesday and the area on the calendar indicating evening, places the card with the symbol indicating there and signs *'Tuesday.'*

Intervenor: *'Who will go swimming with you?'*

Child: *'You.'*

Intervenor: *'No, I will not be here. Who will you go with?'* Hands the child a set of cards representing various Intervenors (family members and others). After a number of interchanges, the child comes to understand and accept the situation.

Child: Choosing card representing father, signs *'father.'*

The use of tactile symbols to represent family members, activities, and so on permits the child to communicate ideas and make decisions.

Example: Making Plans
A teenager, who is profoundly deaf, has mobility vision, and a motor problem involving his left arm and side.

Intervenor: Has just come to work; signs and says, after engaging in the usual social small talk, *'What are your plans for today?'*

Teen: Signs, using a combination of sign and finger-spelling, *'After work, I want to go to Hamilton* (a city twenty-five miles away) *and buy a new computer game.'*

Intervenor: 'I'm sorry, my car is broken. Would you like to take the bus or wait until tomorrow?'

Teen: 'Every time I want to do something your car is broken! It is not fair! I don't believe you! I want to go to Hamilton."

Intervenor: 'I know my car is old and needs a lot of fixing. I don't have money for a new one. I understand you are disappointed. Would you rather wait, take the bus to Hamilton, or do something else? It is up to you. Which?'

Teen: 'No bus; too much money.'

Intervenor: 'Maybe we could go on Thursday if my car is fixed?'

Teen: 'OK.' (grudgingly).

Intervenor: 'What will you do after work today?'

Example: Responsibility for Supper
An adult with some functional vision and hearing, who lives in a group home, talks with her Intervenor.

Intervenor: What are you going to make for supper this afternoon?

Adult: I'm not making supper. I made it Monday. I want to go out to eat.

Intervenor: You know it's your turn. Jannie made supper Tuesday and Marianne made stir-fried chicken yesterday.

Adult: Why don't you make supper?

Intervenor: I go home at 3 pm so I won't be here for supper.

Adult: Then I want to go out! We all could go to the restaurant.

Intervenor: Do you have enough money? I know that both Jannie and Marianne said that they were broke until the end of the month.

Adult: No, I don't have enough money. You could lend me some.

Intervenor: No way! Well, what will you make for supper? How about sweet potato pie?

After many more exchanges, it is decided that fish and chips would be easy to make in the microwave oven.

These types of interchange between an Intervenor and an individual who is deafblind do not simply happen. The author is the first to recognize that creating a Reactive Environment is a difficult, exhausting, and time-consuming task. But it is essential if the individual who is deafblind is to have an opportunity to develop socially and emotionally into a fully functioning adult. You must consciously and continuously create a Reactive, not a Directive Environment.

Parental Involvement in Personal Plan Development and Implementation

If the deafblind individual is to become a functioning member of family and community, his or her family must have an understanding of the goals and objectives of the Personal Plan and be involved at all stages of its development, for the following reasons.

1. In most cases, parents and family members know their infant, child, or youth best.
2. Each family has its own priorities and lifestyle.
3. An appreciation of the infant, child, and youth's strengths and capabilities will not develop within the family unit unless he or she is an involved, contributing member of that unit.
4. Effective communication requires constant practice by all family members and involves much more than taking signing classes. Effective communication requires interaction based upon understanding.
5. The family's expectations must grow as the infant becomes a child, a youth, and finally an interdependent adult.

6. Without family or surrogate family support, the child will experience emotional problems similar to those often experienced by orphans who have no close or caring friends or relatives. These difficulties will be magnified by the isolating impact of sensory deprivation.

A caring family, which is receiving *adequate* support from knowledgeable professionals, is the deafblind individual's greatest asset.

Support for the Primary Caregiver

Throughout this book the importance of the role of the family in providing the support for the deafblind individual will be stressed. It is recognized that the family cannot focus all of its time and energy on the individual who is deafblind. It cannot be repeated too often that a Personal Plan must be written so that its implementation can take place primarily during established family routines. No plan that requires the family to change the majority of its established patterns and relationships will succeed in the long run.

In most cases, in the earlier stages, mother will be the primary caregiver and the most important factor in the infant's life. Without adequate help and support from within the family and from outside agencies, she will not be able to fulfil this important role. Governments and professionals must realize that the family will need help. Mother will need assistance to relieve her of many of the 'housekeeping' chores, thus making available to her the time necessary to devote to her special infant. In these days, where in many families both parents are wage earners, it is doubly important to find assistance both within and outside the family.

Intervention as Parental Relief

Intervention is not parental relief. It is enabling the person who is key to growth and development of the deafblind infant or child to provide appropriate support after she or he has

- had training in methods of handling the infant or child
- participated in the development of the infant or child's Personal Plan
- had help in formulating realistic goals and in recognizing success indicators that show progress
- had instruction in communication development techniques
- had assistance in planning and integrating activities to fit the family's routines.

Mother will also need time for herself and time with other members if she and the family are going to survive. Having a number of visiting social workers and therapists does not provide relief. Scheduling, making cookies, trying to remember what was said, and so on all add to rather than diminish tension and the need for support.

Involvement of Family Members

Family members must be involved in the selection of Intervenors and should participate with the Intervenors as they are trained by the deafblind specialist consultant. (See chapter 16 for detailed information on the role of the consultant.) There are several reasons for this involvement.

1. Both the Intervenors and the family will use the same techniques and have the same expectations.
2. The Intervenors will realize that the family members are knowledgeable and are an essential part of plan design and delivery.
3. The family should be in control of who will be coming into and working in their home on a regular basis.
4. The Intervenor should realize that the family, not the deafblind specialist, will have the final say as to his or her employment.

A Community Support System

The absence of a pool of knowledge in most communities means that specific actions must be taken by the deafblind consultant to identify and educate key people in the community. The make-up of this local support network will differ from one community to the next. The individuals involved will share some common attributes. They will have an understanding of the needs of the family and the family member who is deafblind and will be able to explain to others in the community what these needs are and how they differ from other individuals who are faced with more commonly occurring disabilities. This network must be developed so that it will be available for support when the family requires it between visits by the consultant. In some cases, the network will form part of a service delivery team of medical and therapeutic professionals, social workers, and other community workers. In other cases, the team may be drawn from community and/or church groups to which the family belongs or with which the family feels comfortable. In any case, regardless of the composition of the local support group, the consultant should take on the role of chairperson or case manager.

Additional Points to Consider

1. The school Individual Educational Program (IEP) or Individual Pupil Plan
   (IPP) will form part of the Personal Plan, not the reverse. It is unusual for the
   IEP to contain five-year goals or objectives outside the concerns of the educational program. The pupil who is deafblind, the parents, and the deafblind
   consultant should be part of the team that is developing the IEP. The manager should ensure that the relationship between the school IEP and the Personal Plan is clearly identified and understood by all.
2. The pupil who is deafblind will face many challenges that often are only
   minor inconveniences to their peers who are not challenged by the disability
   of deafblindness. These include, but are not limited to,
   a) obtaining standard texts in an appropriate medium (large-print or Braille,
      as required). Frequently these are not ready to use at the same time as
      they are available to peers who are not challenged by deafblindness, and
      the student who is deafblind may have to operate without timely, first-
      hand exposure to such materials.
   b) obtaining reference materials, such as magazine and newspaper articles,
      library texts, videotapes, and so on. The time and frustration incurred in
      searching for such materials (often finding that other students have
      obtained them first) and the time restrictions placed on reserved texts
      place the student who is deafblind at a severe disadvantage in both read-
      ing the material and relocating specific sections, and they are com-
      pounded if such material must be finger-spelled. (Ask a friend to finger-
      spell the next chapter to you, one letter at a time, and then ask you ques-
      tions about what you have received.)
3. Clear and reasonable decisions must be made about how daily assignments
   will be given and corrected for the student who is deafblind. An assignment
   that may take another class member forty-five minutes can take several
   hours for the student who is deafblind. The problem is not one of being
   unable to process the information or do the assignment; it is one of logistics
   in obtaining non-distorted information in a usable and timely manner and in
   being able to organize such information using the expressive medium available to the student who is deafblind. Is it possible to identify five key questions that will show that the student understands the concepts that have been
   taught rather than assigning the student the fourteen questions that the rest of
   the class will be expected to answer?
4. The method by which the student who is deafblind will be tested must be
   clearly identified prior to the beginning of the course. Simply giving the student 'more time' is not the answer. Expecting a student who is deafblind to

concentrate for three to five hours when the rest of the class writes one- to two-hour examinations is unreasonable. Again, a key question approach should be considered.

5. Sometimes it is suggested that the student take an oral examination. This approach is occasionally objected to because the teacher says that he or she does not know whether it is the Intervenor or the student who is deafblind who is supplying the answer. There are only two possible answers to this objection. Either trust the Intervenor or bring in an Intervenor who knows little about the subject. It should be noted that, particularly in the higher grades, if the teacher has taught so little content that anyone (including the Intervenor) can supply the correct answer, his or her competence as a teacher rather than the competence of the student should be questioned.

6. On many occasions it is advisable for the student who is deafblind to take less than a full course load. Occasionally, parents or a teacher will object to this proposal. The objection will be based upon the supposition that if the student takes less than a full course load, he or she will have 'an easy time' and will get better marks. There is no indication that this is true. Students who take night-school classes, on the whole, do not do better than day students when the factor of motivation is cancelled out. The student's problem is to access sufficient non-distorted information successfully to complete the course. If he or she cannot process it, no amount of extra time will permit success. It might be argued that, if the final examinations required only rote memory, fewer subjects could make a difference, but currently there are few courses that require only regurgitation of selected facts.

7. One teacher should be selected, in consultation with the parents and the student, to act as an advocate for the student together with the consultant and with all other members of the faculty. The careful selection of this staff member, who will do much more than the conventional guidance counsellor, will be one of the determining factors in the student's overall success.

Summary

1. A Personal Plan is designed to meet the needs of a specific individual who is deafblind. It is not the modification or individualization of an existing program.
2. A Personal Plan incorporates all aspects of development, education, and therapy.
3. Most adults who are deafblind can live in and participate as members of the community, provided they receive appropriate support in their younger years and appropriate intervention throughout their lives.

4. Developing a Personal Plan begins with an understanding of the long-term goals. These goals are reflected in the overall level of the Personal Plan developed for a specific individual.
5. A Personal Plan has four required sections and two optional sections.
6. Having a well-written plan lays the groundwork for, but does not guarantee, appropriate implementation.
7. A Personal Plan must be implemented in a Reactive Environment.
8. A developer may overestimate or underestimate the progress that will be made and thus propose inappropriate objectives for the Personal Plan. If the infant, student, or adult fails to attain or surpasses a specific objective, it is not he or she who failed, but the developer, who has failed to anticipate the progress that will be made.

Answers to the Questions

A. You are going to Switzerland for a skiing vacation.
B. You are going to the capital of your country to attend a two-day meeting.
C. You are going to the local store for groceries.
D. You are relocating to Yellowknife in the Northwest Territories, Canada, for three years.

NOTE

1 In the 1982 edition of *Deaf-Blind Infants and Children* (McInnes and Treffry) the program that was developed for an infant or child who was deafblind was referred to as 'An Individuated Program.' Unfortunately, this term was often misinterpreted as providing the child with a modified program that was based upon the needs of some other group. This occurred most often when an attempt at integration placed the infant or child who is deafblind in a preschool or school program designed to meet the needs of a special population who were auditorially or visually challenged. It also occurred when specialists from these fields were relied upon to provide programs. It is hoped that when the term 'Personal Plan' is stressed, the resulting programs will be more comprehensive and designed from the bottom up to meet a specific client's global needs.

REFERENCES

Bloom, Benjamin S., J. Thomas Hastings, and George F. Madaus (1971) *Handbook on Formative and Summative Evaluation of Student Learning.* New York: McGraw-Hill

Callier-Azusa Scale (1966) Callier Center for Communication Disorders, University of Texas at Dallas, 1966 Inwood Road, Dallas, TX 75235

McInnes, J.M., and J.A. Treffry (1982, 1993, 1997) *Deaf-Blind Infants and Children: A Developmental Guide.* Toronto: University of Toronto Press

McInnes, J.M., et al. (1994) *The Developmental Profile for Use with Persons Who Are Deafblind (1994 Edition).* Brantford, ON: Canadian Deafblind and Rubella Association (Ontario Chapter)

3

Intervention

JOHN M. McINNES

Introduction

It has generally been accepted by individuals with congenital or early adventitious deafblindness and their supporters as well as those individuals with acquired deafblindness that there are occasions when interactive support provided by a person who is sighted and hearing is the most practical and efficient way to obtain the information necessary to make decisions and function independently. 'There is a lot of different terminology used to identify people who fulfill this role. Some people call these people guide-communicators, or guide-helps, and some Intervenors' (Sasse 1996). Others use the term interpreter-guide. Rødbroe and Souriau use the term 'Partner' to define the role during the act of communication. 'Partner' is an excellent term, because it combines the concepts of interaction and shared responsibility during that interaction. Regardless of the term, the recognition of the importance of such a person and the role he or she can play in supporting the person with deafblindness has gained wide, one could say 'universal' acceptance.

The term 'Intervenor' (note: 'or' to differentiate from the standard dictionary *intervener* and the accompanying definition, 'as coming between') and the concept of intervention emerged from research by the author and others in the early 1970s. A careful study of a representative group of past and present deafblind individuals showed that those identified as 'successful' had several things in common. The most significant appeared to be that each deafblind person was supported by one or more individuals, including spouses, family members, friends, secretaries, other paid individuals, and volunteers. The study also showed that although these individuals supplied support, they did not make decisions for or direct the deafblind individual. In fact, evidence of success was often seen as the ability to make and carry out decisions.

As Geenens points out in chapter 5, these individuals did the following: provided information to the deafblind person that introduced and broadened the concepts surrounding the words that make up language; facilitated communication between the person who was deafblind and the environment; provided nondistorted information concerning events, actions, and reactions, thus enabling the formation of attitudes and the making of decisions based upon timely and accurate information; supported the deafblind individual in carrying out actions arising from his or her decisions in a timely fashion; and provided feedback that allowed the deafblind person to develop and refine skills, recognize the effect of his or her actions on others, and modify his or her actions before the next attempt. Our study also showed that Intervenors, by any name, supported the individual who is deafblind by an amazingly consistent process that was more influenced by the needs of the individual than the skills of the person providing the support.

Defining Intervention

While the concept of support has generally been accepted, there appears to be considerable confusion concerning the concept when the term 'intervention' is used. The magnitude of this confusion increases as the distance from working directly with the person with deafblindness increases. The concept of intervention can differ according to who is defining it. Professionals often use a definition of the position that incorporates some ultimate criteria or competences, while the individual with deafblindness may see the role as defined by his particular wants and needs. The author believes that both views are incomplete. If one must be chosen, however, he would choose the latter.

Intervention is not a magic cure that will permit the infants, children, youth, and adults with congenital or early adventitious deafblindness to be integrated into an existing program or a community setting. Intervention, by itself, is not the key, nor is the Intervenor the sole answer.

Intervention appears to be a simple concept, easy to explain and easier to implement, and many simplistic phrases have been used to try to explain it. In reality, intervention is the PROCESS that takes place between the person who is deafblind and the person providing support, in such a way that the disability caused by the loss of the effective use of the distance senses of sight and hearing will be minimized.

Intervention is a process, the purpose of which is to enable the deafblind person to establish and maintain maximum control over his or her environment at a level appropriate to physical ability and level of functioning. To repeat: the process of intervention is not defined by the person acting as an Intervenor, but rather by the NEEDS and desires of the person who is deafblind.

The Intervenor is not simply 'the eyes and ears' of the person who is deafblind; such an explanation ignores the real significance of the disability of deafblindness. These phrases are useful when one is trying to explain the concept of intervention to the world at large but are almost totally useless as guidelines for the implementation of such a support system. To suggest that 'Intervenor' is merely another term for interpreter or sighted guide or that an Intervenor is a caregiver like those supplied to individuals who are physically or mentally challenged also shows a lack of understanding of the impairment of deafblindness and the needs of the person who is deafblind.

Intervention as an Operational Concept

A poor, but more correct analogy for intervention would be a combination of services provided by a telephone operator, a taxi driver, and a tourist information centre worker. The telephone operator does not decide whom or when you will call. The operator may assist you to obtain information to make the call or may indicate to you its cost, but he or she does not decide to whom, when, why, or whether it is in your best interests to make the call. The taxi driver does not decide with whom, when, where, or why you will travel. While the driver may occasionally exercise some judgment concerning your safety, suggest the best route to take, and may react either positively or negatively to your behaviour, you are always free to refuse his services. The staff of the tourist information centre has specific information that they know from experience will make your visit more enjoyable. They may show tremendous enthusiasm for certain places and events and try to persuade you to visit them. In the final analysis, however, it is you, not the clerk, who will make the decision. In addition, each of the above individuals will provide a different level of service and information depending on the age and the needs of the individual requesting the service.

For individuals who are deafblind, the Intervenor should be fulfilling the combined functions of the telephone operator, taxi driver, and tourist information centre staff, while at the same time ensuring that the final, age-appropriate decision is left up to the individual with deafblindness. Infants who are not faced with challenging disabilities such as deafblindness make decisions and communicate preferences about people, activities, and things. Regardless of age, individuals who are congenitally or early adventitiously deafblind must be encouraged and supported to acquire the information necessary to make decisions and choices, to be curious about their world, to be 'persons,' not compliant individuals who never get into mischief or say 'NO!' That is what intervention at any level, for any age, is all about.

When intervention is utilized by a person who is deafblind, the process of intervention, *not the role of the Intervenor*, changes with each passing minute, with each repetition of the same activity, with each new activity, and with each change in the world surrounding the person who is deafblind. The type, intensity, frequency, and methods of supplying support will differ greatly according to the needs of each infant, child, youth, and adult. All aspects of intervention will be influenced by the degree of sensory deprivation, the age of onset, other additional disabilities, expectations of the deafblind individual, his or her past experiences, as well as a multitude of other influences, the sum total of which can be described as the individual's needs.

Intervention as a Philosophical Concept

Intervention is also a philosophical concept, which states each person who is deafblind should be provided with sufficient non-distorted information to permit him or her to make decisions and the degree of support necessary to carry out those decisions successfully within a reasonable length of time. Thus, intervention is a function of the interaction between the person who is deafblind and his or her environment. When we say 'successfully within a reasonable length of time,' we are talking about giving the person who is deafblind sufficient support to enable him or her to communicate with his or her environment and the people in it; to do what he or she has decided to do successfully; and to receive sufficient feedback to be able to learn from his or her mistakes through the use of the *Total Communication Approach*. It does not mean that the person who is deafblind will be prevented from making mistakes.

Intervention is not a 'job' that someone 'does' for a person who is deafblind. Intervention is the act of providing that person with a range of information necessary to anticipate events, make appropriate choices, plan future actions, modify skills to improve performance, communicate successfully, and/or apply existing skills and knowledge to interact successfully with the environment.

Confusion Concerning Intervention

Confusion over intervention exists primarily because the emphasis is mistakenly placed on the Intervenor as a person with knowledge and skills rather than on the process. Secondly, it is sometimes assumed that the purpose of intervention is primarily to teach language and motor and self-care skills and to provide care; thus, intervention appears to be the same as that provided by school aides, occupational therapists, or tutors. A third reason for the confusion existing in some quarters results from the fact that in order to obtain necessary funding, stress is placed upon the employment of one or more persons as Intervenors rather than on the process of intervention. Such positions are sometimes funded under other already established job descriptions rather than creating a new category. This approach is fraught with danger. Experience has shown that eventually the individual providing the intervention may be expected to perform according to the established job description that goes with the title rather than as an Intervenor. If this happens, the process of intervention will be endangered or destroyed. In addition, when job cuts are made by class, for example, 'school aide,' the deafblind student may loose his or her intervention with no consideration being given to the special needs created by the disability of deafblindness.

No matter what the reason for the confusion, it must be stressed that *intervention is a process*, and the role of the Intervenor reflects the way that the process meets the needs of the individual who is deafblind regardless of his or her age.

One ultimate goal of every Personal Plan for individuals who are deafblind should be to teach them how to train and utilize their own Intervenors and to control the amount, type, and source of their intervention. Not all individuals who are deafblind will be able to reach the stage where they can independently provide this training for their Intervenors, but all should be encouraged to participate in such training to the best of their present ability.

The Intervenor

An Intervenor is anyone who provides intervention for a person who is deafblind. A member of the family, a volunteer, or a person who is paid, such as a teacher, a secretary, a therapist, or a school aide; in fact, anyone who interacts with a person who is deafblind may provide some degree of intervention. The question is not whether the deafblind person will need and receive intervention. The question is whether such interaction and support will be timely, appropriate, and useful.

Special training, such as that provided by the Intervenor Training Course at George Brown College or the Intervenor for Deafblind Persons Program at Medicine Hat College.[1] In adaptive communication and individualized techniques and methods and in understanding the disability of multi-sensory deprivation will improve the type of intervention provided and its effectiveness. Some Intervenors will attend intensive courses preparing them to work with a range of persons who are deafblind. Others will receive ongoing training from consultants and family members who will prepare them to offer intervention to a specific individual. Intervenors who have received this type of training are not ready to support all deafblind individuals. When they begin providing intervention for a different individual who is deafblind, they will require additional specific training to give them the understanding, specific techniques, and modification of the general methods necessary to meet that individual's evolving needs.

The Role of the Intervenor

The role of the Intervenor cannot be considered in isolation. What the Intervenor does and how it is done will be in direct response to the actions and the needs of the person who is deafblind and the type of support he or she requires at a particular time.

The intervention process can be arbitrarily divided into three types. Intervention providing general support is always present but becomes more evident as the deafblind individual grows older and takes more personal responsibility for making plans and carrying them out. The main focus of General Intervention is the support of the individual who is deafblind. The process of intervention for instructional purposes is described in detail in the model below. A third type of intervention, Social Intervention, takes place at all ages between the deafblind individual and family members or between him or herself and friends or others. The focus of Social Intervention is upon a supportive personal relationship and appropriate social responses. Failure to recognize these distinct types of intervention can result in role confusion for the person acting as an Intervenor, the deafblind person, his or her family, funding agencies, and the general public.

General Intervention

The focus of general or ongoing intervention is the provision of support for the deafblind individual in such a way that the problems caused by deafblindness are reduced to the greatest degree possible. When providing this type of intervention, the Intervenor should respond to the individual who is deafblind and thus empower him or her to exercise control over the activities and interactions taking place. In an attempt to facilitate this role, many suggestions, such as 'do with, not for,' have evolved. Such advice can sometimes seem contradictory or confusing. We will look at some of the most common examples after we have examined other aspects of the general support process.

General Intervention is the process by which a support person provides information to the person who is deafblind that will permit him or her to gain much the same understanding of the world as the non-deafblind individual gains through the use of sight and vision. The Intervenor also provides the information necessary to permit the deafblind person to make informed decisions, act on those decisions, and understand the results of these actions. This information (feedback) concerning the results of the actions of the deafblind person during ongoing routine activities is essential. Such information accomplishes the following.

* It permits the deafblind person to anticipate events.
* It motivates him or her to continue to act. Actions may range from refraining from repeating an action to continuing or modifying the action now or in the future.
* It is essential for skill and attitude modification. An understanding of the success of any attempt at applying a skill is necessary if future attempts are to be improved. Also, unless the deafblind person is able to understand how his or her actions are perceived by others, it is unreasonable to expect that a recognition of, an understanding of, and a compliance with broader societal norms will take place. Compliance without understanding is not acceptable as a basis for long-term behaviour.

The Intervenor's role can also be described in the broadest terms as facilitating contact with and awareness of the environment. Changes in a known environment or in the structure of new environments should be drawn to the deafblind person's attention. If further or more detailed explorations of these changes are sought, it is the responsibility of the Intervenor to support such enquiries. The infant, child, youth, or adult who is deafblind should be supported during attempts to gather, assimilate, and use the same amount and types of information as would be gathered, assimilated, and used by his or her non-challenged peers.

The concept of communication between partners is covered in detail in chapter 4. As an aspect of the general intervention process, the importance of the Intervenor's fostering and supporting communication initiated by the deafblind person, regardless of his or her age, cannot be overemphasized.

During General Intervention the basic objectives of the Intervenor can be summarized as follows: providing support; increasing the deafblind person's level of control over and sense of responsibility for his or her life; and encouraging requests for appropriate assistance. There is little disagreement concerning the role of the Intervenor during the provision of support for individuals with acquired deafblindness or for individuals who are identified as older, high-functioning, congenitally or early adventitiously deafblind. There is considerably more difficulty in understanding this role as it applies to infants, children, youth, and some severely challenged or low-functioning adults. Some confusion arises from the fact that one individual is often called upon to provide all three types of intervention during one activity period. An Intervenor who is a parent or an adult working with an infant, a child, or a youth often sees control as his or her prerogative. We often fail to realize the amount of control over his or her life that a non-disabled individual of the same age exerts. Three of the more effective methods of controlling the situation used by the deafblind individual's peers are changing the subject or redirecting the adult's attention, placing distance between him or herself and the controlling adult by going somewhere else to play, or using physical activity or motion. These three methods of controlling one's life, along with many others, are either not available to the deafblind individual or are available to a less effective degree. The presence of additional disabilities also can lead to a directive rather than a supportive relationship unless specific care is taken to build a reactive environment (see chapter two).

Suggestions for Providing General Intervention

There are many pieces of advice about supporting the individual who is deafblind. They range from 'do with, not for' to 'any activity, no matter how complicated, can become a self-stimulating activity.' Others, such as Dr Geenen's 'Use it or lose it' (see chapter 5) are found throughout the book. Each contains a nugget of good advice that can be modified and applied in most situations.

Approaching a Deafblind Person

Knowing Someone Is There
When you enter a room or return to the 'space' of the deafblind person, make sure that you let him or her know who is there. Everyone who comes into regular contact with a deafblind individual of any age should have a sign, symbol, or other means of recognition. This can range from a distinguishing feature such as glasses or a pigtail to the first letter of a name presented on a specific part of the body or a name finger-spelled. It is absolutely essential to ensure that the deafblind person, particularly an infant or child, knows who is there. This step may be overlooked or ignored if he or she has some residual vision or hearing. This is a serious mistake. It is often the case that the person may not be using his or her distance sense(s) at a given moment or may not be able to integrate information from one or both distance senses while stimulation is being received from the senses of taste, touch, or smell. Perhaps the most common time that this simple act is overlooked is when an Intervenor has been working with the deafblind person and has left to do or get something. Someone else may have interacted with the deafblind individual while the Intervenor was

away, or some environmental cue or time-based routine may lead the deafblind person to expect someone else or to be confused concerning who is now communicating with him or her.

Moving a Deafblind Person
When you wish to have a deafblind person move from his present location to another, these points should be adhered to.

1. Approach, get his or her attention, make sure you are recognized, and then communicate what is going to happen.
2. Do not grab the person's hands or body without first indicating that you are there.
3. If you are communicating hand on hand, always indicate that you are going to communicate by first touching the hands lightly and then allowing time for the deafblind individual to anticipate what is going to happen before you begin to communicate.
4. In most situations, when tactile signing or one-hand finger-spelling is used, the listening hand is on the top and the talking hand is underneath.
5. In all situations, do not grab or hold the deafblind person's hand in such a way that you are preventing hand or arm movement. A light touch is essential.
6. Remember that, even during communication, the Intervenor is providing support rather than control.
7. Lastly, do not move the deafblind person to a new location and walk away. Be sure the person knows where he or she is and when you or someone else will return.

Facilitating Conversation
Sharon Barrey Grassick's well-organized paper, 'CUEmmunication' (1998) is focused on supporting individuals who are deafblind.[2] In an excellent section, 'The Beginnings of Communication,' she deals with initiating communication with an individual who is deafblind and how to communicate with a preverbal deafblind person. The following is an extract from Sharon's paper.

WHERE TO BEGIN

What do you do when you first meet a person who is congenitally deafblind?
How do you introduce yourself?
How do you communicate with a person who is pre-verbal?
Perhaps the most frequently asked question is: Where do you begin?

APPROACH

The concept of approach developed from a firm conviction that the initial contact you make with a person who is congenitally deafblind is critically important – it may even open the gateway to communication and language development ... ...

A person with hearing and vision is given many incidental cues about another person approaching them, before the other person ever says a word or comes within their personal space. A person with hearing and vision will see the other person approaching from quite a distance and may be able to tell by their height or demeanor whether it is a child or an adult. They may be able to tell whether it is a male or a female. They will see the color and style of the hair and the clothing. As the person comes closer they may hear the person speaking to someone else in the background and recognize the voice, and perhaps even guess what kind of a mood the person is in. They can read the facial expression and body language which may indicate how that person is feeling. They will certainly know whether the person is familiar to them or a complete stranger. All of this information, and more, is available to the person with hearing and vision before the advancing person makes any effort whatsoever to communicate their impending arrival.

The person who is deafblind will not have the advantage of this distance information ... We must never assume that a person who is deafblind knows we are approaching or knows who we are once contact is made. The person must be approached appropriately. This means offering useful, meaningful information in the most non-threatening way possible. The simple, but structured, technique of approach can be used with very young children as well as adults.

The following guidelines are recommended to be used consistently by all people who are involved with the person who is deafblind and in all settings:

1. Before making any physical contact with the person, approach from the front, if at all possible, and move to the side as you come closer. This gives the person the opportunity to use whatever residual vision he may have, whether it be central or peripheral vision.
2. Speak in a normal voice as you approach, talking naturally and saying the person's name. This gives the person the opportunity to use whatever residual hearing he may have.

   Come to within about 20 centimeters of his ear, and continue to 'chat' naturally but using good voice inflection and intonation. Never shout. Shouting only distorts sound and may cause discomfort.

   At this close proximity, even if the person is profoundly deaf and/or unable to comprehend speech, he may gain important information from intonation, pitch and/or breath stream. He may also be able to smell shampoo, perfume, after-shave or garlic from last night's dinner! If perfume or after-shave is worn, try to always wear the same kind as this may give the person a valuable cue as to who you are. Do not wear strong perfume or after-shave. This can be very offensive to some people as can the smell of cigarette smoke on hands or breath. Good hygiene is very important, as you will be in close contact with a person who is deafblind.

3. Now you can introduce yourself. Gently place the back of your hand against the back of his hand. Leave it there until he initiates further contact, such as moving his fingers or feeling your hands for rings or a bracelet.

    Be patient. Wait for the person to make the next move. If there is a piece of jewelry that is always worn, or a distinguishing characteristic such as a beard, guide his hand to it each time. If this is done consistently, he will eventually seek the cue himself.

    Never grab or force things into the palms of the hands, as these are the 'eyes' of a person who is deafblind.

4. Say 'Hello.' If he offers a palm you may make a circular movement onto his palm to say 'hello.' This gesture can also be made onto the back of his hand, if he does not offer the palm.

    Some people are labeled 'tactilely defensive' if, at contact, they pull their hands away, retract their hands into fists, or refuse to touch something. 'Tactilely selective' is perhaps a more accurate term.

5. Agree on a sign name to indicate the person. Initially use only one letter or sign. Combined letters or signs may only confuse at this stage.

    Sign 'hello,' and direct his hand to your distinguishing characteristic or personal physical cue.

    A possible sign name would be to finger spell the first letter of his name, e.g., 'hello J,' then guide his hand to point to you and touch your physical cue. Then guide his hand to point to himself and to finger spell 'J.'

    Repeat the procedure.

    [At a later stage you can introduce your sign name in the same way. For example, guide his hand to point to you and to feel you making your sign name; then guide his hand back to point to him and make his sign name; then guide it back to point to you and make your sign name.]

    Always give the person enough time to initiate a response. Sometimes we are too eager to 'help' and we shape or prompt the person's hands into a response before they have had enough time to process their next move. Not only is this frustrating for the person, but it also develops learned helplessness.

6. You can now proceed with an activity. (Consultation with people close to J would have already taken place to establish what kinds of activities he likes.)

    Take J's lead. Respond to any communication attempts. If he indicates preference for a particular activity, respond accordingly. At this stage he may well wait for you to initiate an activity.

7. Give him meaningful information about the forthcoming activity. Never assume that he understands what you expect him to do, or what you plan to do with him. Consistent use of a meaningful object, or cue, presented before the activity can help the person to develop the ability to anticipate that activity.

Make sure that the object, or cue, you choose is meaningful to him, and that everyone involved with him uses the same object, or cue, for that particular activity.

Remember to choose objects for characteristics that will appeal to the individual person being particularly attentive to the tactile characteristics if there is little or no vision.

If it is time for an activity, take a piece of the activity to him. He can then carry the object to the activity to indicate where he is going. If this is done consistently he will build up associations and will begin to anticipate the related activities when presented with the object.

a) If it is time for morning tea, take the empty cup to him for him to carry to the table. Give him a cue as to where he is going and what will happen when he arrives there. Don't just drag him to the table and assume he knows where and why he is going.

b) If it is time to go in the car, take a set of keys to him. He can then carry the keys to the car. If this is done consistently, he will develop an association between the keys and going in the car.

c) The object goes with him and stays with him during the activity, perhaps in a pocket or on the table next to him. When the activity is finished, he can then place the object in a particular container. The container can be the object to indicate the concept of finished.

d) Eventually, he will be able to make a choice, given two objects, as to which activity he would prefer.

e) A zippered waist bag, sometimes called a 'bum bag,' is a great place to keep the objects handy. The bag can be worn to keep the hands free. When the person begins to make his own choices, he can be encouraged to wear the bag himself, to always have the objects available to him. However, discourage play with the particular objects in the bag, as they may lose their symbolic significance if handled frequently without meaning.

If the person likes to have something to explore or play with, an alternative to the contents of the bag could be different objects or textures affixed to the outside of the bag.

f) Natural gestures and iconic signs can be used with the objects, e.g. moving the arms to indicate swimming; hand to mouth to indicate drink; hand on head to indicate a hat for going outside, etc.

g) If the person is in a chair, never move the chair in or out without first indicating what you intend to do, e.g., tap the back of the chair or the handles (if it is a wheelchair).

Always let the person know who is there. Just imagine yourself being propelled through space to an unknown destination by an unknown person!

8. Make a conscious effort to say 'hello' and 'goodbye.' The person who is deafblind will not see you coming or going, nor will he hear you saying 'hello' or 'goodbye,' so you must approach him to give him this information. Give the person who is deafblind the same respect as you would expect from someone who enters or leaves your own home.

9. If you must leave the person for a short period and will be returning to him soon, indicate this by telling him and accompany it by a touch cue (perhaps a gentle squeeze on the shoulder). Whatever cue is used, make sure it is used consistently, and that it differs from what is used to indicate 'goodbye,' when you leave for the day or for an extended period of time.

Always give the person the courtesy of letting him know who you are when you come back to him, even if you have only been away for a minute. It only takes a few seconds to follow the steps outlined above for approach.

Never assume that he knows it is you and don't play games like 'Guess who I am?'

10. Give the individual a reason to trust you and a reason to communicate with you.

11. Approach is really nothing more than good common sense. Use it consistently and it will become automatic. Although it is a structured method, it takes only seconds to apply, so the old excuse, 'We just don't have the time to do it,' just doesn't work here!

What is important in effective communication is not so much the variety of communication methods and number of signs you know, but how you use that knowledge, and respect the communication that is used and understood by the individual who is deafblind. It is what I like to refer to as 'the attitude of communication.'

12. ASSUME NOTHING.

Further Suggestions

Cues and Objects of Reference

It should be remembered that the use of cues and objects of reference, as outlined in Sharon's paper, are only a stage in the development of communication skills, and learned helplessness should not be encouraged by failure to support further development of communication skills.

Facilitating Expressive and Interactive Communication

Two-way communication can be initiated and facilitated by asking questions, such as the following.

What will we do next?
Where is your (coat, shoe, plate, glass)?
Where will we (go, get ... find ...)?
When is Dad coming?
What is it?
Where are we going?
When will we go swimming?
When will you and Mary go to the store?
How do (I, you) make ...?
Why?

Further suggestions for developing dialogue are found in chapter 4.

Continually work to develop two-way communication. If the deafblind person does not seem to use expressive communication, look for body language and help him or her learn the appropriate language patterns to attach to the action. '*Are you angry*' (*sad, unhappy, happy, bored, etc.)?*' Then assist the child to give the '*angry*' or other appropriate sign with feeling.

Don't Talk At, Interact With

Ask questions and assist in forming the response if a response is not forthcoming in a reasonable amount of time. Use questions with even a young child. Structure your questions and responses consistently in the same way, so language groupings may be imitated by the deafblind infant or child.

'Baby Talk' Signing

The deafblind child's peers learn language and communication skills by imitating speech patterns of those about them. The deafblind child must have the opportunity to do the same thing. Provide communication patterns one step above the infant or child's expressive language patterns. If he or she uses single signs or isolated cues expressively, use phrases. If he or she uses phrases, use simple sentences. If he or she uses simple sentences, use compound and complex sentences. Avoid prolonging the manual communication equivalent of 'baby talk.'

Do With, Not For

This is perhaps one of the most used and abused sayings in the field. You do an action when the circumstances are appropriate. In the first example (page 99) Mother draws attention to what she is doing and encourages participation, but she is not expecting the infant to do the whole activity with her. 'Do with' should be more accurately stated as: *'Encourage interactive participation with, rather than do for!'*

A Total Communication Approach

Talk about it before you do it and as you do it and review what you have done. 'Talking about' does not mean that the Intervenor does all the talking. It must involve two-way communication. Again, questions can be used to elicit a response about *'What is going to happen?' 'What will happen next?'* during the activity, and *'What did we do?' 'More?' 'More What?' 'Finished?'* after the activity.

Feedback and Support

Never leave a deafblind individual when he or she is working or practising a skill unless you are absolutely sure that the person can understand how well he or she has performed compared with expectations. If appropriate expectations have yet to be formed, then the Intervenor's input is all the more essential. Feedback after each attempt is a must. Coming back after ten or fifteen minutes is not sufficient in most cases. Intervention is a full-time job, but this does not mean continuous 'hands on' involvement. It means the Intervenor must be available for support upon request.

The Wrong Kind, Not Too Much Intervention

The most difficult skills an Intervenor must learn is to identify the type of intervention that is needed, how best to provide the support for a particular individual, and when simply to be available. Most Intervenors err on the side of directing too much physical interaction, rather than waiting for a request for assistance. Providing information necessary to permit the deafblind individual to act is entirely different from constantly showing the deafblind person a better or the correct way. If in doubt, react rather than act.

There two excellent additional sources of information for providing general support for individuals who are deafblind. Graham Hicks, a deafblind young man working for Sense has produced an excellent monograph titled *Making Contact: A Good Practice Guide* (1996). It contains many excellent suggestions for supporting an individual who is deafblind. Dona Sauerburger's book, *Independence without Sight or Sound: Suggestions for Practitioners Working with Deaf-Blind Adults* (1996) is also a highly regarded source of information for those working with deafblind adults.

Instructional Intervention

Instructional Intervention involves the recognition and use of the three sequences that are taking place.

Presentation Sequence

The Intervenor follows a specific sequence as he or she presents the material to be learned.

Interaction Sequence

There is a recognizable sequence of interaction between the Intervenor and the deafblind individual.

Reaction Sequence

The deafblind individual follows a specific sequence as he or she reacts to the presentation by the Intervenor.

The best way to understand the model that illustrates the processes during instruction is to view it by levels and thus identify the interaction among the three sequences. Figure 3.1 illustrates the model.

Level One

Presentation Sequence (Awareness)
As the Intervenor introduces a new activity, he or she has several objectives in mind.

1. Introduce new language as it applies to the activity. Use it expressively and receptively. This must never be put off to a later stage.
2. Attach previously acquired language, skills, and concepts to the new activity. Most new activities will build upon previously learned concepts and skills and will involve the use of previously acquired expressive and receptive language. The Intervenor should draw the individual's attention to these skills and concepts as they are found in the new activity and assist the individual to identify and use them during the activity. It must not be assumed that the deafblind individual will see how the language, skills, or concepts apply unless he or she is helped to recognize and apply them.
3. Encourage the use of both receptive and expressive language. It is far more important that the repetition of the new activity. There never will be an occa-

An Integrated Approach to Instructional Intervention

LEVELS	PRESENTATION SEQUENCE (Intervenor's action)	INTERACTION SEQUENCE (between client and Intervenor)	REACTION SEQUENCE (expected response from client)
ONE	**AWARENESS** Motivating the individual to want to do the activity and introducing the language connected to the activity.	**HAND OVER HAND** $1 + 1 = 1$ The deafblind individual and the Intervenor function as one.	**RESISTS** the activity **TOLERATES** the activity because of the Intervenor
TWO	**ACQUISITION** Learning the sequences, routines, skills, and attitudes necessary to carry out the activity and linking appropriate receptive and expressive language to all stages in a meaningful way.	**GRADUALLY FADING PROMPT** $1 + 1 = 1\frac{1}{2}$ Moves from 1+1=1 to Intervenor supplying the support required for the deafblind person to be successful during the activity.	**COOPERATES PASSIVELY** Intervenor provides assistance, guidance, etc. **ENJOYS** engaging in the activity with the Intervenor **RESPONDS COOPERATIVELY** shows awareness of the next step, requires prompting
THREE	**APPLICATION** Applying the knowledge, skills, and attitudes successfully to carry out the activity and to solve problems that arise naturally from it.	**INTERVENTION WHEN REQUIRED** $1 + 1 = 2$ Moves gradually from 1+1=1½ through the stages of decision making with support and problem solving to intervention being supplied on request.	**LEADS** through activity with occasional prompting; problem solves with assistance. **IMITATES** variations made in the activity by the Intervenor; problem solves without assistance
FOUR	**TRANSFER AND GENERALIZATION** Carrying out the activity in a variety of situations and combining all or parts of the activity with previous concepts to solve more complex problems and create more complex activities.		**INITIATES** the activity because of enjoyment, confidence in being successful, and anticipated approval.

Figure 3.1   An Integrated Approach to Instructional Intervention

sion when the encouragement of communication should take second place or
be ignored.

4. Motivate the deafblind individual to WANT to engage in the activity. The
activity itself should be enjoyable and should produce enjoyable outcomes.

All activities are not in and of themselves enjoyable. Making a bed can be enjoyable, however, because of the social interaction, and it can also be a precursor to an enjoyable activity following its completion.

The Intervenor should not rush to level two (skill learning) until the deafblind individual is motivated and language has been successfully introduced and attached to the activity.

Interactive Sequence (1 + 1 = 1)

The degree and type of assistance required will be influenced by the relationship between the Intervenor and the deafblind individual, the amount of usable vision and/or hearing, any additional disabilities, and any tactile defensiveness present as well as the deafblind individual's age and level of functioning. In most cases, the initial use of a hand-over-hand approach is recommended, since it assists the deafblind individual who has some usable vision to concentrate on the skill sequence. It is important to remember to involve the deafblind individual in a positive way in all aspects of the age-appropriate activity from beginning to end.

Reactive Sequence (Rejects, Tolerates)

A normal response to the introduction of many new activities for the deafblind individual often is an initial rejection of the activity followed by a toleration of the activity because of the relationship the individual has with the Intervenor, not because of the activity itself. Depending on a number of factors, such as past success, a reactive rather than a directive environment, the relationship with the Intervenor, the amount of residual vision and/or hearing, additional physical disabilities, and so forth, the degree and duration of the rejection and the degree of toleration will vary.

Level Two

Presentation Sequence (Acquisition)

The Intervenor's emphasis will shift to having the deafblind individual learn the routines, skills, and knowledge involved in the process or activity. The **Whole-Whole Approach** will be used to promote understanding and motivation. In the Whole-Whole Approach the individual will be involved in the total routine from beginning to end. Individual sequences that are part of the complete routine will not be taught in isolation. Stress also will continue to be placed on motivating the individual to participate in the activity and on the use of receptive and, particularly, expressive language.

Interaction Sequence 1 + 1 = 1½ (Fading)
The amount of physical support will gradually diminish. Hand over hand will become wrist direction, then elbow support, and finally reach the stage of an undifferentiated physical prompt.

Reaction Sequence (Cooperates Passively, Enjoys, Responds Cooperatively)
The deafblind individual moves gradually from passively cooperating during the activity when directed by the Intervenor to beginning to anticipate the pleasant outcomes of the activity and will gradually begin to show recognition of the next steps in various sequences. It must be stressed that the complete routine, including all subsequences, will be experienced. No attempt will be made to isolate and teach any particular sequence or part of the routine as an end in and of itself. Combining previously acquired concepts and/or skills with the new one was begun in level one through having the individual participate in the activity from beginning to end.

Level Three

Presentation Sequence (Application)
During the Presentation Sequence at Level Three the Intervenor begins to introduce problems to be solved. No more than one problem is presented at any one time, nor are problems introduced every time the activity is engaged in. Sufficient support is always given to ensure that the deafblind infant, child, youth, or adult can solve the problem and complete the activity in a reasonable amount of time.

What is considered 'a reasonable amount of time' will be determined by the complexity of the problem, the degree of visual and hearing losses, additional disabilities, etc. Asking for assistance to identify the problem and seek solutions should be encouraged. Above all, deafblind individuals must not be frustrated by failure to the extent that they begin to see themselves as persons who 'CAN'T!' or that they choose to avoid the activity itself. At this stage, the Intervenor will begin to share, as an equal, in the particular routines or sequences. He or she should introduce the concept of splitting up the work. The Intervenor also can introduce personal variations in the sequences, bring the deafblind person's attention to these, and encourage imitation until the individual's personal preferences are formed.

Interaction Sequence 1 + 1 = 2 (for Levels Three and Four)
The Intervenor's objective will be to encourage the deafblind person to ask for assistance appropriately. This will require constant work on the Intervenor's part.

Intervention will be by communication rather than physical assistance except, of course, when the individual is asking appropriately for physical assistance.

Reaction Sequence (Leads, Imitates)
The deafblind individual takes the lead throughout the activity. He or she may occasionally need direction or prompting particularly when the individual's mind becomes focused on the solving of a particular problem. At this level, he or she understands the process, can divide it into shared tasks [when appropriate] and uses this understanding to imitate variations developed by others.

Level Four

Presentation Sequence (Transfer, Generalization)
The Intervenor helps the deafblind person to apply the skill or knowledge to new locations and situations and continues to provide opportunities to incorporate the knowledge and skill with others previously learned in such a way that the deafblind individual recognizes his or her increased skill and greater understanding.

Reaction Sequence (Initiates)
The Intervenor creates and/or supports an environment in which the deafblind individual can initiate the use of the knowledge or skill and in which he or she receives positive reinforcement and recognition from important persons in his or her life for doing so.

Generalizing the Instructional Intervention Model to All Ages and Levels of Functioning

Infants and Children

The Presentation Sequence (the role of the Intervenor when he or she is interacting with an infant or a child) is easy to identify, whether we are teaching the infant or child the pleasures of playing with blocks or other toys, dropping a block in a tin when a sound is heard, doing up buttons, eating with a spoon, or employing more advanced skills such as doing arithmetic or reading. Language, routines, and skills and knowledge acquisition and use all will be taught more successfully when the Intervenor understands where his or her focus should be and that his or her actions must relate to the infant's or child's response.

The Intervenor's job is to

• respond to follow the infant or child's actions and reactions

- initially motivate the infant or child to want to participate
- stress both spontaneous and directed use of appropriate receptive and expressive language
- begin to teach of a routine and skill and accompanying knowledge and attitude only after the infant or child tolerates the activity and begins to cooperate passively
- help the infant or child to identify problems and find solutions after the basic activity or skill has been mastered
- help the infant or child to compare attempts or efforts to his or her own previous ones and to the efforts of others
- encourage the infant or child to use the skill or pursue the activity in other locations
- promote the combining of the skill, routine, or knowledge with others previously learned.

Adults

Deafblind adults who have some or overall control of their lives should be in a position to identify some or all areas and/or activities that they wish to investigate. However, while they may identify what and when they wish to learn, they have the right to expect that the Intervenor will provide them with

- the necessary language for the activity
- motivation through immediate feedback concerning all attempts made by the deafblind adult, the reactions of others, and so on
- the ability to identify problems that may normally arise
- information concerning how their efforts compare with previous ones, those of others, or a specific model
- support from the Intervenor upon request.

They also have the right to expect the Intervenor to respond to them and follow their lead as to when it is time to proceed from one level of input to the next.

The concept of the infant or child as a partner, as stressed by the European Working Group on Communication, focuses on one of the essential elements of a reactive environment. This concept can be enlarged to encompass all aspects of the Intervenor's interaction with the deafblind individual, regardless of his or her age, level of functioning, or the activity. When this view is taken, the leadership role of the deafblind infant, child, youth, or adult in guiding the Intervenor's level and type of interaction is easily understood. Each can and should be responding to the other's actions willingly and in a predictable fashion.

The author has found that, although the length of time spent at any one level will vary with the age and level of functioning of a deafblind individual, the model will assist the Intervenor to understand his or her role. During a complex activity such as the preparation of a formal dinner, overnight camping, or shopping for a summer wardrobe, the Intervenor may find him or herself acting at several different levels at different times according to the ability of the deafblind person to combine previously learned knowledge and skills with newly required ones.

What the model does not show is that the ultimate goal must be to have the deafblind individual, regardless of his or her age or level of functioning, reach the stage where *he or she will decide appropriately when, with whom, for how long, and how well* he or she will do the activity. This goal will not be reached for all activities with all individuals, but it must be the desired and worked-for outcome for every activity with every individual. Infants can, and do, indicate when they have had enough or want more. They can be taught appropriate communication strategies to supplement and then replace body language. Children and youth must be given the latitude to express their desire to continue or to end an activity. When such action is inappropriate, they must be taught to recognize this and to understand why it is inappropriate.

There are some individuals who may say that the above concept of intervention is too complicated and that they could never do it. *The question is not whether they will use all parts of the process of instructional intervention, but rather how well they will do it.* In other words, will the process be implemented in a way that will provide the best intervention possible, or will it be a question of luck as to whether the needs of the person who is deafblind are met?

Social Intervention

Most of the social skills that non-deafblind persons possess are learned incidentally through our observations of others and their reactions in particular circumstances. Some are learned because our parents or peers take time to indicate what is expected. Unfortunately, the individual who is congenitally or early adventitiously deafblind will be denied the opportunity to learn incidentally or to form relationships to the depth that he or she will care what family or peers 'think' unless specific steps are taken to overcome these problems as they relate to the disability of deafblindness.

Rødbroe and Souriau point out (chapter 4) the importance and the absolute necessity of Social Intervention in the development of communication. It must be emphasized that they point out the importance of and necessity of Social Intervention with congenitally and early adventitiously deafblind persons of any age, and that this is not merely a stage that passes as the infant becomes a child. Intervenors should note, and understand, that time spent interacting with deafblind youth and adults is as, if not more, important than teaching skills or supporting participation in scheduled activities.

The purposes of Social Intervention are to form emotional bonds, communicate the Intervenor's personal response to the actions and responses of the deafblind individual, and communicate family, extended family, and societal expectations in a positive way. Parents and members of family will provide much of the Social Intervention in the early years through play and meeting the infant's or child's needs and during relaxed physical interaction.

If family members must make a choice between participating in Instructional Intervention and Social Intervention, the choice must be the latter. It is far more important that the child learn he is a loved and supported member of the family than that he learn to feed himself a few months sooner. All professionals who are supporting the family must help the parents to realize the importance of providing Social Intervention and support their decision to do so.

Members of the family, the extended family, and other intervenors must take time to establish appropriate social relationships with the deafblind child to the same degree that they would if he or she were not deafblind. Sitting and rocking with the child, playing children's games, participating with the infant or child in physical activities, and taking time to cuddle are some of the many ways Social Intervention can begin at an early age. Such relationships form one of the bases for motivation when new activities are introduced. Activities are often tolerated only because of the person involved, not because of the activity itself. It is not unusual for an individual who has been labelled uncooperative, aggressive, or withdrawn to interact positively with an Intervenor who takes time to establish a social relationship before beginning to implement program activities.

Social skills must be taught through interaction. Loneliness and isolation are identified repeatedly as major effects of deafblindness. Deafblind individuals must be taught age-appropriate social skills that will enable them to initiate and carry on social interaction. It should not be up to the Intervenor to decide whom the deafblind individual interacts with. The Intervenor may provide information concerning the options available in a location and who is present and a few facts about each. The individual who is deafblind must be encouraged and supported to make choices concerning how or with whom he or she wishes to interact. During Instructional Intervention the Intervenor may take the lead. During Social Intervention the Intervenor supplies any necessary information and puts stress on leaving age-appropriate decisions to the deafblind person.

The doorway to understanding, accepting, and developing interpersonal relationships, conforming to societal norms, and understanding societal expectations is through the support provided by the Intervenor. Understanding and responding to society's expectations start with the parents and family and proceed to interactions between the deafblind individual and the Intervenor and through interaction with peers. The job of the family and the Intervenor is to provide opportunities to learn social skills and social opportunities to practise them in a safe and supported environment.

The Ten Commandments of Deafblind Culture

Kerry Wadman, an internationally known member of the deafblind community, has set forth a set of Ten Commandments for Intervenors working with people with acquired deafblindness. They also offer excellent guidance and much to think about for all Intervenors when they are providing a general level of intervention.

For the un-Deafblind missionary, pastor, worker, servant, interpreter, Intervenor, instructor, and otherwise hearing, sighted, mobile. While in the presence of a Deafblind person:

1. Thou shalt put no other Culture above Deafblind Culture.
2. Thou shalt not lose hand contact when communicating with a Deafblind person.
3. Thou shalt communicate Tactile Sign Languages at all times.
4. Thou shalt not be the Deafblind person's Tactile Sign Language Instructor.
5. Thou shalt not be the Deafblind person's English grammar teacher.
6. Thou shalt not be the Deafblind person's Speech Therapist.
7. Thou shalt not be the Deafblind person's comedian telling non-deafblind jokes and puns.
8. Thou shalt not be the Deafblind person's shadow.
9. Thou verily shalt view Deafblind people as unique – not antique couch potatoes.
10. Verily, verily, thou shalt believe that Deafblind human organisms can do all things except see and hear.

One Activity Period, Several Types of Intervention

Often, as will be seen in the following examples, more than one type of intervention is present during a particular time period. In the first example there are instances of General Intervention, Instructional Intervention, and Social Intervention. What is important is that the Intervenor understands which type she is using and thus what she should be looking for as a response.

To illustrate these three types of intervention in practical terms, the following are four examples of appropriate support provided by an Intervenor. Each of the examples represent a set of hypothetical circumstances that reflect parts of many programs that the author has assisted in establishing or has observed while acting as a consultant. While they are based upon the real world, they should not be read as representing a specific program or family.

1. Mother providing intervention during a routine activity
2. A three-year-old at the park with his sister, who is acting as the Intervenor
3. A twelve-year-old in a primary classroom with his Intervenor
4. An eighteen-year-old and her Intervenor discussing what they will do before they leave the house

Mother Providing Intervention during a Routine Activity

Background
Mother's nine-month-old son Jason is deafblind and functioning as if he were profoundly deaf and severely visually impaired. Tests by competent and experienced professionals show him tracking and reaching for objects, but he rarely seems to use his vision in everyday situations. He also has one arm that he has difficulty extending and for which he receives phyisotherapy twice a week.

Morning Routine
It is 7:15 a.m. and time for Mother to change and feed Jason before getting ready to get the family off to school and leave for work herself. Mother enters Jason's room and gently shakes the bed (a large crib) to let Jason know that someone is there. If it had been winter and thus still partially dark, she would have flicked the light before shaking the bed. Mother then takes Jason's hand and touches it to her glasses, her distinguishing feature and at present the cue that is used until the sign '*mother*' is firmly established. Throughout this interaction mother will both use the cue and introduce the sign '*mother*' at every opportunity. She will also be aware of Jason's attempts to initiate communication through body language and facial expression. She will respond to all attempts by indicating that she recognizes what Jason is trying to communicate and by creating and supporting interactive dialogue with him.

She takes Jason's hands and manipulates them to give the signs for '*Jason*' and '*up*,' all the time talking to Jason, as she had with her other children when they were his age. (She will continue both to talk and to communicate tactilely at the same time throughout the activity.) Next, she places her hands under Jason and gently exerts upward pressure several times until she senses that Jason is anticipating being picked up, all the while talking to him. She carries him across the room to the area she has established for toileting and dressing.

She takes a few seconds to introduce a swinging game and to help Jason indicate '*more*' or '*finished*' during the game. When the final '*more*' has been signed and said and '*finished*' means finished, she gently signals that he is going down by false starting once or twice and then lowering him to the changing shelf.

When Jason is resting, securely protected from rolling off by the shelf's sides, Mother takes his hands and forms the sign for '*wait*' and then gets a damp wash-cloth and clean diaper. On returning, she gently takes Jason's hand, pauses, and moves it to her glasses to make sure that he knows that she is there, rather than some other member of the family. She then forms Jason's hand into the correct formation and position for '*mother.*' Even though Jason has some useful vision, there is no guarantee he is using it. She has been told that it is wise to use hand over hand until she is sure he is at a level that ensures he knows who is currently in his world and begins to anticipate what will happen next in his morning routine.

Next, Mother places the wash-cloth in Jason's hands and as she does so she says, 'Mummy is going to change your diaper.' The wash-cloth is the cue that Mother uses to indicate the whole process of changing his diaper. Next, a gentle upward motion of his legs and feet, repeated twice, indicates mother is going to pick up the legs and remove the dirty diaper. She takes the wash-cloth from Jason's hands and then, with Jason's hand resting on top of hers, moves the wash-cloth to the area to be wiped. When the area is clean, still talking to Jason, she signs '*finished*' and she and Jason co-actively place the wash-cloth to one side, manipulating Jason's hands to repeat the '*finished*' sign.

Mother then places the clean diaper briefly in Jason's hands, while she pats the area to be covered. She puts the clean diaper on Jason and, taking Jason's hands, pats the diaper tabs and signs '*finished*' with Jason's hands resting on top of hers. (This is the early beginning of introducing the idea that when hand-on-hand communication is being used, the 'talking hands' will be on the bottom.) She again signals that Jason will be picked up and she picks him up.

If time permits, she may play one or two motor games that emphasize Jason exercising his arm and '*more,*' '*wait,*' '*finished*' signs before heading for breakfast.

Mother gives Jason the '*eat*' sign while saying, 'time to eat.' Then she asks Jason, 'What time?' and Jason makes an attempt to respond with the '*eat*' sign. She assists him to shape his hand correctly and complete the movement to his mouth. She and Jason then proceed to the area in which Jason gets his food and bottle.

Mother has found two important things that make her life and Jason's life easier. She usually does not introduce new foods during the week. She waits until the weekend, when she has more time and is more relaxed. Secondly, in spite of Jason's size, Mother uses the lap position to feed him. This enables her to work on Jason's balance and exercise his arm while carrying out a necessary task. This position also makes it easier to assist Jason in his formation and use of signs and gestures.

She signs and says to Jason, '*Jason and mother sit down. It's time to eat.*' After sitting down and getting comfortable, she again signs and says, '*Time to eat.*' Jason is not a good eater but neither was Jenny, Jason's older sister, who is not disabled. Mother finds that she uses the '*more*' sign frequently when feeding Jason. Once he has had a basic amount of food, she then lets Jason choose between '*more*' and '*finished.*' There was a great celebration last night when Jason spontaneously tried to initiate his modified *more* sign to request more applesauce.

As the breakfast continues, she tries to be constantly aware of Jason's other attempts to initiate communication. She assists him to form the signs with his hands. She is also not above returning to the 'strained peaches' several times, a few minutes after respecting his '*finished.*' She may give him a drink of milk or some of the strained apples that he loves before going back to the peaches. She has found that she must do this in order to get Jason to eat enough, just as she did with Jenny; with Jenny, however, she did not have to talk as much.

Before getting up from the table, Mother takes a few minutes to play a lap game with Jason before she must get ready to go to work. When the final '*finished*' is signed, she and Jason go to her room while she dresses, but not before she signs and uses the cue (a bit of her perfume on a small piece of cloth) that represents her bedroom.

Observation
Mother and Jason's morning routine illustrates several important points.

1. It takes very little extra time to follow the usual morning routine and to work on Jason's Personal Plan at the same time. The total extra time required would be about fifteen to twenty additional minutes maximum.
2. Mother worked on language, body image, balance, the concepts of play and fun, making choices, and bonding. Another member of the family could perform the same function. We would suggest, however, that at Jason's age it should be the same person each day if possible.
3. Because of the support that she and the family receive from a consultant knowledgeable in the area of deafblindness, Mother consistently worked on anticipation, motivation, and communication throughout the morning routine. She presented various parts of the routine at the level appropriate for

Jason. She also worked on Jason's interaction with and understanding of his environment.

4. Much of what mother is doing parallels exactly what she did with her other children in a normal routine. In fact, the major and most important differences are continuing to use her lap rather than a high chair and the stress on eliciting communication from Jason.
5. Most important of all, because of the ongoing support of the consultant she felt that what she was doing with Jason was worthwhile.

A Three-Year-Old at the Park with His Sister, Who Is Acting as an Intervenor

Background
John is a three-year-old child who is deafblind. He has no residual vision and appears to have severe to profound hearing loss. He alerts to his name '*John*' (but will respond equally to Don, Ron, fawn, etc. in exactly the same way) and also responds to 'stop,' 'no,' and 'good boy' when presented verbally. He will not use oral language expressively or respond to any other words receptively, despite extensive efforts in the last two years by both speech therapists (three different ones have been tried) and family members. He has approximately fifty-five signs and gestures that he appears to understand, and of these he will expressively use thirty-two with prompting and he will use fifteen to initiate communication without prompting. He also effectively uses body language and physical actions to initiate communication. The family and supporting professionals are placing a high priority on the development of communication skills (not the acquisition of signs out of context), and there has been a great improvement in the use of expressive language after the introduction of the Total Communication Approach, which stresses interactive communication and dialogue.

John attends a neighbourhood preschool program that is designed to serve all neighbourhood children. It should be noted, however, that when John was enrolled in the program at age two, after two weeks the program director called and told the parents that John was too mentally challenged for them to deal with and also that he would be a danger to himself and others.

After a visit by the consultant, a specialist in the area of deafblindness, it was decided to give him a further trial, provided that he had an Intervenor. He is now well accepted and is benefiting both socially and developmentally from the experience.

Tina, John's twelve-year-old sister, has made a point of getting home from school on every second Thursday, when Susan C., the resource consultant from the Regional Deafblind Resource Centre, visits the family from 4 to 6 p.m. This has proved to be the best time for John's family, since it allows both Mother and Father to leave work a bit early and be home for the consultant's visit. Susan C. has made sure that Tina understands the important role she and her younger sister can play in John's development. Tina has developed a sense of pride in her role, and her parents make sure that her contributions are recognized, while at the same time guarding against expecting too much involvement and constant baby sitting. They realize that Tina must have the opportunity to be with her friends and also to have her own place in the family.

Susan C. fulfils the role of case manager as well as consultant for John's program. She has helped to develop a Personal Plan for John that integrates the therapeutic and preschool programs John is receiving with the overall five-year-goals and yearly objectives. As a consultant, Susan C. also visits John in his preschool program, where she discusses John's progress and demonstrates techniques that will assist the Intervenor, the school's physiotherapist, and his teachers to work more effectively. She makes recommendations for activities that John could do while the other children are engaged in group activities that at present are unsuitable for him. As part of her duties, the consultant provides ongoing training through both discussion and demonstration as well as arranging for John's Intervenor and family members to participate in specialized workshops and communicate with other Intervenors and families in the region. Susan C. also keeps both the Intervenor and the family informed of various sources of useful information and support that are available, such as the DBL (Deafblind List) on the internet.

At the Park

It is Saturday, and John's sister Tina has followed an established routine of asking John to choose among three activities. He can choose the playground at the local park, going for a ride in his wagon, or playing on the swing set in the back yard. The options are presented using symbols that John has come to associate with each activity. John usually initiates the routine and today chooses the playground.

The park is several blocks away. It is much too far for John's limited walking ability. Tina transports John to the park in the two-wheel carrier that she attaches to a bicycle whenever she takes John for a ride. John loves the carrier, and Tina thinks that he often chooses the park because of the ride to and from it in the carrier.

After parking her bicycle and lifting John from the carrier, Tina uses hand-over-hand signs and gestures to give John the choice of using the slide, swing, or wading pool, or playing in the sandbox. She places John's hands on top of her hands as she signs the choices. Then, by reversing the position, with her hand on top of John's she indicates that John should sign an answer. John's signs for '*swing*,' '*pool*,' and '*play*ing' in the sand box are not well formed as yet, and Tina has to be alert to understand his choice and to help him to finish the sign correctly.

John signs '*Slide*.' Tina then signs and says to John, '*John wants to slide?*' and prompts John to sign '*John slide*.' She and John climb to the top of the slide and, with John sitting between her legs, they both slide down. At the bottom, Tina signs to John '*Fun, fun, Tina and John slide. John more slide?*' while at the same time saying 'Was that fun?' 'Tina and John went down the slide.' Do you want to slide more?' John enthusiastically signs '*More*.' Tina, reversing the hand position, signs '*More what?*' With this prompt, John signs '*More slide*.' Tina and John use the slide several more times. John then initiates communication and signs '*Slide finished*' and proceeds to request other activities. Tina and John are becoming well known at the park, and several adults make a point of talking to her and enquiring about how John is doing. Tina was very shy and even somewhat ashamed when people first asked about John. She talked this over with her parents and with the consultant. Susan C. has helped her to understand John's disability and uses his Personal Plan to illustrate how well he is doing. Susan C. sometimes plays the role of Tina and encourages Tina to ask the kinds of questions that she finds hard to answer.

As a result of these sessions Tina now feels more confident and has a sense of pride in John's accomplishments. She has even rented the videotape of the movie *The Miracle Worker* and shown it to her friends. Now, when Tina and John are at the park, two of Tina's friends, Joan and Gail, ask if they can play with John also. Tina is beginning to teach John name signs for them. At first, Tina suggested that Joan be the person with whom John would swing and Gail be the sandbox friend. Gail has a younger brother, Peter, who is John's age, and she and Tina draw John's attention to Peter's presence in the sandbox. Tina helps John to examine tactilely the castle Peter is building and to try to make one of his own. It is obvious to both Tina and her friends that Peter's play is far more advanced than John's. Because of her discussions with the resource consultant, Susan C., and her parents, Tina no longer feels that this is because John is 'retarded.' She is able to explain to her friends how John's ways of learning are different.

Observation

All three types of intervention are being addressed by Tina.

1. Tina is providing John with the opportunity to fulfil his immediate needs for motor activity, socialization, and so on in a variety of ways, all of which are emphasized in his Personal Plan.

2. She is implementing part of John's plan with understanding, because the consultant and her parents have explained to her the importance of the few hours each week that she sets aside for John.
3. She correctly feels that she is doing much more than baby sitting.
4. Tina is carefully giving John choices and assisting him in carrying them out.
5. Without an in-depth knowledge of the 'Whys' of the techniques and methods, she is providing John with the opportunity to *anticipate* what will happen next.
6. Using a positive, warm approach, she is *motivating* him to participate in a variety of activities.
7. She is emphasizing both *receptive and expressive communication* and is encouraging John's overall growth in many areas.
8. Tina is supporting John in deciding which activities he wants to do when.

Tina, like the mother in the first example, is not a trained Intervenor who could work with a variety of children. Because of the visits of the resource consultant, Susan C., and her hands-on demonstrations of the correct techniques and methods to use with John, Tina is gradually learning about John's needs and through discussion is gaining an understanding of how various parts of his Personal Plan are implemented to meet those needs.

In both of these examples, the family members are gaining understanding of the needs of their specific child. Each child is following a Personal Plan that will differ not only because of age differences, but also because of the differing degrees of sensory deprivation. Many of the overall methods, such as the Total Communication Approach, will be employed, but the techniques of employing those methods will differ greatly, according to the needs of the individual.

Next, let us look at two cases from the professional Intervenor's point of view and attempt to identify how the Intervenor combines his or her knowledge of deafblindness with the parents' knowledge of their child and the overall needs of the family to provide adequate intervention for the child or youth who is deafblind.

A Twelve-Year-Old in a Primary Classroom with His Intervenor

Background
Paul is a twelve-year-old boy who is deafblind. He has some residual vision and can identify familiar people at approximately one metre (three-plus feet). He has some usable residual hearing and wears amplification in both ears. He can distinguish among words that differ significantly in sound and length and uses context and situation cues extremely well to 'guess' what a person is trying to

communicate to him verbally. In the appropriate situation he would recognize 'book,' 'look,' and 'took,' but he would not be able to differentiate among them if they were presented in isolation or read from a list. In some cases unexpected behaviours take place when he 'guesses' incorrectly. He has an extensive receptive signing vocabulary and a smaller expressive vocabulary. He can print his name, his Intervenor's first name, and can copy print from a page to his paper in a form that is recognizable but is not on lines or in uniform size. He recognizes approximately 145 symbols representing people and activities, for example, the conventional male and female signs on public washroom doors, printed words for milk, eggs. A few of these symbols are in the form of a picture plus the word (e.g., 'mother' printed on the bottom edge of a Polaroid picture), and some are objects (e.g., the front of a McDonald's fries box).

Paul also has physical malformations of his spine and left leg, which require him to use a wheelchair. He is extremely small for his age. Paul spent almost half of the first three years of his life in hospital or convalescing at home. He has had several serious operations and continues to require frequent visits to various medical specialists.

He attended a preschool program four days a week from the time he was three years old until he was seven years old. The program cooperated closely with the deafblind resource consultant, who visited on a regularly scheduled basis. The consultant provided a Personal Plan for Paul designed to take advantage of the preschool's resources, the therapy that he was receiving, and the resources of the family.

Unfortunately, his early school years were not so productive. Paul was placed in a special class for children who were auditorally challenged, because it had a small teacher-pupil ratio and the teacher knew American Sign Language. This placement was contrary to the recommendations of the resource consultant and the request of the family. After a few months, the resource consultant from the Regional Deafblind Centre was informed that the local school board had its own consultants and her services were no longer required. For the next four years she continued to visit the family occasionally at the parents' request. These visits were viewed by school board personnel as 'interference,' and the consultant was viewed as 'unrealistic.'

Paul made little or no progress in the class designed to meet the needs of a deaf child, and he became a behaviour problem. He was transferred to a program for children who were emotionally disturbed. After a few months, the teacher in this class, together with the school psychologist and the school nurse, recommended that he be placed on tranquilizers, and Paul spent the next two school years in a non-communicating fog.

The last straw occurred when, for no apparent reason, Paul began having the same behaviour problems at home that he was having at school. Paul's family doctor recommended that Paul be taken to a psychiatrist who had experience in working with infants and children who were congenitally and early adventitiously deafblind. On the psychiatrist's advice, Paul was immediately taken off tranquilizers. After many meetings between the parents and the school officials the consultant from the Regional Centre was invited to assist in designing and implementing a Personal Plan for Paul.

In the words of one school superintendent, 'It took a long time but we finally realized that having consultants in deafness, blindness, and behaviour management did not equip us to support Paul. His disability was unique and we needed assistance from specialists in the field of deafblindness.' Because of extrinsic factors, such as his slight size, stairs, the teacher, and access to toilet and bathroom facilities, Paul was placed in a grade three classroom in his local school.

Simply placing Paul in a regular classroom setting accomplished little. After the first few weeks in the previous year's school program the school principal, accompanied by the resource consultant from the Regional Centre approached the Education Authority to obtain funding for intervention for Paul. In the area where Paul's parents live the Education Authority had placed very restrictive upper limits upon the number of dollars that may be accessed by any one child and had a policy against giving any child one-to-one support except for medical reasons. Because of the presentation that was made, however, the policy was modified to include students who were deafblind, and Paul obtained an Intervenor for four days per week while he was in school. The Education Authority felt that it could not give him intervention for five days per week. Although it recognized deafblindness as a unique, low-incidence handicap, it felt that funding limits could not be breached for anyone or any reason.

The family turned to a service club that has a history of supporting individual children according to their needs for additional funding. Again, as a result of a presentation made by the parents and consultant, and because of the support of the school principal, the service club provided funds for intervention for four hours per day for the two days on the weekend and during school holiday periods and two hours per day for four days during the school year.

Paul continued to have problems on the Friday when he had no Intervenor. No one was available to communicate with him on an ongoing basis. The teacher was learning signing but could not give Paul her undivided attention for any extended period of time. Some of the children in the class had developed small basic vocabularies, but it was disruptive when they tried to communicate with Paul during classroom time. It also interfered with their own school work.

A team meeting was held. It was attended by Paul's parents, the school teacher, the principal, Paul's therapist, the Intervenor who worked with Paul in school, and the resource consultant. It was decided that Paul's frustration on the fifth day, when he had no intervention, was doing much greater damage than any benefit he received from attending school, and for a short period he remained at home on Fridays.

Finally, after several attempts over six months, the social service agency of the regional government agreed to fund the fifth day at the school program and an additional eight hours on the weekends. The Education Authority remained adamant that the dollar ceiling on any one child must remain.

The service club members have been so impressed with Paul's progress that they have resolved to fund any future requests for intervention should another deafblind child be identified in their area. They have also convinced their regional association to make it a priority to supply intervention to any person who is congenitally or early adventitiously deafblind.

The Intervenor

Mary G. is Paul's Intervenor. When she graduated from high school, she applied to attend the Intervenor Training Course at George Brown College. She was accepted in the course because of her long record of working as a volunteer with children who had various disabilities. During her field placements she met Paul and his family. She began working with Paul on her own time during the college year and during the summers.

Upon graduation, Mary G. accepted a position with the education authority and became Paul's Intervenor. The education authority involved Paul's parents in the hiring process and they recommended Mary. Before signing a contract with the education authority, Mary G. checked to see that there would be no objection if she continued to provide summer and weekend intervention for Paul. There was some concern expressed that she might experience 'burn-out.' It was decided that she was the best judge and would tailor her involvement (approximately forty-eight hours per week) to prevent 'burn-out.' Mary G. has found that the knowledge she acquired in the Intervenor Course combined with her knowledge of and experience in working with Paul enable her to contribute to the team approach. She understood the principles behind the Personal Plan and the purpose of five-year goals and twelve-month objectives. She was able to discuss Paul's needs with both the parents and the consultant and to benefit from the consultant's suggestions. Mary also assists the family and consultant in training other weekend Intervenors.

A Day with Paul

Mary G. begins her working day at Paul's home. Paul usually meets her at the door, and after the 'Good mornings, how are you's' are finished, she asks about what he did last night after school. She may use this information later in the day to help Paul to develop a story or make a picture. She and Paul then talk about what Paul will do today, using the calendar that they have developed. The calendar has symbols for each major daily activity from breakfast to bedtime. Initially, Paul's calendar was for one day. Next, it contained columns for today and tomorrow only. The resource consultant and mother would like to begin a seven-day (weekly) calendar, but both feel he is not yet ready, since he became confused when it was previously tried. Mary G. suggested that she add one more column, so that she could talk about yesterday, today, and tomorrow, and the planning team agreed. Paul's calendar contains these three columns at present. (See chapter 12 for a full account of calendar development.)

One of the identified five-year goals is to have this calendar become a combination daily planner and diary by the time Paul is sixteen or seventeen. In spite of the 'lost years,' Paul's progress in the last two years gives every indication that this is a realistic goal. Paul has a similar daily calendar at school. Part of each morning routine is to go over the calendar after signing *hello* to the teacher and any fellow classmates who come to his attention while he is hanging up his coat and putting his lunch-box in his locker. The calendar for today was prepared by Paul and his Intervenor before they left the classroom yesterday. Before they get on the school bus, they talk about what they will do today and what he would like to share with members of the class. One reason the Intervenor begins and ends in Paul's home is that the school bus ride is fifty minutes in length, and during that time Paul was receiving little or no stimulation until the Intervenor accompanied him. Another reason was for safety. It was felt that, should an emergency arise, the presence of the Intervenor would be essential for Paul's safety.

The rest of the class begin their morning with 'Show and Tell.' Experience has shown that Paul has difficulty in participating in the activity, and after discussion with the resource consultant and the planning team, it was decided that Paul could use this time more effectively by establishing a morning routine that included calendar-based discussion, expressive vocabulary, and fine-motor activities. Mary G. keeps one ear open to what is going on, and she will invite two or three of the children to share their special news with Paul on a small group or one-to-one basis. Occasionally Paul will have brought something exciting and the teacher will suggest that he take it around and show each member of the class.

This example should not be read as recommending that such activities as 'Show and Tell' are not useful in whole or in part for a child who is deafblind. The example is designed to illustrate that a flexible approach should be taken in utilizing the existing class routines. The student who is deafblind should participate in all or part of every routine from which he can derive benefit. It must be recognized that there are routine activities and parts of activities that provide little or no benefit for the student who is deafblind, and his time would be more effectively spent pursuing alternative individual activities with his Intervenor.

Paul's Personal Program is designed to take advantage of those class activities in which he can participate fully with his Intervenor. These activities range from arithmetic (Paul has good number concepts) to story time and arts and crafts. He copies notes in history and geography with intervention, and he enjoys science. These subjects are reflected in, and form part of, the Goals and Objectives sections of his Personal Plan.

During physical education, Paul participates fully in individual play activities, and some group floor activities. His wheelchair places some limits on his participation. Group ball activities present a problem, as do most team games. When the class is participating in these activities, Paul will do a parallel activity with his Intervenor, and occasionally he will interact with one or two classmates in a modified group activity. The Intervenor modifies the activity to ensure that Paul has a reasonable chance of success.

Initially, it was extremely difficult to get the Education Authority's permission for Paul to participate in physical education classes. It took a presentation to the Education Authority featuring a home video of Paul using playground equipment, horseback riding, swimming, and participating in a community gymnastic class to convince the Education Authority that there was no undue risk involved due to either Paul's physical disabilities or his multi-sensory deprivation. The response of the Educational Authority was predictable. Staff were considering both their own liability and Paul's and other students' safety. They, like many such authorities, realized that as long as each potential activity was assessed, and if necessary modified, prior to Paul's participation, the risks to both Paul and the authority were no greater than those posed by any other student. It must be noted that Paul's parents are required to sign a yearly waiver and to carry liability insurance to cover any accident caused by Paul's disabilities.

Regardless of the subject or activity, the teacher teaches the class just as she would if Paul were not present. Mary G. communicates to Paul what the teacher is saying and draws Paul's attention to things that are happening in the classroom with an explanation when needed. When Paul is interacting with his peers one to one or in a small group, Mary G. makes herself available to assist Paul or his peers to communicate with one another and, if necessary, to assist Paul coactively to make his contribution. In these situations she will also draw Paul's attention to anything happening in the classroom that the other children would notice and find important.

During approximately one-third to one-half of the class time, depending on the activities planned for the class by the teacher, Paul and his Intervenor will carry out individual activities. These activities provide an opportunity to work on some of the behavioural objectives from Paul's Personal Plan, such as sensory integration, use of residual vision and hearing, various life skills, and communication. This individual time also provides an opportunity to do additional work on skills and concepts from the school curriculum that Paul has found difficult as well as to ensure that Paul has sufficient background knowledge to enable him to participate in upcoming lessons as a member of the class.

As the last activity of the day, before getting ready to go home, Paul and his Intervenor will use his school calendar to review what they did today. They will talk about each item on the calendar and may even do a quick review of things that went very well. This discussion is an excellent opportunity to identify any mistaken information that Paul has received. The final part of this calendar activity will be to place symbol cards on the calendar for each of the things they will do in school tomorrow. This activity, one of the goals of which is to promote dialogue and elicit expressive communication from Paul, is one of the most important things he will do during the school day. If it becomes a lengthy process, GOOD! If necessary, the Intervenor, in consultation with the teacher, will cut back on something else.

When Paul and his Intervenor arrive home, they will go over his calendar for the rest of the day as well as review the special things that Paul is going to tell members of his family. As Paul's Intervenor, Mary G. does not deliver messages or discuss happenings at school with the family. The Intervenor should not become a communication tool between or a representative of either the school or the family. She is a professional employed to support Paul so that he can participate successfully in the world around him.

The planning team (the teacher, principal, Intervenor, parents, and resource consultant, plus other invitees) review Paul's Personal Plan objectives at the end of each term. During this review all team members take part in identifying Paul's progress towards each objective. In addition to reviewing Paul's progress, they also discuss the next term. The teacher leads in identifying those aspects of her program that she feels will give Paul an opportunity to work on the specific objectives. The resource consultant makes suggestions as to methods and techniques that would be the most effective. The Intervenor makes suggestions concerning both techniques she has found effective and activities that might be used when she and Paul are working at alternative activities.

It cannot be emphasized too strongly that the teacher is an expert in education and a specialist in her particular grade area. She is not expected to be an expert in working with children who are deafblind. It is the resource consultant who provides this expertise and designs the Personal Plan.

Observation

Paul's programming team is composed of the resource consultant, who acts as case manager, the teacher, the school principal, and Paul's parents. The superintendent of education and Paul's therapist are invited to attend monthly team meetings as often as their schedules permit, and they always receive minutes of each meeting.

1. One of the early questions that had to be addressed was: *To whom is Mary G. (the Intervenor) responsible?* The initial approach by the education authority was that Mary was their employee and, like any school aide, would act under the direction of the teacher. After an in-depth examination of the question, the following decisions were made.

   - The classroom teacher is hired for her expertise in her grade area and is not expected to become an expert in deafblindness.
   - The teacher's responsibility is to the whole class.
   - Mary G's. responsibility is to use the classroom and school resources to implement Paul's Personal Plan without disrupting class or school routines.
   - Mary G. is made responsible to the programming team, which in turn is responsible to the school principal and the educational authority.
   - The classroom teacher is not expected to change either her program nor her method of lesson presentation because of the presence in her class of a child who is deafblind.

2. In this third example the Intervenor is a fully trained professional who is implementing the intervention process in an educational setting. A professionally trained Intervenor is better able to take advantage of the resources available to facilitate the implementation of the Personal Plan in many educational settings.

3. The child who is deafblind will continue to need and receive additional intervention throughout his waking hours. The intervention provided by the educational authority does not take the place of, or negate the need for, intervention for the rest of the child's waking hours, which will be provided by both family members and non-family members who may be volunteers or paid to provide the support.

4. The Intervenor's role and responsibility is to promote communication and to ensure that Paul understands what is happening in the world around him,

both as a result of his actions and as a result of the actions of others. Paul must have sufficient information to understand both the cause and the effects, not just a report of the event itself.

5. A major area of concentration throughout the day is to have Paul use expressive language effectively. A calendar device provides an excellent opportunity to elicit expressive language when the 'partners' (Paul and his Intervenor) share equal responsibility for initiating and carrying out communication.

6. Placing the child in a classroom, program, or school designed to meet the needs of someone with a different challenging condition does not work. Multi-sensory deprivation affects how the child learns not what he is capable of learning. It affects the way the child communicates with his world, not the ability to communicate, and what the child perceives, not the ability to perceive and think.

An Eighteen-Year-Old and Her Intervenor Discussing
What They Will Do before Leaving the House

Background
Janet is an eighteen-year-old girl who is deafblind. She was born with Congenital Rubella Syndrome. She has no usable vision in her right eye and a small area of greatly reduced vision in the corner of her left eye and continuing heart problems. She examines objects by holding them slightly below and to the left of her left eye at a distance of 2 to 3 inches. She has a profound hearing loss. She alerts to loud noises, her name, and 'well done' when loudly spoken directly into her right ear. She is an alert, confident, and attractive young woman. She has an extensive signed vocabulary and reads both one-hand and two-hand finger spelling. She types approximately 30 wpm and prints using a guide.

Several attempts have been made to introduce Braille using both traditional and alternative approaches. Unfortunately, Janet is unable to make the fine tactile distinctions necessary to read Braille successfully. She can recognize the outline of and read the letters of the alphabet, and raised printing has been used with success. The Intervenor prints the message with white glue on dark paper and dusts it with fine sand. The glue dries quickly and Janet can read the note using a combination of vision and tactile information. She also can read notes printed with black marker on white paper but tires quickly when attempting to do so.

Janet, in consultation with her advocate and her consultant, designs her own Personal Plan. She has kept her history up to date and does a good job of describing her present level of functioning. Setting five-year goals continues to be an interesting experience for all concerned. Janet's ideas range widely and much discussion is required to identify goals that she, her parents, and her consultant agree are realistic. The discussion arising from these interchanges of opinion are extremely valuable to everyone involved. She and the consultant work together with the Intervenor to identify specific objectives in various areas and decide how success can be measured. One of her cluster of objectives is in the area of education. After much discussion, it has been decided that simply obtaining 'high marks' does not adequately describe what she wishes to accomplish.

The Intervenor

Anne H., Janet's Intervenor, is a graduate of the Intervenor for Deafblind Persons Program at Medicine Hat College. She works with Janet thirty hours in each week. Janet, with the help of her parents, negotiates with Anne H. a week or two in advance as to when she will use the thirty hours. This negotiation is also an important part of Janet's Personal Plan. The long-range goal is to have Janet take total responsibility for hiring, scheduling, and evaluating her Intervenors, and she is beginning to work with Anne to learn how to use the *Intervenors Self Evaluation Guide* (McInnes 1996) as a basis for understanding the role of an Intervenor and evaluating their effectiveness. At the present time the focus is upon Janet's arranging for intervention to support her out-of-school activities.

Janet has other Intervenors both in school, provided by the Education Authority, and out of school. Members of her family (mother, dad, brother Bob) and a girlfriend provide approximately twenty hours per week of intervention. The Education Authority provides six hours per day, Monday to Friday, when school is in session. The Social Services Regional Office provides funds for forty hours per week, of which Anne H. provides thirty. Thus, at present Janet has adequate intervention available if her family and her girlfriend do not have other plans. As she grows older, Janet will require more non-family (paid) intervention. Mothers, fathers, and even brothers are not particularly welcome as permanent fixtures in groups of young adults.

Janet has shown the ability to function at her age level both academically and socially and is very aware of the expectations that her peers hold for themselves, each other, and her as well as those held by her parents, members of her extended family, and society in general. Janet's emotional stability is often endangered when an appropriate level of intervention is not available. It cannot be stated too often, or too strongly, that the higher the level of functioning of the person who is congenitally or early adventitiously deafblind the greater the need for an adequate level of stimulation, communication, and social interaction. In our experience such stimulation and continuous feedback from an ever expanding world can be provided only by the process of intervention, not by technology.

Making Plans

Anne H. (Janet's Intervenor) has arrived at nine o'clock on Saturday morning. Janet asks if she would like a cup of coffee. After Janet gets Anne her coffee, they sit at the kitchen table and Anne asks Janet '*What's new?*' This has become a weekend ritual. After each updates the other on what has happened since they last were together, Janet will discuss with Anne H. what she wishes to do for the weekend. This will have been discussed the previous week, and Janet's review of what she is going to do makes sure that there are no misunderstandings, changes of mind, or unforeseen problems that will require changes in plans.

Occasionally, Anne H. will have to explain that the changes Janet wishes to make in the use of the twenty-four hours of intervention available on the weekend are not possible because Anne has other personal commitments. Initially this caused pouting, withdrawal, and even temper tantrums. Janet has gradually come to accept that others also have plans and that she cannot always arrange the world the way she would like it. She is learning to compromise and to respect the wishes and rights of others and to accept her personal responsibility to arrive at workable compromises.

Anne H. speaks as she finger-spells, gestures, and signs to Janet. She can remember the discussions during her Intervenor training classes when the necessity of speaking to a person who was profoundly deaf was questioned by members of the class. Many reasons were given by the instructor and the one that she remembers most clearly had to do with 'atmosphere' and how this approach differed from that used in the community of the deaf. After working with Janet for the last six months, she no longer needs convincing that this Total Communication Approach using adopted sign language makes a difference.

Anne H. is more than just eyes and ears for Janet. She has become a friend and confidant. Janet's age and level of functioning make this one of the most challenging aspects of the position. It is particularly challenging when Janet is with her girlfriends. Unless Anne H. is careful, her twenty-two years of age can be almost as big a barrier as if she were a parent, to someone of Janet's age. Anne grew up in a different setting from Janet's and has very decided personal and religious views. She has learned to reconcile her personal views with her responsibilities as an Intervenor when conversations turn to areas she would not personally discuss with casual friends. She and Janet have had many discussions about this and have come to agree that Anne can hold different views while still effectively intervening for Janet. If Janet wishes to know what Anne H thinks, she asks.

Today Janet is meeting three friends at the mall. Anne H. and Janet say '*Hi,*' and after introductions Anne H. backs off while the four girls huddle and discuss what they are going to do. Two of the three girls know how to finger-spell and sign into Janet's hands. When one of the girls wants to know how to sign 'cute,' Anne H. provides the sign without comment. A shopper stops and looks disapprovingly at the group. One of the girls makes a comment to the others that they are not doing anything wrong and wonders what she is looking at. Anne takes Janet's hand and quickly signs what her friend has said. Janet tries to ask her friend what she meant, but her friend cannot read Janet's signs. Anne quietly speaks the words as Janet signs them. The other girls begin to offer their opinions. One says, 'I don't know why she didn't take a picture!' Anne H. knows that Janet will be asking questions and wanting to discuss the incident on the way home.

Observation

1. The Intervenor is placing the responsibility on the person who is deafblind to make the plans. The Intervenor may offer suggestions to try to enlarge the available choices, but the individual who is deafblind, not the Intervenor, should make the final decision and that decision should be respected.
2. The Intervenor provides the support necessary for the individual who is deafblind to interact with peers and avoids becoming the centre of attention. The Intervenor makes every effort to ensure that Janet is receiving the same information from the environment that is being consciously noticed by her friends.
3. The transition that is taking place in the relationship between the Intervenor and an adult who is functioning at Janet's level is extremely difficult. In more than one case, the only solution has been to suggest that the Intervenor move on and have the person who is deafblind take a very active and visible part in the hiring of the replacement.
4. Janet appears to be ready to begin evaluating her Intervenor's performance. The shift is being made from the role of the person receiving the support to the role of the employer. Both the employee and employer will have to learn how to play new roles if the same intervenor continues to provide support.

Additional Considerations

Every Intervenor and professional working with the family of a person who is deafblind should read, and spend time discussing, the Ten Commandments laid out by Norman Brown and Gini Cloke (chapter 8). It clearly enunciates the parents' expectations and what they wish to receive from supporting professionals. No Intervenor, or any other professional, should fail to follow this advice every day.

The most difficult part of the role that an Intervenor has to play when working with a person who is congenitally or early adventitiously deafblind is not the provision of care for an infant who is deafblind or for an individual who is deafblind and has a number of severe disabilities. The most difficult role for the Intervenor to play is to begin working with an individual who is deafblind and who is moving from dependence to independence. While no infant, child, youth, or adult with deafblindness should be seen as dependent, age and disabilities often mask the inappropriate treatment of the individual as dependent and no real effort is made to promote the move from such dependence to real independence as represented by being allowed to make a mess, to make a less appropriate choice, to make a mistake, or to say 'NO!'

The Intervenor who begins working with and promoting a real move from 'childlike independence' through 'teen independence and even rebelliousness, to adult independence and finally to interdependence with choice, understanding consequences, and responsibility is taking on a task that will require him or her to promote his or her demotion and create his or her own boss. This is the real challenge for an Intervenor and should be attempted only by the select few who have the self-confidence equal to the task. Whether we call them friends or Intervenors, whether they are family members, volunteers, or paid professionals, without them an active, interesting, fulfilling life is impossible for the person who is congenitally or early adventitiously deafblind at any age. Helen Keller stated, 'My life is a chronicle of friendships. My friends – all those about me – create my world anew each day. Without their loving care all the courage I could summon would not be sufficient to keep my heart strong for life.'

Summary

1. Intervention is a process that is defined according to the needs of the infant or child who is deafblind.
2. The process changes as the needs of the infant or child change.
3. Three types of Intervention occurs often within the same activity period.
4. There are certain guidelines and competences that will assist anyone providing intervention to do a more effective job.
5. Each of the three types of intervention has its own underlying goals and methods for achieving those goals.

NOTES

1 The George Brown College of Applied Arts and Technology (P.O. Box 1015, Station B, Toronto, ON M5T 2T9) and Medicine Hat College (299 College Drive

SE, Medicine Hat, SK T1A 3Y6) offer a two-year Intervenor Program. They are two of very few such programs offered throughout the world and they provide in-depth training to work with persons who have either congenital or acquired deafblindness.
2 A manuscript in process. Sharon may be reached by email at grassick@iinet.net.au

REFERENCES

Hicks, Graham (1996) *Making Contact: A Good Practice Guide.* Sense, 11–13 Clifton Terrace, Finsbury Park, London, U.K. N4 3SR
McInnes, J.M., ed. (1996) *Intervenor Self-Evaluation Guide (1996 Edition).* Brantford, ON: Canadian Deafblind and Rubella Association (Ontario Chapter)
Sasse, Hugh (1996) The Deafblind List FAQ, 10 July
Sauerburger, Dona (1993) *Independence without Sight or Sound: Suggestions for Practitioners Working with Deaf-Blind Adults.* New York: American Foundation for the Blind. Purchase from AFB, c/o American Book Center, Brooklyn Navy Yard, Building #3, Brooklyn, NY 11205. ISBN 0-89128-246-7 (print); ISBN 0-89128-933-X (Braille)

4

Communication

I. RØDBROE and J. SOURIAU

Introduction

The Focus Group

The focus of this chapter is the development of communication with the group of people identified as congenitally or early adventitiously deafblind. The population of this focus group is very heterogeneous as regards

- degree of visual and hearing impairment
- cognitive capacities
- additional impairments
- the onset of intervention
- and the quality of services available.

Nevertheless, the way we address this topic will cover the whole variety of congenitally deafblind people as regards differences in capacities and ages, including infants, children, youth, and adults. The road you have to follow as a partner in communication will be the same one. (In this text, we use the word *partner* to refer to any person – family member, teacher, etc. – who is in the position of interacting with a deafblind person in a communicative way.) In some cases there will be more hindrances on the road, since additional impairments and deprivation will make the communicative journey challenging. At times it may seem that you are not moving anywhere; at other times, passing one of the hindrances you meet will implement progress that you at first did not consider possible. For some deafblind people the journey on the communication road will bring them far towards advanced goals; for others the road will be rather short.

As you always travel with a partner, you might discover that together you can make even the short road broad and full of shared experiences.

The History of Deafblind Education

Developing strategies for intervention of communication has always been a main focus for partners of deafblind people. In the 1960s the main educational goal was to teach the deafblind person a symbolic linguistic system (e.g., sign language or speech). The educational strategies being used were influenced by learning theories (*behaviouristic approach*). The teaching strategies were mainly adult directed, and much emphasis was put on developing communication systems and methods that could support and facilitate the development of language. Deafblind children did learn signs but they were rarely used in a communicative way, for example, to share feelings, experiences and information with partners. A search for new theories to give partners the missing link to develop communication based on *reciprocal social togetherness* started in the late 1980s. In the 1970s attention to attachment theories presented by Bowlby (1969) was common ground and considered very important. The relationship between access to proximity (the caregiver) and the initiatives of the child was emphasized in this theory and considered crucial to all development. Using *attachment theories* in intervention did facilitate the initiatives of the child to explore the world, because access to the partner was obtainable (Nafstad 1989). The spin-off effect on the development of communication was not experienced as expected.

From the 1970s on, research in early development of communication with infants and their mothers was carried out all over the world. The results of that research became the missing link for partners of deafblind people. The development of communication and language was now seen as an ongoing process that develops in interaction with the physical and human environment from birth onward. According to the new approach that rose from this new knowledge, the intervention strategies of communication must start at focusing on establishing the social interaction and the pre-linguistic communication that are the prerequisites to the development of more advanced forms of communication as language. This strategy is based on child-directed intervention. The child from birth on is considered to be a competent partner as well as an active contributor to his own development of communication. The role of the partner is to facilitate and to support the development of communication based on the initiatives of the child. When a mother supports new functions, she does what the child cannot yet do. She gradually takes away the supporting framework when the child masters the task on his own. The mother makes it look like her child can, for instance, take turns in interaction long before the child masters this function. In this chapter we shall describe how clinical practice with deafblind people has been linked to the new scientific literature on early communication and the development of language.

Communication Is a Basic Need

Parents and professionals working with deafblind people agree that the main goal of all intervention is to give the deafblind person a **Life of Quality**. Essential and basic to a Life of Quality for all human beings is that you experience the following:

- being important to other people
- having influence on the way you live your own life
- being able to share your experiences with somebody (Lindstrom 1994).

These essential needs can be fulfilled only through communication. Thus, intervention on communication should be given the highest priority in all deafblind programs.

Besides the fact that communication is vital to the basic needs of human beings, communication can be called the main entrance to all aspects of development. You build up emotional, personal relationships, and you widen the world by means of your ability to communicate about the world with your partner. Thus communication is vital for being human and for learning.

Lack of Natural Context

Deafblindness is an extreme disability as regards lack of access to the physical and human environment because of the serious impairment of both distance senses. Partners must make the environment accessible, meaningful, and interesting for the deafblind person. This access, meaning, and interest must operate from the perspective of the deafblind person. For each individual deafblind person 'the natural environment' in which he can develop and learn has to be constructed by his partners in a way that will meet his specific needs. This means that deafblind people all their lives will be dependent on their partners' knowledge, intuition, and creativity, which are the prerequisites to creating the extreme conditions in which deafblind people can learn and develop. No natural context for developing communication is available for this disability group.

A consequence of these extreme conditions for congenitally deafblind people is that without intervention communication is not going to emerge. This problem will continue through the different stages of development, which means that the deafblind person will not reach a stage of further development without the intervention of his partners.

Chapter Content

We shall address the different aspects of development of communication as follows:

1. A presentation of the core strategies of intervention
2. An overall description of how communication develops
3. A more detailed description of different important stages in the development of communication with practical examples from our own practice
4. A description of the specific challenges we meet in developing communication with congenitally deafblind people

Core Strategies of Intervention

Creating a Natural Context for Communicative Development

The intervention on communication should be based on the natural way all children learn to communicate. This means that we have to create the same kind of communicative events that exist in normal development, but arranged in a different way. Natural learning conditions are characterized as follows:

- They are initiated and controlled by the child.
- The partner of interaction is observant, reactive, and responsible for the expansion.
- The natural way of learning is to play. Play is characterized by shared affections, curiosity, and discovery through exploration.

The individual program for developing communication for each deafblind person is based on on-line assessment. By on-line assessment we mean the following: The way we plan a communicative event with our deafblind partner is always based on what we already know about our partner's capacities, his likes and dislikes, his ways of expressing attention and initiative and his ways of perceiving information and expressing himself in communicative acts. This information gives us important cues to plan the events in a qualified way. Within the events, however, we shall always be on the lookout for new information that can add and change the cues we already have. The only one who can tell us how to intervene in the right way is our deafblind partner. Thus, every time we are together with our deafblind partner we might learn something new about him and the way he learns, which might change the next event.

Use the Strong Channels and Try to Instrument the Residual Senses

When we communicate with a deafblind person we always make use of the strong channels. In the case of deafblindness the most efficient channels will be movement, touch, airflow, vibration, smell, and taste. Most deafblind people have residual hearing and/or vision, and, of course, our goal is to make functional use of every possible channel, however weak it might be. The more channels that a person will be able to use the more flexible he will be in new and complex situations, which again means the greater his possibilities will be to develop new and more advanced functions.

When a deafblind person is learning new functions that are not yet automatic, he or she must use the strongest channels, but at the same time we must always be on the lookout for using the weaker senses in addition. This might create the possibility of making functional use of the weaker sense, at first together with the strong sense and maybe later on its own, whenever needed. Making functional use of residual hearing and vision with deafblind people always happens in interaction with the environment and always with the support of stronger senses. This phenomenon is called **instrumentation** (Bullinger 1994).

Sensitivity and Child-Directed Intervention

The role of the communicative partner has changed as a result of the new intervention strategies based on creating a natural learning environment to develop communication. Of course, the partner must plan *frames of activities* during the day, but within these frames he must be ready to be very sensitive to the contributions of the deafblind partner and let them direct him in following and at the same time challenging his partner. All communicative acts are created by both partners in a dynamic way. This means that both partners in communication must be aware of the contribution of the other partner and ready to react to them in a way that keeps the **interactional exchanges** going. The partner of the deafblind person is responsible for expansion and further development. This means that he must know or have access to supervision on how different advances can be supported in communicative development. The partner's job will be to discover and then support new emerging competences in communication and never to try to train competences that are not ready to emerge (cf. Vygotsky 1962; proximal zone of development).

Repetition and Novelty

Probably the most challenging job of the partner is to be able always to regulate the tension of the child so that the attention, motivation, and curiosity of the child is kept as a basis to sustain and expand the communicative events.

Regulating the tension of your partner is of course reciprocal, but again the responsibility of the *regulation* must be greater on the part of the more competent partner. The regulation involves a lot of dilemmas in the communicative acts. On one hand, you have to make use of recognition by the use of repetition to create conditions that will help the deafblind person to have an overview and to support the cognitive development. On the other hand, you have to add novelty to a well-known act in order not to make it dull and thereby loose the interest of your partner. This regulation is very much based on the experiences, intuition, and creativity of the partner. *It will never be possible to create a program indicating when and what to do in communicative events.* What we shall do in the following is to make this problem and challenge explicit to the partners in communication and to give ideas and examples of important principles of how to regulate and expand within communicative acts. This will give the partner some tools to add to his own sensitivity and creativity.

Using Activities to Develop Communication

Any Activity from the Deafblind Person Can Be Used in a Communicative Way
Communication can take place using very different forms of utterances on the part of both partners, from non-verbal 'emotional' body expressions to signs or words. Any activity by a child (or any prelinguistic person) can become social and communicative by the way the partner reacts to that activity. If an activity is either not observed or even, if so, is not reacted to as an initiative to communicate, it will not be developed into an utterance within a communicative act. Again, the responsibility of turning the child's utterances into contributions within communicative acts is that of the partner. Of course, because of the very nature of deafblindness, the child will have difficulties seeing a partner's face and hearing the reaction when the partner attempts to predict, see, and react to activities that often are very different from those seen in normal infants. To begin to make an activity communicative the partner has to discover the activity, and therefore, it is often necessary to know the deafblind child well, so that you have some idea of what to expect. Then the partner must see the activity as an initiative to communication, make an interpretation of the utterance, and react to it in a way that can be perceived. From the reaction of one partner the other partner will get a response, which will indicate if the interpretation was

correct. This response can be the initiative to continue the communicative act (Bjerkan 1996).

Example: The child performs the sign for food. The partner reacts by giving the child food. The child eats the food. In this case the sign is responded to as a signal for food and no communication is taking place.

The child performs the sign for food. The partner reacts by placing his hand on top of that of the child (responds to the sign).The partner answers with the child's hand on top of his 'you food.' The child smiles and starts moving his mouth. In this case the sign is used in a communicative way and the communicative episode can go on.

The partners of deafblind people have to play different roles in communicative development. At first the role will be the role every mother plays when communicating with her baby. She shares affection, she looks at her baby as a competent partner, and she supports the development of new milestones. Later, the partner will take the role of a playmate who explores, discovers, and shares the experiences of the world with his peers. At all times, the professional partner will be an explorer of the competences of his deafblind partner. He will learn to be as competent a partner as possible to any deafblind partner and more specifically to the deafblind partner he is sharing the development of communication with.

How Communication Develops

Communication Is a Co-Created Process

When starting to communicate, none of the partners in the dyad knows in advance how the communicative episode will develop, how much time it will be sustained, how topics will change over time, how the emotional flow will be regulated, and how the communicative tools will be used. This is true for any conversation: it can be observed in a baby-mother interactive episode or in a conversation between two linguistically fully fledged adults. Both partners contribute to the success of communicative episodes. For instance, in the case of a congenitally deafblind child, changing the topic could be moving from tapping to jumping; changing tools could be using gestures followed by vocal utterances. During the episodes, the competent partner answers the child's initiative by sharing these different aspects and also by challenging him with surprise, new topics, or a more sophisticated use of communicative tools. In this way it can be said that communication is co-created, which means that a communicative episode is an on-line process of adaptation to each other within which intentions and emotions are shared and negotiated (Nadel and Camaioni 1993).

It Happens in Social-Interactive Play

It happens in social-interactive play as topics for communicative acts where utterances of the child are used. There is no possibility for a child to develop communicative competences without interacting with a partner. This partner can be either a peer or a more competent adult. At the very early stages of development, successful interactions between peers are almost impossible because the children are likely unable to sustain their own attention and to adapt to their partners. The role of the so-called 'competent' adult consists in using the child's utterances in order to make them communicative. For instance, researches on early development of 'labels' (Barret, Harris, and Chasin 1991) show that most of the first labels used by the children are learned in contexts where the adult has named the object that is the child's focus of attention (not the ones that the adult wants to teach). Utterances of the child can be movements, vocalizations, *deictic gestures* (pointing at, looking at, etc.), signed or vocal words, and so on. They give the adult an indication of what is in the child's mind. At the earliest stage of development, typical ways to react in a communicative way to these utterances are to match them (by making similar movements), to attune to them (by doing something that expresses that the emotional state is shared), or to imitate their contours using another modality (e.g., using vocalizations imitating the dynamic shape of a movement) (Fogel 1993). In this way, there is a high probability that the child will answer the adult back, so completing a communicative act (Bjerkan 1996), which is the starting point of a playful communicative episode within which variations, challenges, and surprises will take place. The more child directed these episodes are, the more efficient they are in giving the child opportunities for sustaining the interaction and acquiring new competences.

Communication Exists and Develops at a Pre-verbal Stage

Communication exists and develops at a pre-verbal stage of development and is a prerequisite for using emerging competences (like symbols, signs, pictograms) During pre-verbal stages of development, partners do experience that communication is really taking place, although language is not used as a tool to implement it. Just think of a mother looking at her baby, who is looking at her face and drawing her attention with eye movements; the mother answers back with head and eye movements accompanied by vocalizations; and the baby goes on, sharing the emotion and already experiencing a turn-taking format. If we admit that communication requires three dimensions: sharing emotions, addressing the same topic, and using tools and channels accessible to both partners, we can consider this mother-child interaction as communicative. Let us compare the above situation with another typical one, where mother and child look together at a picture book. In this situation the child will have to shift his or her gaze from the book (the topic) to the mother's face (expressing the emotional state) and to use his or her voice / hearing system to deal with the utterances. By contrast, in the first situation (face-to-face interaction), all aspects are concentrated on the faces: the topic is the movements of the face (eye movements, mouth movement linked to the vocalizations, and head movements), the mother's emotion can be checked by looking at her face without gaze shifting and the tool / channel system is also the face movements, perceived mainly through the visual system. The perception of the vocalizations of the mother by the child is supported by the visual and tactile cues that are synchronized with them. In both situations communication is going on, but in the picture book situation more sophisticated skills are required.

We can also describe the face-to-face interaction as a development of a previous experience: the close body contact between mother and child. This contact provides both partners with *kinaesthetic* and tactile cues, thus making possible the sharing of emotional states and providing the child with security. So, face-to-face interaction (which is embedded in a global body contact) is another way to experience this closeness, using more distant senses and a differently organized time structure (turn taking).

Thus, from the very beginning of the life, communicative skills are emerging and building up. Examples of making communication more sophisticated are as follows.

Aspects Related to the Partner
The ability to shift attention from the topic to the partner, to use movements geared to drawing his attention (e.g., by pointing), or to implement communicative actions without the presence of the partner (like writing or reading letters).

Aspects Related to the Topic
The building up of joint attention to topics in the external world (e.g., looking together at the same object) and progressively being able to refer to objects that are not present and within reach.

Aspects Related to the Tool/Channel System
The introduction of new kinds of utterances: movements with symbolic value,

tactile/visual pictograms, words (signed or spoken), semantically or linguistically organized chains of words.

Neurological, Cognitive, and Social Conditions for Developing Communication

In all human beings, the maturation of the brain is a condition that determines the development of the capacities. A child cannot acquire a new skill if the necessary neurological equipment has not yet been built up through maturation. Nevertheless, maturation is not enough. Functions, in order to emerge and develop, have to be instrumented in communicative contexts. For instance, the lack of context within which vision is socially used can prevent a child with a normal visual equipment from developing a visual function (Portalier 1990). We know also that the *wiring process* in the brain needs to be nourished by stimulation: the visual area of the *cortex* will not be wired if there is no visual stimulation conveyed through the eye. Moreover, this wiring process is also dependent on whether or not the physical stimuli supporting the maturation of the nervous system are loaded with emotion (Trevarthen 1993). There is obviously an interaction between the *neurological maturation* of the brain and the use of emerging functions in a communicative context.

Another process through which new skills develop is '*automatization.*' For instance, over repetitive communicative episodes, the child can 'automatize' processes (such as following the attention focus of the partner, mastering body movements, vocalizations, signs), which in turn liberates resources for concentrating in more advanced emerging skills. In the case of individuals who are congenitally deafblind, it can be that physical and neurological conditions are so limited that the more sophisticated formats of communication (e.g., using speech or sign language in a communicative way) may not be reached. Whatever level is reached, however, communication can be rich and creative. Card playing could be a metaphor for communicative life: some people play simple card games (e.g., the French 'belote'), other ones play more 'sophisticated' ones (e.g., 'bridge'), but all can enjoy playing cards because of all the cognitive and emotional variations that can be experienced in each of the systems. By the same token, at any level of communicative competence, communication can be nourished by the variety of physical and emotional contexts within which it can be used, thus enhancing the repertoire of activities experienced in a communicative way and the repertoire of actions/symbols/words that can be used within the structure of the communicative level obtained by a person who is congenitally deafblind. This is an extremely important condition for a life of quality. Families and staff should not stop offering new challenges and experiences to their deafblind partners on the grounds that the highest possible communicative competence has been reached, thereby making further development impossible. Human beings cannot fly, which does not prevent them from walking around the world and making new acquaintances if they wish to.

What Is Communication For and About?

Understanding orders or asking for food are only very small and specific aspects of communication. What people enjoy about communication is communicating, which means sharing affects and experiences. By naming, commenting on, asking for, or about, and so on, one gains understanding of the world, influences other persons and events, and fosters continuing interaction. If, on the other hand, partners systematically interpret children's utterances as asking for something rather than as thinking about something that can be shared, we run a high risk of making the communicative act rigid and thus preventing more sophisticated development. Utterances should not be interpreted literally but should be given expansion related to the child state of mind. For example, asking for coffee does not mean necessarily that a child wants coffee; he may want to evoke the situation, the social interaction, or even a chance to rest.

Another aspect of communicative development is the impact of communicative experiences on supporting the child's interest and ability to go on thinking and mastering emotions and communicative tools when on his own. The objects and the utterances that are shared during communicative episodes are emotionally loaded, which supports the child in playing and exploring on his own these themes and symbolic or linguistic tools. Symbolic play (e.g., 'doll's tea party') contains actions and utterances that previously were parts of communicative episodes or shared events. Symbolic play is a way to master new skills and to develop imagination, creativity, and exploration. Although symbolic play is not much seen in congenitally deafblind children (at least in its most sophisticated form), there are many examples of children using symbolic elements of the environment (objects of reference, pictures, items of the calendar) to express to themselves their own emotional concerns (e.g., sitting down smiling next to the Friday part of the calendar when thinking of the prospect of going home). This individual follow-up of interactive episodes can bring new development to the next 'conversations.'

Communication and Language Develop within Play

*Communication and language cannot be taught on the basis of **frustration/ reward** procedures; they develop within playing contexts.* Communication requires a sustained and organized attention to a partner, a topic, and a message. In this way, it is a process that is much more complicated than each of the elements. In the field of deafblind education, often attention has been given mainly to the message, especially in a coded form (signs, pictograms, objects of reference, etc.) and less to the process itself. Besides, as many congenitally deafblind people seemed to lack motivation for communicating, frustration/reward procedures influenced by learning theories have been used, for instance, giving the child a piece of cake after he has produced the sign for *'cake.'* There is a danger in using this kind of method, because it gives the child an experience of communication restricted to using a semantic element to obtain an object, whereas the kind of communication everybody enjoys is what happens between two (or more) human beings who are sharing feelings and interests. There is very little probability of obtaining a sustained and joyful communicative episode if only a frustration/reward procedure, is used. Moreover, this procedure, which is meant to compensate for a lack of interest, is likely to be counterproductive, since it does not help the child to shift from the interest in gaining a piece of cake to the interest in communicating. There is a danger that children learn that they will get interest from an adult only in situations when they ask for something. Thus, it is a priority that children not be restricted to experiencing communicative attention only for practical reasons. From the very beginning of the life, communication is used to express and explore the pleasure of being together. The practical aspect of communication (asking for a piece of cake) is only an aspect (limited) of the functions of communication. Besides, it is during the playful episodes of communication that new communication skills are more easily acquired.

Communication Is Developing as Long as the Flow of Interaction Is Not Broken

Communication is developing as long as the flow of interaction is not broken by the introduction of a new element too early (e.g., objects of reference or signs). Correlatively, openings should always have been looked for to introduce new and more advances elements.

During the first years of the life, maturation of the brain and social interactions allow the child to experience communication episodes in an increasingly sophisticated way, which means that competent partners are able to be sensitive to emerging possibilities in the child and to challenge him with new tools (verbal or non-verbal utterances). It can be very difficult, during communication with deafblind children, to introduce these new elements, since all the functions that make communication possible have to be implemented mainly through the tactile channel. The hands are involved in checking the partner's emotional state, exploring the shared object of interest, and receiving utterances. Thus, the flow of interaction can very easily be interrupted if the adult breaks into the child's action at the wrong time. The partner has to be careful to introduce a new element (a sign, an object of reference) without breaking the flow of interaction, which means that he has to be ready to use the 'window' offered by the child for using his hand to convey a message or introduce a new shared object. A communicative episode looks like a musical game within which a new element must contribute to making the music go on instead of interrupting it. Fortunately, there are possibilities of intervention by either accompanying the child's movement or waiting until the moment when he or she gives back attention to the partner. We can feel that a movement addressed to the child has been wrongly timed when he withdraws his hand or becomes more tense.

Many Aspects of Communicative Development Are Not Related to Age

Many aspects of communicative development are not related to the age of the individual but can be observed in both adults and children who are deafblind. In this chapter, we often use the word 'children' when referring to infants, children, youths, and adults with congenital deafblindness. The processes that are described usually take place at the beginning of the life. Nevertheless, all the aspects that are addressed concern the congenitally deafblind of any age. Possibilities exist in adults of developing new skills or of using them in various contexts. The structure of the communicative episodes depends on the existing competences rather than on the age. Of course, there are differences between children and adults. In general, adults have accumulated more experiences and are at a different stage of brain maturation. Nevertheless, there are many evidences of communicative episodes whose structure is the same in interactions with children as it is in those with adults, a similarity that reflects the fact that the same level of competence has been reached by people of different ages. It follows that people in contact with adults (families, professionals, friends) face the same challenges as those who are in contact with children.

Frameworks for Communicative Events with Congenitally Deafblind People

In deafblind education we use different methods for developing communication, for instance, objects of reference, calendars, photos, relief, pictograms, pictosigns, pictogrammed words, sign language, writing, Braille, finger-spelling, and speech. The methods are being used according to the traditions of the schools and the centres and also on the basis of the capacities of the deafblind learners.

Very often we use more than one system for one deafblind person and they can change over time. We use different systems because they support each other and also because doing so provides the deafblind person with options that can be chosen according to different situations. What we would like to emphasize here is how these methods can be used in a communicative way.

In what follows we shall give a description of the different stages in the development of communication and through practical examples try to show how some of the communication methods can be used within communicative acts.

Primary Intersubjectivity

As stated before, communication develops in social interactive play. The development of interpersonal togetherness or *intersubjectivity* starts within the face-to-face interaction called *primary intersubjectivity* (Trevarthen and Hubley 1978). In this basic pattern of interaction the partners start sharing emotions and attention with each other and exchanges of utterances between the two partners emerge, which at this stage consist mainly of emotional and affective expressions and body movements. The world outside is not yet involved or a part of the interaction. The attention of the child and the space within which the interaction takes place cannot yet include more elements than the two partners involved in the interaction. Communication has to be established, sustained, and automatic between two people before the world (the third element) can be a part of the interactive play as it is in secondary interaction. In communicative acts within primary intersubjectivity, the emotions shared, the topic addressed, and the utterances being used are emerging from the togetherness between the two partners.

As mentioned earlier, the attention of the child in the face-to-face interaction is monitored in the global body contact of the mother and the baby. Research shows that all babies are biologically preprogrammed for social togetherness. For instance, babies are born with preferences of vision and hearing designed to attract the attention of the baby to the face and the voice of the mother, and they are born with the capacity for body expressions of vitality as contributions to communication.

Deafblind children who have either impaired vision and hearing or no vision and/or hearing at all seem to have the same interest in faces as seeing and hearing children if, in addition to visual and hearing cues, their partner uses other channels, such as airflow and touch. In the natural interaction between mothers and their deafblind children, we see that the mothers intuitively use touch (e.g., kisses on the cheek) and airflow in greeting rituals to attract the attention of their deafblind children, and often this activity leads to the exploration of their mother's face by the hands of the children (Daelman et al. 1996).

When deafness precludes the use of only sound to attract attention to the voice, vibrations and airflow take on an important role for deafblind children. Perhaps attention should be given at that early stage to attracting attention to the hands of the mother as well as her face by presenting the hands close to the face, almost as a part of the face. In the future hands will play the main role as substitutes for eyes and ears. Hearing children babble as play with the speech organs. All children babble with voice and hands, but what is not responded to (or perceived) decays. Deafblind children should babble with their hands on their own and together with their partner to prepare them for 'speaking' as well. Tactile interest in the faces and hands of partners is essential for deafblind children, since it might make it possible, at a later stage of communicative development, to read facial expressions or speech (*Tadoma*) and signs.

What makes the activities of the child social in these early stages of development is that they attract the attention of the adult and trigger the adult to react. That process gives the child the feedback that he is socially 'seen' and is able to influence his partner, which triggers more and new activity from the child, and a good circle has started. One of the ways the adult reacts is by immediate imitation. Papousek (1981) describes how mothers imitate their babies' vocalizing or face-making. This imitation is not a boring repetition, because mothers introduce small variations, which take place within a turn-taking framework. The imitation game with mother and baby at the same time creates a 'theme' where the interaction pattern turn-taking can be supported by accompanying the activity using another channel. For instance, the child moves his arm and the adult accompanies the movement by using voice. This way of reacting to the activity of the child in an amodal way is called 'affective attunement' by Daniel Stern (1985). These ways of reacting make it possible to make the activity of the child social, to support interactive patterns, and to attune to the emotional state of the child.

The expansion within primary intersubjectivity is that the reactions of the adult are delayed in time, which stimulates the child to act again in order to bring the adult back into the game. The gap between the activity of the child and the reaction of the adult expands gradually. In the beginning the adult is the one who reacts to the activity of the child. Progressively, it is possible for the adult to be the initiator and the child to start to alternate between the roles of initiator and responder, which means that the *reciprocity* within communicative acts is being built up. At this stage, when initiating, the adult must keep to the child's existing repertoire of activities or to small variations in that repertoire. The communicative events in this stage of communicative development consist of daily routine situations, such as feeding, bathing, and play. In all cultures all over the world social games exists. Mothers play these games, which develop the rules of social togetherness, guided by intuition and tradition. At the same time, these games and daily routine situations create optimal conditions for communicative utterances to emerge.

Example: Mother is changing the nappy of her deafblind infant. This activity has happened many times during the day and a routine situation has been built up (repetition of the same sequence). Before going to the bathroom, mother tickles her baby with the nappy on the breast. They play a tickling game where the child shows expectation just before the mother starts to tickle again by holding the breath and positioning the body for the tickling. Mother triggers the baby by making breaks between the tickling. When they come to the bathroom, other games have been developed, for instance, a peek-a-boo game with the trousers. The child expects the game and shows anticipation by putting his hands on his face where mother usually puts the trousers. Communicative utterances have been developed in the game and are answered and expanded by the mother. The objects being used, like the nappy and the trousers, are being loaded with emotions, which makes it possible later to use these objects as shared objects in the interaction and as objects of reference used not only to indicate an activity but in a communicative way.

The interaction between the two partners is regulated at first by the adult and later by both partners. Video recordings have made it possible for us to watch on a micro level how small details in the interaction can either break the flow of the interaction or sustain it. We think that it is necessary to be able to look at the interactions on a micro level to be able to intervene in them effectively. If the interaction is distorted on a micro level, this distortion will be transferred to the interaction patterns of togetherness, which again will be transferred to later stages of communicative development.

At this stage, further development means that the attention of the child can be kept for longer and longer periods and that the space of interaction is expanded, which makes it possible to facilitate the reciprocity and use different themes with many variations within these themes. Again, this will lead to a stage where the time and the space of interaction will allow more advantageous elements to be introduced as objects.

What we look for in intervention is effective ways to sustain interactions (Daelman et al. 1996). At first, social togetherness is regulated by the adult answering the activity of the child, trying to attune to the affective mood of the child and trying to tune into the tempo, the rhythm, and the intensity of the child. Immediate imitation is a very effective way of responding, as mentioned above. When you interact with partners who may do so in a way that is very different from your usual way of interacting, imitation can be a big support in developing your own competence as a partner. When you imitate a person, you will experience in your own body the tempo, the rhythm, and the intensity of the other, which makes it easier for you to adapt to him or her. Later on, when you are attuned to each other, you will have to find a way to keep the attention and the interest of your partner. This applies to both partners. It could be called regulating the interaction so that it continues for as long as possible.

Regulating interactive play means that you are always looking for ways to introduce variations to keep the interest of your partner. At the same time, you have to be alert for variations suggested by your partner and respond to him or her. The variations can be within the musical aspects of interaction, like changing the tempo, the rhythm, and the intensity of the interaction (Halland and Hauge). Variations may also be introduced, for instance, a clapping game or new themes such as changing from a clapping game to a jumping game. The art in creating these co-creative events is in the awareness of both partners of each one other and that each one finds the right moment to introduce variations and new elements. If the variations are introduced too early or are too complicated, the flow can be broken. In face-to-face interaction, elements from communication systems, such as objects of reference and signs, should not be introduced if they break the flow.

Example: Susan is playing at the switchback with the teacher. Susan is blind but has some residual hearing. The teacher puts her on the top of the switchback, hugs her and taps her legs in a rhythmical way indicating the start of her slide and at the same time accompanying the tapping with her voice synchronically. Then the teacher moves back, but keeps talking to sustain the contact. When Susan slides down to the teacher, she gets the expected hugging game, and at the same time the teacher says, 'you slide,' again and again. After a few hugs Susan puts one hand to the face of her teacher, listening to 'you slide' again and again. Susan laughs and moves her legs where they were tapped.

If the teacher had introduced signs for sliding, she would have had to take Susan's hands away from the hugging game, and the flow in the act would probably have been broken. By using more than one communication system (speech and signs), you offer a choice to the deafblind child, a choice that will depend on the situation itself. In this case, the teacher and Susan can keep the flow in the interactive play and communicate at the same time.

Regulation of proximity within the interactive play is crucial. Of course, communication with deafblind people has to be close, but it is essential that the deafblind person is the one who decides how close and when to be close. If this decision is not respected by the partners, the deafblind person will direct all his or her energy towards regaining control, and the flow of the interaction will break down. When we watch mothers communicating with their deafblind children, we can see that they are able not to invade their children's personal space. Professionals must learn from this. We must knock at the door before entering, and we must wait for our deafblind partner to give a signal inviting us to come nearer. This point is even more essential when one works with the adult population. In a partnership, each partner has equal control over his or her personal space. If this control is threatened, not only will effective, interactive communication be threatened, it will be difficult to establish and almost impossible to maintain. In addition, the person who is deafblind will focus his or her attention on regaining control rather than on interaction and may even use physical force in an attempt to re-establish control.

In primary intersubjectivity, objects are not yet included in the interaction. In some cases, however, we have found that it has been necessary to use an object loaded with emotions (from the viewpoint of the deafblind child) to achieve basic contact in face-to-face interaction. This object can, for instance, be the bottle. In these cases a sensitive way of trying to share the object by immediate imitation can lead to a shift of the attention on the part of the child. In the beginning, the attention of the child is on the bottle, and gradually the attention may shift from the bottle to the adult who is trying to share the activity and the attention of the child. One might say that the bottle or the object instruments the basic contact in face-to-face interaction.

Secondary Intersubjectivity

There is no sudden jump from one stage of development to the next. **Secondary intersubjectivity** starts when the world is introduced in communicative acts. This means that it is possible to sustain face-to-face interaction and at the same time pay attention to a third element. This element will be the new topic of conversation. At first, the new element is often a part of the communicative act itself as a shared object used within a shared activity. Later, the topic will belong to the world outside the communicative act itself, but it must be shared by the communicative partners. The partners thus need to be able to give joint attention to something in the world and at the same time keep the flow of their communicative act. The communicative act is now more complex, and it is essential for the flow that the basic face-to-face interaction is working automatically. This will release attention and perceptual capacities and free them for new options (the third element).

Since the content of the interaction is still the shared affective togetherness that has been built up in face-to-face interaction, these first shared objects must already have been loaded with affect by the child. Thus, the object can be part of the adult, such as glasses or necklaces, or perhaps – even better – an object that is part of the child, such as a favourite toy, a bottle, a cup, or a dummy. In interactive play with these objects loaded with emotions the adult acts upon the object as the child does, more or less simultaneously. Gradually, the interaction pattern becomes stretched in time and space. The adult supports the 'give and take' pattern by making it look as if the child gives the object. She acts with the object as the child does. The child takes back the object because it is his. Thus, at the start of the 'give-and-take' game the child is only taking, whereas the adult makes it look as if he is giving as well. Gradually, the adult makes small variations in the way she acts with the object. The child's experience is that he or she gets the object back and that the adult will show him new ways of acting with the object. That process will empower real reciprocity, where the child gradually lets go of the object and gradually masters the 'give-and take' game. This giving place to the partner in interaction has to be formatted in relation to objects.

In our experience new objects that can be introduced by the partner at this early stage of secondary intersubjectivity without breaking the flow of interaction are objects that in a way are extending the face of the adult and the near senses, such as a flute or a carnival pipe. Even hats or other items that can be placed in the face or on the body will be interesting for the child, since it probably will be experienced as a part of a person the child already knows and pays attention to.

It is especially important for functionally blind, deafblind children to be aware of the significance of sharing objects. If you arrange to have two objects that are identical, when the child is playing with his or her favourite toy, you can share the activity by imitating what the child is doing, gently touching the child with your object, so that he or she is aware that you are reacting to that activity. Gradually, variations will be introduced by both partners, and the objects will be exchanged by the partners participating in the interaction.

Interactive play with objects between partners will include the social games that all mothers in all cultures play with their children. They play expectation games, 'hide-and-seek' games, 'give-and-take' games, and imitation games, all with the purpose of making togetherness joyful and predictable, but with unpredictable variations to keep the attention and interest of the child (regulation of tension). At the same time, those social games will give the natural frame of developing the **interactional patterns** that are needed in communication. When the child's experience is that the way the adult reacts to his or her object is similar to the way the child reacts to his or her object, this will empower the representation of the adult as one who is of the same kind as him or herself, which is a prerequisite for transfer of roles and the feeling of empathy.

The last and most complex of the patterns of social togetherness is joint attention to a third element that has not already been loaded with affect in the *dyad* and is outside the *dyadic joint space*. Mothers of non-impaired infants structure this pattern so that they obtain mutual joint attention by following the attention the child already pays to an object/event outside the dyad. In this way joint attention is acquired. In other words, at first, the mother looks for attention cues from her baby, and then she follows that attention and shares it with her baby. One of the major challenges for partners working with deafblind people is that cues that are easy to follow, such as head-turning and directional gaze, are weak, non-persistent, or not present in deafblind people. This means that partners of deafblind people have to look for attention cues that are more difficult to predict, to discover, and therefore to react to. For instance, the attention to sound (active listening) will often look like passivity and therefore often not be reacted to by the partner in a way that leads to joint attention. When the child's attention is maintained tactilely, it can be very difficult to see when the child needs time and no intrusion from the adult because he or she is building up an image of the object and when there is an opening to share attention to the object. Sometimes it is possible to share the attention by using another channel, for instance, by accompanying the tactile exploration by sounds following the movements in a synchronic way or answering the movement as in a dialogue.

Example: Simon is playing the piano. He explores the instrument tactilely and enjoys exploring the different sounds and vibrations he can produce. After a while his teacher tries to join him, answering his play by imitating the tempo, rhythm, and intensity of his play. Simon is immediately aware and pushes the teacher gently away. She stays in position, so close that Simon knows that she is still there but without sharing his activity. After a short while she tries to join him again. This time he accepts the closeness and interaction and even smiles a bit when she follows the variations he makes. The play continues, and the teacher starts to make variations as well. Between these variations Simon puts his hands on top of those of the teacher 'looking at' her hand movements. Then Simon pushes the teacher away again in a more determined way. This action is respected by the teacher, and Simon continues exploring the activity and the piano.

Mastering joint attention is the most complex of the patterns of togetherness and is necessary for developing communication on a linguistic level. The child must be able to attract the attention of his partner, lead the attention of the partner to the third element, check that the partner shares his attention, re-establish the contact, and exchange utterances. When functions and situations are very complex, deafblind people need more than one channel to be functioning at the same time. For instance, the visual channel can be used for contact and perceiving the utterances (signs), and the tactile channel can be used for leading the attention of the adult to the object by tactile pointing (leading the hand of the partner to the object). For all congenitally deafblind people it will be necessary to include the tactile channel in complex situations like joint attention. If the utterances are maintained through the tactile channel, for example, tactile sign language, different parts of the body can take care of the contact (legs), leading the attention to the third element (left hand), signing (right hand), listening (left hand goes back to the partner). Mastering joint attention for congenitally deafblind people requires a much greater cognitive capacity than seeing hearing people need, who can get simultaneous information on different channels and who can easily alternate their gaze between an object/event of interest and the partner.

In our experience the first third element (content or subject of the conversation) that deafblind children share will be a topic already loaded with affect. If, for instance, the deafblind child is interacting with a stranger and the caregiver is available, the child often wants to share this wonderful experience with his or her caregiver or he simply wants to say: 'Look what I am doing together with another person.' This is a situation where communication is needed and where the child's motivation to communicate is high.

Another situation that often may lead to joint attention on the initiative of the deafblind child occurs when a very motivating activity is broken after some time but before the deafblind child is ready to leave the activity. Again, the child needs to attract the attention of the adult to objects from the activity and thereby take the initiative to communicate that he or she wants to continue.

Different gestures are used by both partners in communication actively to direct the attention of the other partner to outside entities. These distal gestures are called *deictic gestures* and can take the form of pointing, showing, offering, giving, and requesting by opening the hand or moving the hand up and down (Nadel and Camaioni 1996). These gestures are supported by the mother when she follows the attention of her child. She creates mutual attention by looking and pointing at the object/event that is the focus of the attention of the child and reacts emotionally to it. With blind or visually impaired children the pointing has to be performed or supported by the tactile channel. These distal gestures can be either *imperative* (meaning that they are used in a instrumental way by the child, who uses the pointing to obtain desired objects/events; they do not include joint attention), or they can be *declarative* (meaning that the child intends to share attention to a common focus and therefore to include joint attention). When the child uses declarative gestures, he or she intends to communicate with his or her partner. Camaioni suggests that the underlying differences between being able to use deictic gestures in either a non-social way (imperative) or a social way (declarative) concern the fact that the child must have experienced that his or her partners can and are willing to share the same object/event in order to be able to develop an understanding of others as psychological subjects with whom one may share experience in a communicative way. The way the partner interprets and reacts to the deictic gestures is crucial. The partner must answer as if the child had the intention of sharing (declarative) wherever possible to support the development of this essential aspect of communication.

Emergence of Symbolic Aspects of Communication

Progressively, children, youth, and adults make communication more symbolic. When trying to communicate intentions or interests, the child uses 'body language.' This body language includes movements that are geared towards drawing the partner's attention (pointing at, touching, taking the adult hand to) and also towards producing an equivalent of the experience the child is thinking about. The last part of a video presented at the European Course on Communication in June 1996 is very good example of this.

Example: Thomas is playing with the tunnel together with his teacher. The teacher goes into the tunnel and Thomas enjoys following her. During this play Thomas experiences the voice of the teacher by putting his ear close to the tunnel, and the teacher responds to his attention by patting his ear in synchrony with using her voice. Later, Thomas puts his arm around the tunnel to feel the movement of the teacher in the tunnel. When the teacher comes out of the tunnel, she wants to change to another game and suggests playing with a ball. Thomas is not yet ready to switch; he wants to continue the game with the tunnel. This situation makes it necessary for Thomas to get the attention of his teacher and to communicate to her that he wants to go on with the tunnel game. Thomas does so in the following way:

– He takes the hand of the teacher and points at the tunnel. Could be interpreted: 'I want to go back to the game that took place here.' The teacher doesn't understand.
– He then points to his ear where he felt the patting of the teacher. Could be interpreted: 'I want the game that I felt here.' The teacher doesn't understand.

– He then makes a movement with his arm like the one he made when he felt
the teacher in the tunnel. Could be interpreted: 'I want the game that felt like
this.' The teacher repeats this movement with her own arm, and then she
understands. She answers: 'You want to go back into the tunnel,' and Thomas laughs. At last he is understood.

In this example Thomas points to the place where the event took place, and he
produces two embodied signs experienced during the experience.

In a parallel way, people who live with congenitally deafblind people have
their own intentions; they are willing to provide them with information and
comments about future or past events in order to give them the potential to
anticipate and to get an overview of their own life. For instance, using *objects
of reference* and signals is part of the traditional culture of deafblind education.
When a deafblind child is presented with an object of reference (e.g., a '*sponge*'
representing '*having a bath*'), the adult's intention is

- to trigger the child's related activity (e.g., going to the bathroom); in this case
it works as a signal
- and/or to help him to build an image of this activity; in this case it is used as
a symbol.

In many facilities for deafblind people, you can also find 'calendars,' frame-
works within which various kinds of object (things, pictures, pictograms,
words, etc.) are stored in an organized way in order to represent the different
activities of the day or of the week. There are many kinds of calendars, whose
form depends on the local tradition of the institution and on the functional level
of the deafblind people who use them.

Objects of reference and calendars are often understood as the first way to
communicate with deafblind children. It is true that they provide them with an
overview of how their own lives are organized, and they help the staff and families to express their intentions to their deafblind partners. In this way they are
very useful, because they allow deafblind people to predict what is happening
and to be informed, which greatly contributes to their feeling of security. Yet
the way these devices are used is a very important aspect of their communicative value. Let us look at some characteristics that can help us to use them in as
communicative a way as possible :

- Perceptual qualities. When an object of reference is selected, it should be
easy and interesting for the child to touch or look at. Attention must be paid

to the sensory capacities of the child and, above all, to how he uses them – for instance, many deafblind people prefer scratchy surfaces to soft ones. Also, in spite of good residual vision, it can happen that a child is more interested in tactile features, which may reflect the way his senses are instrumented. Thus, it can be useful to provide these children with objects with tactile and visual qualities, so they can explore them in different ways over time as their perceptual skills develop. The more interesting an object is to the child, the more chance there is that he will remember it and share it.

- Affective qualities. It can be very useful to use what the child prefers in an activity to select an object of reference. For instance, if, while bathing, the child has a lot of fun feeling the *sponge* on his body during play episodes with his mother, this *sponge* could be the right choice for an object of refer-ence. Of course, in this case the object is not scratchy, but it triggers the memory of the interesting, emotional, and communicative part of the bath : playing with mum with the sponge. This is an example of a child-directed choosing strategy.

- Communicative quality. An object of reference can be used effectively to suggest a communicative episode. For instance, the *sponge* can be shown to the child in a teasing way by mimicking the funny part of the bath. There is then a chance that a sustained communicative episode will take place. Of course, during these episodes, more sophisticated systems of communication can be introduced, as long as they do not break the flow of the interaction. The combination of physical and affective qualities of an object can make this kind of episode attractive to the child. It is assumed, however, that this child has already acquired the capacity to share an object with a partner (what we have called secondary intersubjectivity), or at least, it can be a context to help it to emerge.

This communicative way of using objects of reference (or more sophisticated tools, such as pictures, pictograms) can lead to further development in the cog-nitive and affective area. The more an object of reference (or a picture, a picto-gram, etc.) is loaded with physical, affective, and communicative qualities, the more it is likely to trigger an interest from the child in situations when he is on his own. It is helpful when these objects are available for him to explore and play with on his own. Such autonomous symbolic activity, at this stage of development, would be difficult without a physical medium that can be played with. In addition, shared symbolic play can offer the child his or her first expe-rience of a narrative, which is a cognitive and affective structure helping to organize the different small elements that constitute a shared event so that they can be recalled and described in an organized way.

Introducing Semantics and Linguistics

So far, we have expressed how important it is that during the pre-verbal stages, communication develops as co-created dialogues on topics that can be either the partners' body expressions or objects of the external world. We also have addressed the emergence of symbolic skills as an aspect of communicative episodes or as a an autonomous activity. Part of the expansion of communicative and symbolic skills rests on using new media which are increasingly complicated and increasingly culturally designed instead of being private codes or rituals.

Deafblind people and their partners have designed or borrowed many systems in order to meet their communicative needs in various contexts. Let us mention sign language (tactile or visual), speech (that can also be perceived tactilely using the Tadoma method), finger-spelling, written words or Braille, pictograms (pictosigns and pictogrammed words), pictures (visual or tactile), objects of reference, and so forth. Various forms of these systems exist all over the world and new versions will probably result from the creativity of users.

It is a challenge for deafblind people and their partners progressively to master the use of these systems in order to improve their quality of communication and to acquire new tools for thinking. These systems are not always used the way they are by people who are not deafblind. For instance, graphic forms are used in *dialogic ways*, which means that 'conversations' are taking place using graphic forms (pictograms) instead of the usual conversational ones (speech or sign language). Moreover, it happens very often that spoken or signed language develops after the use of graphic forms (pictures, pictograms, etc.). Thus, it is impossible to decide on the best system of communication for deafblind people, since many elements are involved: the specific profile of development of each individual, the cognitive and sensory capacities, the stage of development, the cultural or institutional context, the immediate goal, and so on.

Mastering a fully fledged linguistic system is a goal that all try to achieve in deafblind education, but it cannot always be realized. Fortunately, the quality of life and the quality of communication does not depend only on reaching that goal. We have already emphasized how important pre-verbal communication is for a Life of Quality. Two pitfalls could contribute negatively to this quality:

- having too high expectations for language development and thus not broadening the use of prelinguistic capacities in a communicative way
- not offering deafblind people the tools that they would like and be able to use in order to have more control over their lives and on the world.

In other words, the dangers are either to over-expect or to deprive. In order to try to avoid such dangers, it is necessary to get a more precise description of how these different tricks or systems of communication are functionally used.

First, it is important to mention that items that usually belong to a linguistic system can be used in a prelinguistic way, which can solve the problem of communicating accurately or thinking about the world. Let us use again the *sponge* example. If this object of reference is no longer necessary for the child to refer to the bath situation, and if a graphic form (like a drawing or a pictogram) has been successfully substituted, this pictogram could be used in a sentence-like sequence of pictograms ([tonight] [sponge] [Mary]). In this case, they could be designed so that the child understands something that could be expressed with the sentence: 'Tonight, it is Mary who will take care of my bath.' The child uses a cognitive strategy allowing him or her to match an interpretation of these three pictograms with a situation he knows. To do so he or she must have some understanding of each of the items and a capacity to infer from them a new meaning that is different from each of the items. The result could be the same, however, if the pictograms were organized in a different order. This successful example of comprehension of a graphic utterance is the result of a semantic competence rather than a linguistic one, because no grammatical structure has been used. Of course, in this example the pictograms have not been actually presented in a fully linguistic form, but even if the same utterance had been produced in a perfectly correct sign language, it does not mean that the child would have understood it on the basis of its specifically linguistic form. The child can create some meaning without mastering the grammar of the language in use. In this case, by putting together two or three words (or a word and the context), he or she is able to build an adequate interpretation of the utterance and to react appropriately from a communicative point of view.

The items used in symbolic communication have different degrees of symbolic value. At one end of the continuum, the items are very close to the perceived reality, and at the other end, they are totally conventional: objects of reference, tactile or visual drawings, photos, tactile or visual pictograms, pictogrammed words (words with pictograms inside), pictosigns (pictograms representing signs instead of forms), spoken or signed words, written words, and Braille. Many congenitally deafblind people are able to use some of the items in a semantic and pragmatic way, which means by processing different levels of informations (the items, the physical situation, the habits of the partner). It is true also that this capacity can be trained either in situations of daily life or in special sessions geared towards helping the child to match symbolic items with contents or to process more complicated information, such as sequences of items. But the success of these sessions is dependent on the quality of the communicative and emotional involvement of both partners, quality that can derive from the here and now situation (i.e., the quality of the interaction itself) as well as from the themes that are shared. The motivation of the deafblind child, in order to be sustained, requires from the partner the same capacities that were described at the beginning of the communicative life: sensitivity, creativity, and challenge. Special mention should be made of concepts related to emotions, which cannot be taught without seizing, during communicative episodes, the emotional states of the child in order to 'name' them. For instance, the only way to help a child to build up the concept of 'sadness' is to seize an occasion when he or she feels sad and to make him or her feel (using body expression) that this sadness has been perceived; on that basis it will be possible to 'name' this 'sadness,' which contributes to the child's awareness and categorization of feelings.

It is necessary to have some knowledge of the features of the various systems of communication that are usually used with congenitally deafblind people in order to make the most of them according to the stage of development, the sensory capacities, the information-processing skills and the here-and-now conditions of the situation. First, they belong to different linguistic systems. Oral speech, finger-spelling, written language, Braille, pictogrammed words, and pictograms are based on the grammar of the oral language of the country in which they are used. On the other hand, sign language and pictosigns are structured according to the grammar of the sign language of the country. Problems occur when the grammar of the system used for conversations is different from normal grammatical structure, as is the case when sign language is used in conversations and Braille or normal writing is used in texts. (Similar difficulties are encountered in the education of congenitally deaf people.) Another typical developmental feature of congenitally deafblind people is that many of them more easily process graphic communication (drawings, pictograms) than speech or sign language, especially because written information can be contrasted and remain available as long as necessary for the person to process it, whereas the elements of sign language or speech are transient and less contrasted. In addition, graphic communication, even though presented according to normal grammatical structures, allows enough time for semantic strategies to be used when grammatical ones are not available. These difficulties have led to the use of systems that are usually specific to writing as a way of conversing. Finger-spelling offers a successful compromise by using all the elements of the written language (letters instead of phonemes) in conversations. Written conversations are also realized through sentences in pictograms or in normal written language. Objects of reference, drawings, pictograms, or sequences of pictograms are also used in daily life to exchange information. Many kinds of situations could be described that reflect the creativity and the mutual adaptation of congenitally deafblind people and their partners. Obviously, there is no unique way, and it is impossible to suggest a strategy that would be right for everybody. Nevertheless, it is useful to keep in mind a principle that is relevant all over development: *Communication systems should be used so that they do not break the flow of interaction.*

We can mention two illustrations of this principle. (1) At the first stages of development children withdraw because an adult's utterance has been wrongly timed. (2) Deafblind people with high communication skills can prefer using sign language in conversations and meetings, rather than finger-spelling or Braille translation, because the speed and the expressiveness of sign language are more appropriate to the flow of emotions that usually takes place in any conversation. To add to the complexity, it is not unusual for youth and adults with congenital or acquired deafblindness to combine finger-spelling and signing to convey a single thought. Thus, partners continually must compromise. Yet this need to compromise is a pervasive element of all the communicative situations in human life.

Supporting language acquisition in congenitally deafblind people consists in helping them to make the most of their symbolic, semantic, and linguistic capacities. The level that can be reached is different for each person, but at each level there is potential to be creative in the use of these capacities in real life. The symbolic function also can develop in activities other than those geared towards developing communication as such. Craft and artistic activities, for example, can provide deafblind people with opportunities to share their emotions or their vision of the world without using words. Proposing a wide set of options for these creative activities offers more situations for identifying the strong interests and abilities of each individual. Moreover, these activities open a very wide field for exploration. This non-linguistic form of sharing is extensively used by people without disabilities, and it should be supported in deafblind people, whose linguistic capacities are impaired.

Cognitive and Information Processing Problems in Communicative Development of Deafblind People

Specific Challenges

At the beginning of their lives, all human beings progressively build up a system through which their different senses are used in a coordinated way. None of the senses can be considered separately from the others. This coordination allows humans to develop efficient ways to meet their communicative needs while acting in the world. For instance, when two adults are collaborating on a shared task, they can use their hands for the task itself, their hearing for exchanging information (technical or emotional), and their vision to check alternately the action and the partner. This kind of coordination, which assigns different channels to different tasks in a coordinated way, is the result of both maturation and practice (Ratner and Bruner 1977), and processing action and language in a parallel way is a very important aspect of communicative development.

From that point of view, people with congenital deafblindness have to face specific challenges. A very important one is the fact that tasks that could be carried out simultaneously (e.g., hearing to get the verbal utterances and vision for joint attention) have to be implemented either sequentially through the same channel or in unusual and unexpected ways. For instance, we have observed the following behaviours:

- using residual vision/hearing for contact and hands for exploring
- using one hand for contact and the other one for the object
- using hands to explore an object and feet to keep contact with partner's face.

In all these situations, there is a risk that the utterances from the partner will break in on the flow of the other focuses of attention. If the tactile channel is the only one available, therefore, the deafblind person has to use his hands to explore the shared object, to feel the emotional state of the partner, and to receive or produce utterances. This sequential organization is very demanding and can delay progression to the secondary intersubjectivity stage. The situation eases at the primary intersubjectivity stage because contact, topic, and utterance can be processed through the same channel. For instance, by touching the face a child can check the emotional state of his or her partner, explore the topic (the face itself), and pick up the utterances (movements of the face, such as smiling, blowing, or vocalizing).

Because of this very specific situation, the partners of deafblind people have to be careful in observing the channels that are actually used in order to respond and challenge without breaking the interaction. Introducing an object into the dialogue and then introducing signs can be complicated. We have observed an effective way to introduce an object: the adult, after communicative episodes with a totally deafblind child involving tactile face exploration, uses a whistle. This object, being as easy to reach as the mouth and producing also sound, vibration, and blowing, is naturally accepted by the child, who shapes his or her hand according to the shape of this object, obviously enjoying this new experience, which has both the same features as the previous one (without object) and new ones.

The difficulty of coordinating attention to the emotional state of the partner, to the state of the world, and to verbal (or non-verbal) utterances is present at all stages of development. It is a challenge for deafblind people's partners at the start of life, but it is also a challenge for interpreters for deafblind people who are asked to bring to the deafblind person not only the verbal utterances of the person they speak with, but also the emotional reactions and a description of the physical environment. Again, only on-line sensitivity makes it possible to find out where and when the 'windows' are opened by the deafblind person for introducing all these elements in a coordinated way. Video-analysis is a good way to improve the skills of families and professionals in this area.

Summary

In this chapter we have addressed the main aspects of development of communication with congenitally deafblind people. We have emphasized the fact that mastering the rules of pre-verbal dialogue is a prerequisite for using symbolic systems in a communicative way. They describe natural strategies and contexts that make it possible to support communicative competences in congenitally deafblind children.

1. The core strategies of intervention are as follows:
   a) Creating a natural context where strong channels are used in order to support the instrumentation of the residual senses is important.
   b) Adult sensitivity to child's utterances and the balanced use of repetition and novelty in playful contexts are also crucial ways to make the child active in his own communicative development.
2. Communication develops as a co-created process that happens in social-interactive play, where utterances of the child are used as topics for communicative acts.

REFERENCES

Barret, M., M. Harris, and J. Chasin (1991) 'Early Lexical Development and Maternal Speech.' *Journal of Child Language* 18, 21–40
Bjerkan, B. (1996) 'Aspects of "Communication" in Relation to Contact with Congenitally Deaf-Blind Persons.' In *Bilingualism and Literacy Concerning Deafness and Deaf-Blindness: Proceedings of an International Workshop, 10th–13th November 1994*, ed. A.M. Vonen, K. Arnesen, R.T. Enerstvedt, and A.V. Nafstad. Oslo: Skadalen Resource Centre
Bowlby, John (1969). *Attachment and Loss*, Vol. 1. *Attachment*, London: Hogarth Press

Bullinger, André (1994) 'Le concept d'instrumentation: son intérêt pour l'approche des différents déficits.' In *Le Développement de l'Enfant: Approches Comparatives*, ed. Michel Deleau and Annick Weil Barrais. Paris. PUF

Daelman, M., A. Nafstad, L. Rodbroe, T. Visser, and J. Souriau (1996) *The Emergence of Communication. Contact and Interaction patterns. Persons with Deafblindness.* Video, IAEDB Working Group on Communication. Suresnes, France: CNEFEI

Fogel, Alan (1993). 'Co-regulation and Framing.' In Nadel and Camaioni, eds (1993)

Halland, Tonsberg G., and T. Strand Hauge. 'The Musical Nature of Prelinguistic Interaction.'

Lindstrom, Bengt (1994). *The Essence of Existence.* 'On the Quality of Life of Children in the Nordic Countries – Theory and Practice in Public Health.' Göteborg, Sweden: *NHV Rapport* 3, 63–75

Nadel, Jacqueline, and Luigia Camaioni, eds (1993) *New Perspectives In Early Communicative Development.* London: Routledge.

Nafstad, A.V.(1989) *Space of Interaction.* Publication No. 9. Dronninglund, Denmark: Nordic Staff Training Centre for Deafblind Services

Papousek, M., and H. Papousek (1981) *Advances in Infancy Research.* Norwood, NJ: Ablex

Portalier, Serge (1990) 'L'instrumentation visuelle. Naître de parents aveugles,' *Le Journal des Psychologues* 84, 30–3

Ratner, Nancy, and Jerome Bruner (1977) 'Games, Social Exchange and the Acquisition of Language.' *Journal of Child Language* 5, 391–401

Stern, Daniel (1985) *The Interpersonal World of the Infant.* New York: Basic Books

Trevarthen, C. (1993) 'The Function of Emotions in Early Infant Communication and Development.' In Nadel and Camaioni, eds (1993)

Trevarthen, C., and P. Hubley (1978) 'Secondary Intersubjectivity.' In *Action, Gesture and Symbol: The Emergence of Language,* ed A. Lock. London: Academic Press

Vygotsky, L.S. (1962) *Thought and Language,* Cambridge, MA: M.I.T. Press

5

Neurobiological Development and Cognition in the Deafblind

DOUGLAS L. GEENENS, DO

I think of you as a profound thinker who because of your handicap has seen some aspects of life more clearly and truly
Karl Menninger, MD, to Helen Keller, 10 April 1951

Introduction

Cognition is a term that refers to thought or thinking. Broadly defined, it reflects the operations of the brain enabling the individual to process the stimuli that impinge on him and program his behaviour to enhance his survival and well-being. Although cognitive development is relatively well understood in the general population, its application to the disabled is not. In a deafblind cohort, the process of cognitive development is typically skewed by the severe limitations in achieving language. This obstacle is the primary limiting variable in the cognitive development of deafblind individuals. The lack of adequate distance senses greatly reduces the input to the brain. At a minimum, this will modify cognition, since information supplied through the remaining channels will be utilized differently and more intensively. The resulting altered behaviour will be perceived by others as deviant and will colour their interaction with the deafblind person, which will have an impact on his or her social and emotional development. Cognition also conjures many associations such as *IQ*, ability to learn, education, productivity, and so on. Thus, the typical questions raised around cognitive development in deafblind children are both common and difficult to answer. The two most relevant questions are: What is their potential? How do we measure it? In this chapter I set out to answer these two fundamental questions.

The ability to assess cognitive skills in a deafblind population is at best limited, if not impossible, because so many of these children have developed without the ability to use effective language, which has thereby limited their exposure to information. Indeed, facility with language is one of the best indices of intelligence (Lenneberg 1967) and thus cognitive development. There are numerous, more recent theories that argue that language is but one measure and that other parameters of 'intelligence' can be measured, for example, Test of Raven's Progressive Matrices and Gardner's theory of multiple intelligences; none the less, the ability to obtain information is the most relevant issue, and language is the primary avenue.

Current instruments used to assess cognitive functioning of deafblind individuals are a measure simply of their developmental progress without effective language, rather than of their innate abilities. Thus the usefulness of these instruments is limited to developmental achievement, not as a measure of potential. False assumptions based on preconceived notions about cognitive ability and strengths lead inevitably to low expectations.

There is a marked lack of research in the area of cognitive development in deafblind persons because of the low frequency of deafblindness, the widely and falsely held belief that these individuals are mentally retarded, and lack of funding. The misallocation of resources for deafblind children to schools for the deaf or blind limits their exposure to effective language development, since these are not simply deaf children who are blind, or blind children who are deaf. The need for specialized services for this unique population, assuring access to effective language, is the cornerstone for cognitive and conceptual development for the deafblind.

The Development of Intelligence

Intelligence is an abstract concept that is generally measured by the volume of information we know. Specific abilities, such as the abilities to reason, learn, solve problems, and manipulate symbols are characteristic of intelligence. Intelligence is a rich and multidimensional concept that defies easy definition; common to all definitions, however, is the idea that intelligence is positively related to success in the world (Wedding and Cody 1995). In other words, intelligence enhances the effectiveness of adaptation to the environment, and intelligent people are likely to maximize the outcomes of their interactions with the world. A person is identified as intelligent by formal or informal observation of that person's behaviour across a sample of situations. Most often the behavioural sample takes the form of standardized testing or the assessment of specific abilities with clearly defined procedures and tasks. Intelligence, however, is always an inference; it is not intelligence but rather intelligent behaviour that is observed.

Some aspects of intelligence can be quantified in the form of an intelligence quotient (IQ) score. As it is used today, an IQ score is an expression of how well a person performed on a standardized intelligence test in comparison with others of the same age group. Equally important, however, is the evaluation of *adaptive intelligence*, or the extent to which measured intelligence has been effectively used in the pursuit of everyday goals. An essential part of adaptive intelligence consists of non-*intellective* factors such as motivation, perseverance, and determination. Both of these components, IQ and adaptive effectiveness, must be evaluated if intelligence is to be assessed adequately. Assessment requires that test results always be interpreted in the context of a person's current situation and circumstances. IQ scores are influenced by educational opportunities, socio-economic status, and cultural background. Professionals are likely to label individuals wrongly if they are not sensitive to these issues and confuse testing with the broader and more useful practice of assessment.

There are multiple variables that may effect IQ, including age and genetics. The impact of age on IQ is a relevant issue because prior to the age of eight IQ is considered unstable, owing to the incomplete development of language (Wedding and Cody 1995). IQ also increases up to ages sixteen to eighteen, and at any given age a large sample of normal children attain scores that are distributed in conformity with a Gaussian curve (see figure 5.1). For deafblind individuals, incomplete language development is virtually universal and may span their lifetime.

There is little question that heredity affects intelligence. The studies of *monozygotic* and *dizygotic* twins raised in the same or in different families have put this matter in a clearer light. Such studies have shown that identical twins reared together or apart are more alike in intelligence than non-identical twins brought up in the same household. There can be no doubt, therefore, that genetic endowment is a most important variable in estimating one's intellectual capacity. Piercy (1967) has estimated the ratio of hereditary and environmental components of intelligence to be from 6:4 to 8:2. There is also convincing evidence that early learning may greatly modify the level of ability that is finally obtained. In the absence of systematic assessment, the best estimate of a child's IQ is the regressed average of the parents' IQs (Wedding and Cody 1995).

The most common and destructive myth about deafblind individuals is that they are mentally retarded. This is fostered by their lack of language development and their stereotyped behaviours, which often mimic those of mentally retarded or autistic individuals. The diagnosis of mental retardation requires that three essential criteria be met:

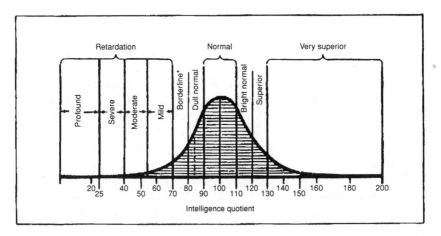

Figure 5.1   The Distribution of IQ Scores in the General Population

1. IQ score < 70
2. deficits in adaptive behaviour
3. onset before age eighteen.

This formal definition excludes individuals with cognitive impairment resulting from head trauma or brain injury (American Psychiatric Association 1994). The idea of mental retardation as it pertains to most deafblind individuals is acquired, not inherited. That is, most deafblind children are not exposed sufficiently to the necessary elements for language or communication with the outside world because of their significant sensory disabilities. If this is the foundation from which a person is built, he/she has little chance of becoming 'intelligent.'

Current Theories in Cognitive Development

A broad review of cognitive theory is beyond the scope and purpose of this chapter. A basic review of Piaget's cognitive theory as it applies to the deaf-blind allows for an illustration of the developmental hurdles these individuals face. It should be noted that Piaget's theories of cognitive development have undergone much criticism over the past twenty years, and when he did venture an opinion about the cognitive development of the blind, it turned out to be, for the most part, wrong. (He also felt that Helen Keller was the 'exception to the rule.') Despite the above noted criticism, Piaget's theories offer some funda-mental processes that are readily accepted. A primary component of his theories is that each stage has a distinct pattern of organization and must be completed before moving on to the next.

Piaget described the first two years of life as constituting the sensorimotor period of development. At the start of this period, the infant comes into the world with certain sensory capabilities and a repertoire of reflex responses to inner and outer stimuli. Experiences of the infant during the sensorimotor phase consist of direct, physical interactions with the environment. The interplay of these innate, internally driven experiences with the outer, externally driven ones creates a dynamic stage in which the infant can effect his/her environment and vice versa. Initially, these experiences are with their own body and then are externalized. With the development of locomotion, as long as audition and vision are intact, infants begin to predict and anticipate their effects on their environment. Although Piaget focuses on cognitive development, the process that he describes also has implications for social and emotional development. For deafblind infants, one cannot underestimate the obstacles present, not only in successfully completing this stage of development, but even in participating in it.

The next developmental stage is what Piaget calls pre-operational thinking and ranges from ages two to six. It is characterized by the understanding of associations of events, but only from one's own perspective. Although an egocentric method of understanding, it provides individuals with unique information about themselves and may be a time when they begin to formulate their own identity within their environment. With deafblind children, it is very difficult to differentiate self from environment because the visual and auditory cues are obscured or absent. The sense of utter dependency on an environment poorly understood creates an atmosphere of apprehension and uncertainty, contributing to developmental stagnation. Utilizing compensatory sensory input in a supportive, safe environment can, in part, positively alter this stage of development.

Concrete operational thinking ranges from ages six to eleven. This stage is characterized by reasoning through imagined events. Children can think through 'what if' problems. Many deafblind children do not reach this stage of development because of conceptual delays. Cognition can be adequate, but contextual understanding with the ability to anticipate consequences is an advanced level of development for deafblind individuals.

Formal operations is the final cognitive development stage and is characterized by the ability to think abstractly.

Piaget provided an extensive line of evidence suggesting that infants who have yet to acquire language set out to solve problems by manipulating objects and following them visually. Achieving the concept of object permanence, that is, the realization that objects do not vanish into nothingness when they are out of sight but must be 'someplace' and therefore that search for them will be fruitful, takes place during the first year of life. (The difficulty encountered by blind children in achieving object permanence is due to the absence of vision.) These achievements are the fruit of problem solving and of thinking of a relatively high order, yet of non-verbal thinking. Piaget further proposed that only gradually do verbal symbols supplant visual images and real objects as the data on which the mind operates. Even at the stage of concrete operations, reached by most children by the age they start school, thinking is still largely non-verbal. But as the child learns to operate on verbal symbols that have no physical referents, that is, reaches the stage of logical operations, language becomes more inextricably linked with thinking.

The largest body of research on cognitive development that is somewhat applicable to deafblind children is the cognitive development of deaf children. Observations of deaf infants and toddlers suggest that development proceeds normally through the sensorimotor stage, except in the area of vocal imitation (Best and Roberts 1976). This would be the first glaring difference between the cognitive development of deaf children and deafblind children. The ability to compensate for hearing loss with vision allows the deaf child to participate in and complete the sensorimotor stage with limited insult. Deafblind children have inadequate compensatory mechanisms and thus are significantly impaired in their ability to participate and complete this stage of development.

Studies concerning the preoperational years (ages two to six) of deaf children are relatively scarce, but the research suggests that nonlinguistic differences begin to appear towards the end of this stage (Furth 1964; Youniss and Furth 1965). This suggests that even a single sensory handicap may have detrimental effects on cognitive development beyond that of communication.

Studies that deal with the concrete operational stage show significant developmental delays, ranging from two to eight years. Properties of concrete operational thinking may not be achieved until late adolescence. Thus, the developmental lags present early in life tend to increase and broaden, compared with norms.

Luria (1976) postulates that problem solving of whatever type (perceptual, constructive, arithmetic, psycholinguistic, or logical) proceeds in four steps.

1. The specification of a problem and the conditions in which it has arisen
2. A plan of action or strategy for the solution of the problem is formulated, which requires that certain linguistic activities be simultaneously initiated in orderly sequence
3. The execution, including implementation and control of the plan
4. Checking or comparison of the results against the original plan to see if it was adequate.

These postulated mechanisms apply more directly to conceptual development, a broader, more complex mode of understanding rarely achieved by deafblind individuals. The concept of understanding is, in fact, unidimensional and can be as simple as knowing a definition. This level of cognitive development can be reached readily by deafblind children and adults. The more advanced level of cognitive development, 'realization' is multidimensional and encompasses not only understanding, but experience and emotion. It is this level of sophistication that is so difficult to accomplish for those working with deafblind individuals, because of the barriers that exist.

Neurobiological Correlates to Cognitive Development

To understand the phenomenon of intellectual and cognitive development, it is helpful to have some idea of how cognition is normally organized and sustained by the brain. As stated previously, hearing and sight are the dominant distance receptors supplying humans with data about their environment. Sight is the main spatial receptor enabling simultaneous processing of many stimuli; complex visual patterns can be apprehended in *milliseconds*. Sight is continuous, but it can be turned off at will by closing the eyes or averting the gaze. Active visual scanning seeks out information and integrates the disparate inputs from the other senses. Sight is the principal medium used to construct knowledge of the environment and differentiate oneself from it. It directs behaviour by providing feedback about the consequences of acts on the environment and, in particular, on others, for example, empathy.

Audition requires time. Complex sounds, such as words, require tens or hundreds of milliseconds in order to gain meaning. Hearing cannot be turned off, even during sleep, but is discontinuous, since the listener has little or no control over the production of sound by persons and objects in his environment. Hearing does not require active scanning, although its resolution can be enhanced by selective attention to one set of acoustic signals over others occurring simultaneously. Hearing is the main channel for processing oral language, a human's most sophisticated vehicle for interpersonal communication, for conveying complex information about events remote in time or space, and for many aspects of thinking.

The process of thought is primarily a function of the cortex, the outer part of the brain. In lower species, for instance, primates, the cortex is much less developed, diminishing the ability to learn or apply knowledge. A human being has an extremely well developed cortex (esp. frontal lobes), which allows for typical cognitive development. Most of the information we have on the functions of the frontal lobes has been gathered from study of people who have suffered head injury or other neurological insult that has compromised their frontal

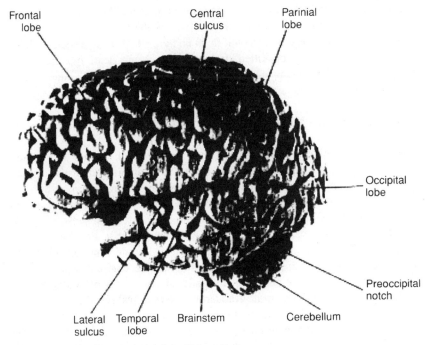

Figure 5.2   The Major Lobes of the Human Brain

lobes, that is, strokes and *dementias*. Persons who have experienced cortical disease, especially involving the frontal lobes, have decreased ability to learn, decreased abstraction ability, conceptual difficulties, and other undesirable personality traits such as irritability and behavioural *disinhibition*.

The primary function of the brain is to allow the organism to interact with the environment. To this end, human neurological systems have evolved multiple sensory systems geared towards providing us with information about our environment. There are proximal senses (touch, smell, taste), which allow us to analyse information that is close at hand. There are distance senses (sight, sound) which allow us to analyse information that is further away. The distance senses allow the organism to predict and anticipate consequences.

There are other brain regions that may effect our cognitive strengths and abilities. The left cerebral cortex typically is involved in analytical functions such as language. The right cerebral cortex is typically involved in visual-spatial concepts and creativity. The parietal lobes may also be involved in conceptual orientation. Thus, cognition is a diffuse process involving multiple parts of the brain and many brain functions.

If one accepts evolutionary theory in the development of human beings, natural selection of sight and sound have evolved as the primary discriminatory senses that are necessary for survival. In an uncivilized, primitive society, deafblind individuals would be killed. Individuals who are deafblind are at the mercy of their environment for safety, and without access to language, remain victims of a society who neglects their needs.

Sensory Deprivation and Brain Development

There is a body of scientific research that involves both animal and human responses to sensory deprivation. The single most significant distinguishing feature of all nervous tissue is that it is designed to change in response to external stimulation. It is this capacity that allows the brain to be responsive to the environment. All experience is filtered through senses. All sensory signals initiate a cascade of cellular and molecular processes that alter neurochemistry, *cytoarchitecture*, and ultimately brain structure and function. This process of creating some internal representation of the external world (information) depends upon the pattern of intensity and frequency of neural activity produced by 'sensing.' The more frequently a certain pattern of neural activation occurs, the more indelible is the internal representation. Experience thus creates a processing template through which all new input is filtered (Perry et al. 1995). The more often a neural network is activated, the more there will be use-dependent internalization of new information needed to promote survival (Cragg 1975).

In the developing brain, undifferentiated neural systems are critically dependent upon sets of environmental cues to organize appropriately. The brain develops in a sequential and hierarchical fashion, from primitive to complex. Each area develops and organizes, and becomes fully functional at different times during childhood. During such 'critical periods' the areas are sensitive to organizing experiences. Disruptions in these experience-dependent *neurochemical* signals during a critical period may lead to abnormalities that are irreversible (Perry et al. 1995).

The simple and unavoidable result of this sequential neurodevelopment is that the organizing, sensitive brain of an infant or a young child is more malleable to experience than a mature brain (plasticity). While experience may alter the behaviour of an adult, experience literally provides the organizing framework for an infant or child. Because the brain is most plastic in early childhood, the child is most vulnerable to variance of experience during this time.

Deprivation of critical experiences during development may be the most destructive force, not allowing for maximal growth to occur. Ironically, while rarely studied in humans, the neurodevelopmental impact of extremes of sensory deprivation is the subject of hundreds of animal studies. A review of animal research reveals three global and reproducible phenomena in response to sensory deprivation:

1. alternative sensory adaptation
2. anatomic and physiologic changes
3. a narrow window-critical period during which specific experience is required for optimal organization and development of the part of the brain mediating a specific function.

Primary sensory modalities (sight, sound, smell, touch) have been those most extensively. For example, *somatosensory* deprivation was performed on newborn and adult rats, and then their ability to function through a rectangular maze was measured approximately eighty days later. Newborn rats consistently performed better than the adult rats, suggesting that early sensory deprivation induced compensatory changes in other sensory systems (Volgyi, et al. 1993). Visual deprivation or blinding in infancy results in anterograde transneuronal degeneration in the lateral geniculate body and occipital cortex. Geniculate neurons are smaller; occipital neurons have shorter, deformed apical dendrites and are less densely packed. Uniocular deprivation alters the columnar organization of the occipital cortex; columns receiving their input from the deprived eye shrink, while those receiving signals from the normal eye expand (Wiesel, et al.).

In another study, newborn rats were monocularly enucleated (blinded in one eye), and the contralateral changes in the visual cortex were studied. Early monocular enucleation exerted a significant compensatory change in the contralateral visual cortex (Toldi et al. 1994).

The anatomical and physiological changes induced by sensory deprivation have been well documented. Male rats were placed in complete darkness from birth to thirty days, followed by either death or a thirty-five day rehabilitation under controlled lighting conditions. Rats raised in complete darkness showed morphological changes in the optic nerve (Fukui et al. 1991).

Four infant monkeys were binocularly deprived of vision (both eyes) through their first year of life. They were permitted visually guided behaviour in their second year of life. Upon examination of the brain, early visual deprivation permanently reduced the number of visually responsive cell groups in the parietal association cortex (Carlson 1990).

To examine the impact of dark rearing on the time course of development, cats were monocularly deprived at various postnatal stages. For cats that were reared normally for the first six to nine weeks of life, then placed in darkness until five months of age, the time course for the 'critical period' was slowed significantly. Neural plasticity (the ability of the brain to change) also was studied. 'Normal cats' were more plastic at younger ages, and dark-reared cats were more plastic at older ages. This study suggests that visual input accelerates neural growth and plasticity, while total darkness decelerates it (Mower 1991).

Information about the anatomic changes in the nervous system of humans that arise as a consequence of early loss of vision is, of course, much more sparse than it is for other animals. One clear example is the permanent impairment of visual acuity in the strabismic eye of children with an uncorrected squint. Input from the non-fixating eye is thought to be suppressed, thus avoiding diplopia (double vision). It is assumed that this effect reflects *maldevelopment* of the visual cortex, since kittens with experimental strabismus have a decreased number of occipital neurons that respond to binocular stimulation, whereas the complement of monocularly driven cells is normal (Wiesel and Hubel 1974). Patients with astigmatism for whom corrective lenses were prescribed after six years of age had permanent loss of visual acuity limited to the affected meridian, a situation that did not develop in a child prescribed glasses by age three, suggesting the importance of early identification and intervention in changing what could be permanent neurological damage.

Psychological Testing and Deafblindness

Assessment tools utilized in the evaluation of deafblind children encompass a variety of developmental scales for the severely handicapped. Although validation has, in part, involved deafblind individuals, these instruments typically measure outcome or developmental progress, not innate potential, intelligence, or cognitive ability. Many authors increasingly question the validity of psychologic test results as a means for measuring children's cognitive competence and for making predictions about competence at maturity (Goslin 1968). We know little about the organization of the brain in the deafblind individual; thus, tests that give a rounded and representative view of the spectrum of their cognitive skills still need to be designed. A major consequence of these serious sensory handicaps is a profoundly different life experience and drastic informational impoverishment.

It may be helpful to review psychological testing results of deaf individuals and blind individuals separately. Vernon (1967) reviewed thirty-one studies in which a variety of non-verbal test instruments and been used with over 8,000 deaf children. Since deaf children performed as well as normal children despite their minimal verbal skills, he concluded that the deaf have no intellectual impairment. Furth (1966, 1973) performed a series of experiments designed to tap the problem-solving skills of the deaf. The deaf did just as well as the hearing in many of the tasks, but they did lag behind suburban middle-class students, although they were not behind hearing students from a rural background. He concluded that both groups, the deaf and rural students, suffered from experiential deprivation.

A number of other writers have reviewed results of psychological testing in deaf and hearing-impaired children, stressing the poor correlation between academic achievement and scores on non-verbal tests of intelligence. These findings in the deaf raise a central question of epistemology: the relation between language and thought. The competence of the deaf for non-verbal test items confirms that some aspects of cognition do not require language as a mediating symbol system. In fact, impaired verbal processes may serve as a vehicle for other types of thinking.

Very few investigators have tested verbal items in deaf populations. Kates, Kates, and Michael (1962) had deaf and hearing students sort a series of objects and words into classes of their own choosing and asked them to verbalize about the relationship between paired words. They found that deaf students were delayed in verbalization but not in categorization. The deaf had difficulty attaching new words to old categories and therefore ended up with more categories than the hearing.

O'Connor and Hermelin (1976) reasoned that if deaf students store verbal material visually, items should be equally accessible for read-out from any direction; therefore, the deaf should repeat items backward with fewer errors than those who store them acoustically, that is serially. In an experiment testing the recall of strings of six letters presented visually one by one, they did find that the deaf's backward recall was somewhat better than that of the hearing, but they concluded that the deaf tagged items for both spatial position and temporal order. Therefore, it appeared too simple that a straightforward visual storage model could account for the superior performance of the deaf.

The bulk of the material just reviewed leads to the somewhat perplexing conclusion that, provided one does not tap areas where the deaf are known to be incompetent, they will not be found incompetent. According to Furth, any deficit in an area where the deaf should by rights be incompetent can be ascribed to a developmental delay rather than to a cognitive deficit, or to experiential deprivation that will be made up, at least partially, with time.

The question one can ask is: Competent or incompetent for what? In the routine situations of daily life and in familiar social situations, the deaf are competent. But are they competent to deal with the intricacies of complex social relations, with abstract verbal problems, or with the red tape required by many of society's institutions? The answer is no.

The assumption that tests ostensibly not dependent on learning information and not requiring verbal instruction or a verbal solution are necessarily solved non-verbally may not always be warranted. For instance, the norms for the deaf on the Hiskey-Nebraska Test of Learning Aptitude are two years behind those of norms. Is this because they know less, or have they adopted alternative strategies of learning?

Many of the issues that arose concerning psychological testing of the deaf pertain to the blind as well. What is the purpose of testing the blind? Comparing them with norms seems irrelevant, since their life experience is so totally different. There is little to suggest that standard psychological tests have the power to forecast a blind person's ability to get along in the world of the sighted, where high mobility and drive for independence may be more relevant than verbal IQ. Even short-term prediction may be invalid, since the blind lag behind the sighted in many areas, starting from infantile skills, such as midline hand play, reaching for objects, sound localization, crawling, and independent walking, and going on to more conventional skills, such as maze learning, concept formation including that of conservation, verbal reasoning, and social maturity. Gillman, Gillman, and Goddard (1974) argue that overlooking maturational lags, especially those affecting social development in the preschool years, and deficiencies detected later with psychologic testing may be unwise. One would not want to foreclose opportunity for a blind or deafblind child because of a false diagnosis of mental retardation. One might assume that testing using the verbal scales is valid in blind individuals because their language development can be normal, if not precocious. One cannot assume, however, that the words used by a blind child, even if appropriate, have the same connotation and reference for him as for the seeing. Quite the contrary, many of his words will have smaller semantic fields that only partially overlap those of the sighted. On verbal tests, blind children often score better than norms on tasks that require verbal memory, since the blind must remember if they are to function adequately. They also do well on vocabulary, but tend to encounter difficulty with conceptual information, mostly because of their impoverished sensory experience. In comparisons of congenitally blind with adventitiously blind adults, the congenitally blind typically score lower, although within the normal range. This is thought to represent some compromise in concept formation.

Hayes (1962) stresses that test results at the time of entrance into school may be deceptive, perhaps because of the widely divergent experiences of blind children at home, some having been grossly overprotected and given few opportunities for incidental learning and for expanding their horizons. He gives several examples of children whose scores rose by 50 or more IQ points between elementary school and high school; another example of the recurrent theme stressing the information deprivation suffered by the blind.

One of the crucial variables that will determine how well a blind person will function is his or her spatial sense. Orientation is the prelude to independent mobility, which will mean so much to the blind child or adult. Orientation in the absence of vision depends on a well-developed body scheme, on a good sense of timing, and on noticing sound echoes and localizing them with reference to oneself. To be mobile, the blind person must be bold and constantly alert and attentive and be able to call on his memories of the environment in which he finds himself. A good sense of timing facilitates independent ambulation, yet it may be deficient in those blind since early life. Spigelman (1976) made the observation that in both rat and man, early blinded individuals and blindfolded norms localize sound less accurately in space than do late blinded persons. This finding suggests that even a brief period with functional sight, during which the infant can develop visually guided manual behaviour and a sense of space, may play a decisive role for later development. This is another reason to treat age at blinding as a relevant variable when test results for the blind are evaluated. A major drawback of psychological testing limited to the verbal dimension is that the correlation between verbal skills and spatial skills is not necessarily high.

A number of non-verbal batteries have been developed for the blind, but most have not been extensively standardized. Miller (1977) tested sixty congenitally legally blind adult males with the Haptic Intelligence Scale for Adult Blind, the Wechsler Adult Intelligence Scale (WAIS), and several other tests designed to sample concept formation, body scheme, and personality traits. The factor that explained the largest portion of the variance was a non-verbal ability factor. It included subtests of non-verbal, perceptual, and organizational characteristics, such as speed and accuracy of performance, and judgment. It is not surprising that level of useful vision had a strong loading on the factor.

Millar (1975) compared normal and congenitally blind children on a test of memory for positions traced along a maze hidden by a curtain. She found that seeing and blind children used different strategies for recall; the blind relied on haptic (somatosensory) memory, which decays with time and is interfered with by subsequent movements, rather than on verbal coding and rehearsal; the sighted used visual representations that did not penalize backward recall. They visualized the entire path they had followed quasi-simultaneously, whereas the blind relied on sequential memory of touch and movement.

Information concerning test results for the blind would be markedly enhanced if two variables were better controlled: age at onset of blindness and severity of visual loss. Even brief visual experience may affect test performance, even though children blinded before age five years retain essentially no visual imagery (Lowenfeld 1975). For instance, Warren (1977) describes several studies showing that children blinded as a result of retinoblastoma performed better than children with congenital blindness. Others indicate that, among the legally blind, those with usable vision performed differently, although not necessarily better, than the totally blind. In the absence of validated research regarding the use of psychological testing in a deafblind cohort, one most extrapolate for deaf or blind populations from the information available. In review of the previous paragraphs, there are several identifiable and generalizable findings.

Deaf or blind individuals appear to compensate for their sensory disabilities with the other distance sense. This process leads to a different style of learning that may not be identifiable on standard psychological tests. For deafblind individuals, compensation is significantly limited, therefore invalidating the idea that conclusions drawn from a deaf or blind cohort can be utilized in the assessment of a deafblind individual. One cannot assume that the disability of deafblindness is simply a summation of strengths and weaknesses of the deaf or blind.

Current Assessment Tools for the Deafblind

There are no valid instruments for the cognitive assessment of deafblind individuals. The extent to which existing instruments assess cognitive development is limited to developmental achievement at the time the instrument is administered. There are several instruments used in the developmental assessment of deafblind individuals. The Callier-Azusa Scale and the Functional Skills Screening Inventory (FSSI) are two commonly used instruments.

The Callier-Azusa Scale is an instrument designed for the assessment of developmental level of deafblind, multihandicapped students. There are multiple subscales with an ordinal sequence of developmental steps provided. Specific scales include motor development, perceptual development, daily living skills, language, and socialization. This instrument has, in part, been studied in deafblind populations. It has some psychometric validity and reliability. Its usefulness is limited to the developmental level subjects have achieved. It does not assess cognitive potential or intelligence in deafblind or severely handicapped individuals. Inter-rater reliability suggests that this instrument can be used by observers who have not completed college, observers with less than two years of experience with the deafblind, and observers who have had no prior experience with the Callier-Azusa Scale itself (Day and Stillman 1975).

The Functional Skills Screening Inventory (FSSI) is a domain-referenced behavioural checklist designed to be used in natural settings to assess critical living and working skills in persons with moderate to severe handicapping conditions. It can be used to assess current level of functioning, identify placement needs and options, identify and prioritize training needs and goals, document progression in training, and facilitate transition to adult living. It can be used with individuals aged six years through adulthood. There are 343 items that are either a functional skill that contributes to an individual's ability to live and work independently or a problem behaviour that hinders this accomplishment. The items are divided into eight content areas and twenty-seven subscales, including basic skills and concepts, communication, personal care, homemaking, work skills and concepts, community, and social awareness. This instrument can be used by professionals, paraprofessionals, and family members. It is limited to developmental level achieved and does not assess cognitive potential or intelligence of the deafblind.

Patterns of Cognitive Development in the Deafblind

Cognitive development in deafblind individuals is dependent on multiple variables, including the severity of the sensory disability, age of onset of the sensory disability, and the environmental input.

The deafblind disability is a spectrum disability that encompasses varying degrees of visual and auditory compromise. Generally speaking, the more severe the compromise, the more slowly cognitive development occurs. As stated previously, the primary goal in achieving growth in the cognitive domain is the development of language, which allows the deafblind individuals to interact with their environment. Auditory and visual pathways are the evolutionary means to accomplish this. Compensatory mechanisms can be utilized and maximized, except in the most severe cases. Individuals who are totally blind and profoundly deaf have the greatest hurdle to overcome in cognitive development.

Age of onset of deafblindness is also a significant variable to consider in cognitive development. It is generally accepted that it is better to have had access to information at any point in life than to have had it obscured from the beginning. Distortion of information is a significant problem for people who have not had an opportunity to experience their environment with their total sensory capacity. For those with adventitious deafblindness, cognitive development can occur along a normal spectrum until the specific event occurs. Hindrance to further cognitive growth lies along the social/emotional spectrum and involves dealing with loss and the individual's ability to develop alternative means for communication (Braille and sign).

Cognitive development in the deafblind differs from that in norms in that the typical pattern of methodical, systematic, and predictable development does not occur. The most obvious observation about developmental patterns in the deafblind is that it occurs in 'spurts and plateaus.' Although the reasons are unknown, this inconsistent pattern is probably related to the effort it takes to obtain information. This effort is so great that these individuals cannot sustain their efforts over time. Thus, it is typical to observe periods of rapid information processing, followed by periods of latency, where individuals may further process the acquired information or seek respite in silence and solitude.

Abstract concepts are often totally missed because the context in which events happen is unfamiliar or foreign, not only because of limited life experience, but because delays in the acquisition of abstract thinking are typical and expected. As is the case in the Piagetian model, concrete thinking precedes abstract thinking. In fact, the ability to abstract and formulate conceptions, anticipate, and so on, may not be reached, depending on the severity of the sensory disability, the general cognitive ability of the individual, and the interventions utilized.

Another area of cognitive difference between deafblind individuals and norms is processing time. The barriers that interfere with information acquisition necessitate longer periods of time to incorporate and process information for understanding. This variable in itself contributes to the tortuous course of cognitive development as well as the limited understanding.

The natural course of cognitive development in deafblind individuals is the process of integrating fragments of concrete and conceptual information. Without a means for this integrating phenomenon (e.g., an Intervenor), there is limited likelihood of meaningful cognitive development.

The longer people can make use of distance senses, the better adapted to a life without them they can become. Orientation to the external environment with some memory or knowledge facilitates ongoing cognitive growth.

The environmental variable is a most powerful one that society can control. A stimulating environment can provide an atmosphere of growth and enhancement. Conversely, an environment of limited or no stimulation creates an atmosphere of regression and stagnation. The spectrum illness of deafblindness presents itself for environmental intervention, since these individuals are in need of a 'pathway' through which they may interact with their environment. An Intervenor is the method of choice to create this pathway.

The Role of the Intervenor

The Intervenor is more than an interpreter, a translator of language (see chapter 3). An Intervenor conveys information from the environment, not only in the sense of language, but in context. This contextual translation is what makes cognitive development in the deafblind different. The Intervenor formulates incoming information and presents it in a way that is meaningful to the deafblind person. Understanding that their life experience is qualitatively and quantitatively different, an Intervenor tries to incorporate societal norms and experience with the literal interpretation of the language. This process aids not only the cognitive development but the conceptual development as well.

The extensive and dynamic interplay between cognitive development and emotional development plays itself out with the Intervenor. This relationship, whether with a parent, friend, stranger, provides fertile ground for the development of trust, companionship, familiarity, and security.

In infancy intervention is much like typical parenting, where intuition and meeting the child's needs are what drives the interaction.

At early stages of cognitive development (toddlerhood) intervention consists of pairing behavioural and tactile responses with signing. Consistency of response is very important, so that toddlers can begin to anticipate that their actions will be met with predictable responses. As they begin to feel comfortable, an increase in curiosity and seeking will be observed as they attempt to master their environment.

One of the interesting observations made by this author is that despite significant developmental delays, these children often struggle with the same conflicts that age-appropriate norms do, for example, adolescents with peer acceptance. Thus, the Intervenor must be vigilant to the concerns of the child or adolescent and help them cope with the issues at hand.

Throughout the developmental process, defining is an important aspect of further cognitive development. Ideally, conceptual understanding will follow as the deafblind child may ask questions. If the inquisitive characteristics are not seen despite some level of understanding, the Intervenor may need to be more assertive in delivering information. Clearly, the relationship with the Intervenor is exceedingly important to the cognitive and emotional development of the deafblind individual.

Proposed Course of Action

The current method of assessment and intervention in deafblindness must undergo dramatic change if deafblind individuals are to maximize their capabilities. The focus of change should be balanced across many fronts, including education, funding/politics, assessment/research, family, and the Intervenor model itself.

Educational intervention should take the form of Intervenors in the classroom. There will likely be much resistance on the part of educational systems because of the expense. The deafblind child needs the constant feedback provided, so that the educational experience is comprehensive and well rounded. Children are sent to school for two major purposes: learning and socialization. Socialization is a component of education that is poorly addressed even in mainstreamed settings. Intervenors help to put the educational material in a social context that facilitates growth.

One must also wonder if traditional educational programs can address the needs of the deafblind (see chapter 2). Curriculums generally are based on critical, basic concepts that the child who is deafblind may not have had the opportunity to experience because of the unique skills and time required for him to acquire them. Therefore, specialized curriculums would be appropriate for this population. Typical classroom education with a single lecturer seems somewhat reductionist when one looks at the overall needs of the deafblind individual. It would seem that a vocational/apprenticeship model combined with a heavy emphasis on language and communication (Braille and sign language) would be the most beneficial. A commonly overlooked detail is that in order to read Braille, one must be able to use language (e.g., English). If deafblind children and adults cannot read Braille, their access to information is severely limited and is dependent on input from others. Braille literacy allows for continuous access to information within the individual's discretion, and helps them to avoid hours and hours of 'nothingness.'

The Intervenor model must be embraced by agencies at the local and state level as the most effective treatment strategy. Funding that is now typically funnelled through schools for the deaf or for the blind is often misappropriated for less effective interventions.

Utilization of the Intervenor model must start with the family. Upon early identification of a deafblind child, intervention should begin immediately. The fundamental rule in working with deafblind children is: If you don't put the language in, it can't come out. A trained Intervenor should meet regularly with the parents to educate them as to the needs of their deafblind child. Assessments of the sensory deficits, for instance, audiograms, should occur. Sensory aids such as cochlear implants and hearing aids or glasses should be initiated. Speech and language should also begin in infancy, through the Intervenor's always talking and always signing. Utilization of tactile proprioception, such as touching the voice box, teaching children to read lips, and pairing a sign with an object, will greatly enhance language development at an early age. In children who are blind, motivating the child to use vision, for example, light boxes or coloured lights, can facilitate use of residual vision. Early cane use, such as learning to use a push toy, combined with orientation and mobility training will help the child conquer the fear of moving about. Emphasis on adequate stimulation of all of the infant's senses, pairing behavioural and tactile responses with signs, and so on should begin early. Creating an atmosphere of hope and encouragement will help to fight the disillusionment and hopelessness that often afflict parents. Teaching parents as Intervenors, at least for children of younger ages, will dramatically reduce the cost.

New instruments must be developed to assess more accurately the cognitive development and potential of the deafblind. Variables that are often not considered in the assessment phase include age of onset, severity, and environmental intervention. A greater understanding about brain development and the impact of sensory deprivation on the human brain may fuel new and innovative interventions. An open mind about alternative cognitive mechanisms and strengths may stimulate new research that maximizes the deafblind individual's strengths and does not exploit their weaknesses.

Finally, the most effective strategy in cognitive development for the deafblind is the Intervenor model. It serves the needs of the deafblind individual and facilitates growth across multiple domains, including cognitive, social, and emotional development.

Case Studies

The purpose of this section is to share with the reader typical stories of individuals who are deafblind. The intent of the author is to stimulate an atmosphere of hope and understanding as we observe how the influence of intervention can change the lives of deafblind persons.

Case Study 1

Baby A was born to a sixteen-year-old mother at thirty weeks' gestation with a birth weight of 2 lbs, 14 oz. APGAR scores (an early measure of vital functioning in a newborn's life) were 5 and 8, at one and five minutes, respectively. Owing to prematurity, the infant's lungs were poorly developed (this is known as hyaline membrane disease and often results in respiratory distress syndrome), and she was placed on oxygen to assure viability. The utilization of oxygen in prematurity, especially in large amounts, may result in retrolental fibroplasia, now called retinitis of prematurity. This condition often leads to blindness. With prematurity many other complications frequently follow. This child's medical problems included sepsis (infection in the blood), intracranial hemorrhage (bleeding in the brain), hyperbilirubinemia (liver metabolic problems), hypocalcemia (low calcium level), seizures, thrombocytopenia (low platelet count), patent ductus arteriosis (an abnormal opening in the heart), osteomyelitis (bone infection), gastrointestinal bleeding, and cardiac arrest.

These complications were treated aggressively during the first two months of Baby A's life with a variety of medical and surgical interventions. As a result of high doses of antibiotics, known to be ototoxic, the infant also became deaf.

As is the case with most deafblind children, her sensory deficits were not discovered until later. She was placed in foster care for several months and subsequently adopted at five months of age (the family was advised not to adopt, owing to this child's developmental status). Now known to be deaf, she was severely developmentally delayed and showed hypotonia (poor muscle tone), clumsiness, failure to thrive, and tactile defensiveness. The parents intuitively helped the infant to overcome her tactile defensiveness by keeping her naked much of the time and allowing her to rest skin to skin on the chest of the father. She also received her first hearing aid at 6.5 months of age.

By the age of one year, this child was being called mentally retarded by professionals. Because of her identified disabilities, she began to receive auditory training, speech and language therapy, and sign language training in the first year of life. (They did not yet know she was blind, but the parents suspected something else was wrong.) She showed little organized movement or programmed locomotion.

As Baby A progressed through toddlerhood, it was noted that she often fell and limited her activity in darkness. At age seven she was diagnosed as deafblind. Throughout her development, she was frequently tested with repeated results of mild mental retardation or borderline intellectual functioning. She was labelled severely mentally handicapped.

Although she did not know it, Mother was providing essential Intervenor services, helping her child to interact with her environment through these important years. Because of this intervention and the assistance of typical deaf services, language had been established to some degree.

Baby A received her primary education in the public school system, with marginal results, along with consistent Intervenor services at home. At age ten she moved to a specialized school for deaf children in the United States, where she resided for four years. At age twelve she received a cochlear implant, which further facilitated language development. At the school she completed two academic years in one year. At age fourteen she returned home and received ongoing Intervenor services both at home and abroad. Currently, she is attending high school and taking college courses. She has a 4.0 GPA in both. She also has a part-time job with the Chamber of Commerce.

Case Study 2

Baby B was born at twenty-five weeks' gestation with a birth weight of 1 lb,

7 oz. Like Baby A, he received large amounts of oxygen to combat poorly developed lungs and suffered retinitis of prematurity, for which he received an experimental medication that resulted in deafness. Additional complications included renal failure and patent ductus arteriosis. In contrast to the previous case, this child was identified as blind, and then identified as deaf at four months of age. (Note that he was called deaf and blind, not deafblind.) Mother sought out professional consultation, but received only routine help with traditional speech and language therapy and occupational therapy. The child did not receive his first hearing aid until age five. Later, it was determined to be too weak.

He attended school via the Department of Mental Retardation from two and a half years until the age of four; he then was educated via the public school system until age eight. No Intervenor services were rendered. From public schools he moved to a residential school for the blind, where, the mother was led to believe, her son could be taught. She reports this to be the worst placement of all.

At the age of nine this boy rarely sat up and his only point of orientation was down. He had acquired no daily living skills or language and had suffered severe experiential deprivation. He was aggressive and marginally functional by any measures.

Mother received Intervenor education at this time that consisted of one week's training. Within one week, this boy had begun to develop toilet skills and better eating habits and was beginning to use sign language. The mother then spent two years effectively intervening for her son. He is now fourteen and is able to sign some sentences and to take care of most of his daily living skills, and he is learning new things daily. Since his old, 'too weak' hearing aid has been replaced with a more powerful one, he can hear certain noises.

Summary

1. Deafblindness represents an infrequent, but extreme form of disability that leaves its victims at the mercy of their environment.
2. Society has been largely unable to handle the severity and complexity of this problem. In response to the feelings of hopelessness that accompany deafblindness is an equally hopeless solution: labelling these children as mentally retarded or severely mentally handicapped.
3. Society must look beyond the external inadequacies and understand that such children may have cognitive potential beyond expectation, but they cannot access information via evolutionary pathways. As a result of these barriers, children are predisposed to 'experiential deprivation' leading to informational impoverishment.

4. Early identification and intervention can alter the course of cognitive development by utilizing the innate 'plasticity' of the human brain, thus facilitating neural growth during 'critical periods,' minimizing permanent neurological damage, and maximizing compensatory change.
5. The qualitative and quantitative differential experience of the deafblind may, in fact, create opportunities for novel cognitive experience and training that will allow for optimal adaptation in a world of sighted and hearing people. These 'alternative' cognitive strategies must be evaluated and studied and looked upon not as somehow inadequate or remedial, but as adaptive and functional.
6. The Intervenor model provides the most consistent method of cognitive intervention, since it provides contextual material to an impoverished being, beyond that of functional language. It is this 'pathway' that will lead the deafblind to a functional and productive life experience.

The author would like to thank Sally Ruemmler, mother, advocate, and Intervenor consultant, for sharing her seventeen years of experience, breadth of knowledge, and time, in contributing to this manuscript.

REFERENCES

Adams, R.D., and M. Victor (1985) *Principles of Neurology*. 3rd edition. New York: McGraw-Hill
American Psychiatric Association (1994) *The Diagnostic and Statistical Manual of Mental Disorders*. 4th edition. Washington, DC: American Psychiatric Association
Best, B., and G. Roberts (1976) 'Early Cognitive Development in Hearing Impaired Children.' *American Annals of the Deaf* 121, 560–4
Carlson, S. (1990) 'Visually Guided Behaviour of Monkeys after Early Binocular Visual Deprivation.' *International Journal of Neuroscience* (England) 50 (3–4), 185–94
Cragg, B.G. (1975) 'The Development of Synapses in Kitten Visual Cortex during Visual Deprivation.' *Experimental Neurology* 46, 445–51
Day, P., and R. Stillman (1975) 'Inter-observer Reliability of the Callier-Azusa Scale.' Unpublished manuscript. University of Texas at Dallas
Fukui, H.G., and K.S. Bedi (1991) 'Quantitative Study of the Development of Neurons and Synapses in Rats Reared in the Dark during Early Postnatal Life.' *Journal of Anatomy* 174, 49–60
Furth, H.G. (1964) 'Research with the Deaf: Implications for Language and Cognition.' *Psychological Bulletin* 62, 145–64
– (1966) *Thinking without Language. Psychological Implications of Deafness*. New York: Free Press

– (1973) *Deafness and Learning. A Psychosocial Approach*. Belmont, CA: Wadsworth

Gillman, A.E., D.R. Goddard, and C.A. Belmont (1974) 'The Outcome of a 20-year Study of Blind Children Two Years Old and Younger. A Preliminary Survey.' *New Outlook Blind* 68, 1–7

Goslin, D.A. (1968) 'Standardized Ability Test and Testing.' *Science* 159, 851–5

Hayes, S.P. (1962) 'Measuring the Intelligence of the Blind.' In *Blindness: Modern Approaches to the Unseen Environment*, ed. by P.A. Zahl. New York: Harper

Kates, S.L., W.N. Kates, and J. Michael (1962) 'Cognitive Processes in Deaf and Hearing Adolescents and Adults.' *Psychology Monograph* 76 (32) 1–34

Lenneberg, E.H. (1967) *Biological Foundations of Language*. New York: Wiley

Lowenfeld, B. (1975) *The Changing Status of the Blind. Separation to Integration*. Springfield, IL: Charles C. Thomas

Luria, A.R. (1976) *Cognitive Development: Its Cultural and Social Foundations*. Cambridge, MA: Harvard University Press

Millar, S. (1975) 'Spatial Memory by Blind and Sighted Children.' *British Journal of Psychology* 66, 449–59

Mower, G.D. (1991) 'The Effect of Dark Rearing on the Time Course of the Critical Period in the Cat Visual Cortex.' *Brain Research, Developmental Brain Research* (Netherlands) 58, 151–8

O'Connor, N., and Hermelin B. (1976) 'Backward and Forward Recall by Deaf and Hearing Children.' *Quarterly Journal of Experimental Psychology* 28, 83–92

Perry B., R. Pollard, L. Toi et al. (1995) 'Childhood Trauma: The Neurobiology of Adaptation and Use-Dependent Development of the Brain: How States Become Traits.' *Infant Mental Health Journal* (in press)

Piercy, M. (1967) 'Neurological Aspects of Intelligence. In *Handbook of Clinical Neurology*, Vol. 3: *Disorders of Higher Nervous Activity*, ed. P.J. Vinken and G.W. Bruyn. Amsterdam: North-Holland

Spiegelman, M.N. (1976) 'A Comparative Study of the Effects of Early Blindness on the Development of Auditory-Spatial Learning.' In *The Effects of Blindness and Other Impairments on Early Development*, ed. Z.S. Jastrzembska. New York: American Foundation for the Blind

Toldi, J., I. Rojik, and O. Fehar (1994) 'Neonatal Monocular Enucleation-Induced Cross-Modal Effects Observed in the Cortex of Adult Rats.' *Neuroscience* 62, 105–14

Volgyi, B., T. Farkas, and J. Toldi (1993) 'Compensation of a Sensory Deficit Inflicted upon Newborn and Adult Animals: A Behavioural Study.' *Neuroreport* 4, 827–9

Warren, D.H. (1977) *Blindness and Early Childhood Development*. New York: American Foundation for the Blind

Wedding D., and S. Cody (1995) *Intellectual and Neuropsychological Assessment. Behavior and Medicine,* ed. D. Wedding. St. Louis, MO: Mosby

174   Douglas L. Geenens

Wiesel T.N., and D.H. Hubel (1974) 'Ordered Arrangement of Orientation Columns in
    Monkeys Lacking Visual Experience.' J Comp Neurol (USA) 158(3), 307–18
Willerman, L. (1978) 'The Influence of Transitivity on Learning in Hearing and Deaf
    Children.' *Child Development* 36, 533–8
Youniss J., and H.G. Furth (1965) 'The Influence of Transitivity on Learning in Hearing
    and Deaf Children.' *Child Development* 36, 533–8

6

Social Relationships and Behaviour

GARY BRIDGETT

Introduction

An introduction to this chapter requires an explanation of the perspective of the author and of the intended scope of the work. I am a teacher. Consequently the ideas presented here are those which I have found relevant as a teacher and more specifically as a teacher of children who are deafblind. The content of the chapter is neither the result of clinical study nor the product of an exhaustive examination of previously published literature. Being a teacher, I have found that my writing is directed towards teachers. Where this causes problems for some readers, it is my hope that individual teachers will be consulted for clarification. Teachers, being the most numerous and available professionals to interact with families of children who are deafblind will in turn make this work accessible to the widest possible audience.

The topic of the social and emotional development of deafblind individuals is so broad that, in order to have a useful discussion of the relevant issues, it is necessary to frame the discussion within certain limits. The issues of values, civic responsibility, and personal fulfilment are as relevant to the deafblind individual as they are to other members of society. These issues, however, while undoubtedly presenting special difficulties for persons with deafblindness, will be faced only by the individual who has established a stable self-image, is socially aware, and has had sufficient opportunities to experience, identify, and reflect upon a range of human emotions.

Congenital or early adventitious deafblindness presents specific obstacles to the acquisition of these prerequisites. Our discussion will focus on these obstacles and on techniques that may be helpful in overcoming them.

Emotional Bonding

When we use the hyphenated term 'social-emotional' we are stating a great deal about how we understand emotions. Our feelings are to a great extent directed outward towards others. Even when we are angry with ourselves or proud of ourselves, the emotion is likely an indication of our understanding of how others regard us. If we had no relationship to others, our feelings would be limited to the fulfilment of physical needs.

The social-emotional starting point for all infants is the establishment of a bond with their mother. Attachment to a mother figure is a biological event that arises within the first few weeks of life. Through repeated experiences of need satisfaction the infant comes to associate the mother with comfort and pleasure.(Need satisfaction must be understood in the broadest terms as inclusive of all innate infant drives.) This association comes about through the infant's ability to establish recognition of familiarity. Constant perceptual qualities, such as smells, mother's voice, touch, taste, visual regard of mother's face, and physical positioning, are factors that help to build this association. These experiences, coupled with the joy experienced through the intangible qualities of nurturing and love, provide the foundation for future social-emotional development.

Emergence of Self

The newborn infant exists in a predominantly reflexive world. Concepts about the content of experience must be built moment by moment, day by day. The self as an experience of the unifying principal of conscious experience is a reflective concept. Establishing a sense of self requires the ability to organize sensory information, emotions, and thought processes under a single umbrella concept that we can identify as 'I.' This ability develops slowly over the first few years of life and continues to be refined throughout our lives. Deafblind infants, as we shall see, are greatly disadvantaged in this endeavour.

Awareness of the Environment and Options

The socially-emotionally adapted individual will make choices that express personality. These choices are made from the variety of opportunities that a free society offers. All aspects of life, from work to recreation to creative and spiritual thought, are the scope of these decisions. Accessibility is not universal, however, and, in fact, individuals can be limited by many different factors (political, cultural, legal, etc.). Regardless of these limitations, the precondition of all choice making is awareness of options. It is essential that teachers of deaf-blind individuals utilize methods that will assist in maximizing awareness of the environment and of its possibilities.

Management of Emotions

Regardless of personal choices, we continue to live in a social reality. Individuals interact and there are patterns to those interactions; as a society we have evolved a set rules of behaviour in regard to them. Some rules are formalized in laws, while others are culturally transmitted. Further, peer groups, family traditions, and social conventions define increasingly subtle degrees of behavioural conformity.

Emotions often precipitate an individual's confrontation of these norms. Although we see breaches of conduct each day, we are more likely to see individuals demonstrate restraint in the acting out of their emotions. Thus, each of us to a greater or lesser degree practises a form of emotional management. Society has an interest in this ongoing management and has fostered techniques either to help individuals control their emotional behaviour (counselling, organized religion, socialization in school) or to coerce individuals into restraining themselves (police, courts, jails).

We have outlined certain preconditions of what we shall call social/emotional adjustment. They are the ability to form emotional bonds, an awareness of self, an awareness of environmental choices, and the ability to manage emotions and/or behaviour. Before we attempt a discussion of pedagogical techniques that will be appropriate to fostering these preconditions in children with deafblindness, it will be helpful to look at a model of the structural components that underlie development of these skills.

Anne Nafstad has authored an article published by the Nordic Staff Training Center for Deafblind Services entitled *Space of Interaction*. In this insightful article, Nafstad has described interactions that underlie social/emotional development. The interactions indicated are reflective of the work by John Bowlby in *Attachment and Loss*. In that text, Bowlby cites research from Ainsworth's study of attachment behaviour in Ugandan mothers and their infants: 'Soon after an infant is able to crawl, he does not always remain close to his mother. On the contrary, he makes little excursions away from her, exploring other objects and people and, if allowed to do so, he may even go out of her sight. From time to time, however, he returns to her, as though to assure himself she is still there' (1969, 74). This movement of the child away from and back to the mother is central to the interactional structures described by Nafstad. Bowlby asserts that these attachment behaviours continue throughout childhood, adolescence, and adulthood, although the focal point of the attachment changes as one enters different phases of life.

Aspects of Early Bonding

Bonding

We have stated that establishing an emotional bond is the first step in social development. It is important that we define what this means in practical terms. Nafstad (1992) has identified two basic qualities of bonding: sharing and attachment. *Sharing* is described by Nafstad as 'mutual attention or mutual experience' and as 'the experience of being with others' (1992, 24). *Attachment* is said to be 'a consequence of the primary experience of sharing' (ibid.). These two qualities of bonding are clearly linked, but whether or not all sharing has attachment as its consequence is left somewhat unclear. As well, we are not told anything about how long or how many sharing experiences are required to produce the effect of attachment. We might qualify these definitions by suggesting that mutual pleasurable experiences, over a period of time, will lead to attachment. This process is what we understand as bonding.

Although we usually understand bonding as an invisible quality of our interactions with students, Nafstad indicates that bonding may be observed if 'The congenitally deaf-blind person seeks, or seeks to maintain, social close-contact for the sake of close-contact itself' (ibid.). Later in our discussion we shall see how this seeking to maintain social close-contact is a primary function through which the student establishes a fixed point or *locus of security* from which he or she may safely explore the world.

Lifesphere and Landscape

Nafstad tells us that *lifesphere* is 'that part of you, you are familiar with, of which you are in control, and in which you plan your activities. The lifesphere has a centre and a periphery. We orientate from the centre out to the periphery and back to the centre again (ibid., 15).' This concept is useful to the teacher in that it provides a framework for educational progress. Teaching is the process of expanding the lifesphere. By definition then, we must create educational experiences that will assist the student to gain familiarity with, and control of, new aspects of the world.

Nafstad also explains that 'The *landscape* exists "objectively" for each one of us' (ibid.) We can understand landscape as the physical world and therefore as limitless.

From these definitions we can see that lifesphere is a term describing a psychological 'comfort zone' that expands throughout our lifetime. We can learn about the landscape in a factual sense, but until that knowledge becomes relevant through some type of familiarity, it will not be part our lifesphere. Familiarity seems to be defined by our ability to manipulate and make use of the knowledge. I may be aware of a language called 'Russian,' but until I am able to speak or understand that language, it remains in my landscape.

Pendulum Movement

In order to understand the significance of the preceding terminology and definitions, we must appreciate the dynamic relationship among the indicated functions.

Through sharing we discover that there is something inherently good or satisfying in being with another. This leads us to attempt to maintain that social close-contact. Through our efforts to maintain the closeness, we begin to experience control (if the 'other' recognizes and reacts positively to our efforts). From the secure position of being-with, we may choose to direct our attention to the immediate landscape and to explore, thus expanding our lifesphere. Whenever we venture too far or too long into the landscape, we may retreat to the security of being-with.

This moving outward to the periphery followed by a return to the centre repeated over and over in ever-expanding explorations is the essence of individual social/emotional development. This psychological moving back and forth is called *pendulum movement*.

The Mother Bond

At birth the congenitally deafblind child is as close to being on an equal footing with the child who is not disabled as he or she ever will be. Both children exist in a largely undifferentiated sensory state. The newborn's first experiences should be the tactile, olfactory, and gustatory sensations of breast feeding and of cradling support. Unfortunately, the deafblind infant's experience often quickly diverges from that of the healthy baby. Medical interventions often take precedence over family considerations. As well, the new parents will face a set of problems for which they have never been prepared. At a time when these parents should be enjoying the culmination of nine months of preparation and anticipation, they will be swept into a whole new world of medical specialists, social workers, and emotions they don't readily understand.

These factors have great potential to disrupt the infant's early opportunities to establish bonds with the mother or principal caregiver. It is very important that these issues be addressed as quickly as possible after the birth of the child so that adverse effects are minimized. This can be done through enlightened hospital procedures that promote proximity and interaction between mother and child, even in cases where medical procedures are necessary. Additionally, support services personnel who are familiar with the developmental issues relevant to deafblind infants and who are able sensitively to assist parents with the necessary emotional learning that confronts them should be involved as soon as possible.

The deafblind child's need for intervention begins at birth. Vision and hearing are the principal senses that give us information from a distance, and these senses make possible the early following of mother as she moves about the infant's immediate environment. This visual and auditory following takes on greater significance when seen as a precursor to mobility and development of 'pendulum movement.' Also, without these senses the deafblind infant effectively has no early warning system and, as a result, experiences occur immediately on the body. The deafblind infant will need compensatory strategies if he or she is to avoid establishing patterns of startle behaviour that will complicate future interactions.

The child whose distance senses are intact is generally approached in a sensorily 'soft' manner; prior to picking up or physically handling an infant in any way, we tend to announce our presence through auditory and visual cues (eye contact, facial proximity, verbal greetings, and baby talk). These distance sense cues become part of the complex of repetitive and comforting sensations that announce for the infant the experience of proximity to the mother. The vocal dynamics and visually presented behavioural mannerisms of the mother transmit personality traits that are comforting in their recognizability. Although we may not assume that the infant is fully cognizant of all of the qualities that we might have as adults, we can suggest that a process occurs in which these sensory impressions are being organized in the baby's mind and are the building blocks of early perceptual and cognitive development. The infant begins to respond with pleasure to the mother's approaches and signals. These responses are recognized and enjoyed by the mother and are reinforced through tactile expressions such as cuddling and stroking. This reciprocal attentiveness provides the foundation for development of attachment behaviour or bonding.

When we consider the role of vision and hearing in the development of attachment behaviour, it becomes very clear that the deafblind infant is at a severe disadvantage. The deafblind baby must be presented with alternative sensory impressions that will allow for the possibility of parallel development. The principal caregiver may utilize a pleasant scent that is consistently worn during interactions with the deafblind child. A gentle touch on a specific part of the baby's body followed by a brief pause can also announce the presence of the caregiver. Movements through space can be less startling if gentle 'false starts' are built into the interaction routines. These techniques will also provide the child with opportunities to establish residual visual and auditory functions, since potential 'markers' are built into the regular sequence of experience. These 'markers' give the baby a chance to recognize that there is something interesting to attend to auditorily and/or visually.

Further specific techniques that can be used in providing these alternative sensory impressions can be found in works dealing with infant development, such as *Deaf-blind Infants and Children* (McInnes and Treffry 1982). Since the focus of this chapter is the process of social-emotional development, we must be content with having indicated the starting points of both healthy and deviant development.

Awareness of Self and Other

Self-Awareness

The deafblind infant will show little interest in the external world. Even with the best of planning, the infant's moment-to-moment existence will consist of those perceptions arising inside or immediately beside him. The consequence of this condition cannot be overemphasized. The deafblind individual lacks dis-tance senses. (Although the majority of assessed individuals that a professional in the field might encounter will have varying degrees of residual sight and hearing, the degree of distortion experienced through these residual abilities and the inability to integrate the sensory information received through these faulty senses mitigates against their natural development.) Whereas the natural condition of infancy is highly social, with the earliest developmental achieve-ments being oriented towards the proximity of the mother, the infant who lacks distance senses begins life in isolation. This isolation and its consequences for development in all areas is the central issue for parents and professionals.

The deafblind infant will not see or hear rattles or mobiles that respond to body movements. The connection between action and reaction that underlies so much of early development will go unnoticed. The experience of cause and effect in which we are the causative agent is critical to the discovery that we have some degree of control. Effecting change in the environment around us becomes a critical experience in terms of both our awareness of ourselves (intention) and awareness of the world as a source of interest (creativity). Again we see that sensory isolation from the mother and the resultant delay in establishing the interactional sequence characteristic of the mother/infant bond has a severe impact on the deafblind infant's opportunities to experience a connection with the world outside.

In spite of the difficulties presented, infant-stimulation workers must understand the impact of deafblindness upon the developmental needs of infants and assist parents to establish compensatory strategies to foster interactional social and object experiences. As preschool and school-age teachers we must attempt to emulate the caregiver's relationship with the child such that we can function as a locus of security within the physical environment of the educational setting. This must be established through the 'sharing' experience that Nafstad has described. The resulting attachment to the teacher provides the child with the security necessary to attend to events that arise externally.

Emergence of Emotions

We must briefly back up and examine further the role of the interaction between parent and infant in establishing the beginnings of emotional awareness. At some undefined point an infant moves from experiencing emotions reflexively in relation to physical needs to experiencing emotions socially during times of caregiving and attention giving. As stated, the attendant parent smiles, sings, maintains facial proximity, and generally begins to engage the infant in ways that elicit pleasurable expressions from the baby. Without presupposing a cause-and-effect principle that places the parent as the agent of the infant's subjective state, we can safely indicate that there is an interchange between the two in which these early socially rewarding experiences emerge. This interchange may be the beginning of the experience of 'sharing' as defined by Nafstad. There is a quality of action/response to the process in which the participants modify the outward expressions of their subjective inner state in a communicative-like dialogue.

Other-Awareness

In the beginning of the 'sharing' described by Nafstad the child may not discriminate sensations belonging to his body as opposed to a world that is 'other.' The child may have established sensation-based behaviours that function to control sensory input. These self-stimulatory behaviours are protective in nature in that they maintain a minimal level of cognitive function in the face of constant sensory deprivation. As well, these behaviours serve to override the confused mass of sensations arising from incomplete residual vision and hearing and from tactile sensations arising from manipulation by caregivers. It is necessary to establish within the child an awareness of the world as 'other' and to coincidentally demonstrate the experience of control of the 'other.' In order to accomplish this, Van Dijk of the Netherland's Sint Michielgestel Institute has included among his curricular strategies the phenomenon of *resonance*. Using this technique, the teacher joins the child in an action from the child's behavioural repertoire. Within this sharing experience the teacher seeks to identify an indicative action on the part of the child that signifies 'start' and/or 'stop.' With repetition it is hoped that the child will recognize the sequence of interaction and begin to participate purposefully in the turn-taking or 'conversational' nature of the interaction.

Resonance activities, according to Stillman and Battle, 'Have multiple purposes: to elicit the child's attention to and participation in interactions with others, to develop the child's understanding of how his actions can effect the environment, and to encourage the child's formation of positive relationships with others' (1984, 163). Resonance activities are both a starting point that allows us entry into the world of the deafblind child and a bridge over which the child may begin to reach outward into the 'landscape.' As teachers we must recognize that it is the child who takes this step. We may provide the security that makes the step possible, and we may create sensorially interesting phenomena in the landscape that is proximally immediate to the child, but it is the child who must determine the moments in which it is safe to venture outward.

Awareness of the Environment

In the beginning, the child who is emerging from a world of self-stimulatory sensations will direct attention only to those objects that satisfy the basic needs of nourishment and maintenance of the self-stimulation. Our goal as teachers is to direct the child gently to other qualities of experience, such as sequence and discrimination of attributes such as texture, shape, and function. These qualities cannot be explained, they must be experienced. At the W. Ross Macdonald School in Brantford, Ontario, the most often heard phrase is 'Do with, not for.' This maxim provides a great many insights in a nutshell. The child must physically (or possibly more accurately, motorically) experience all aspects of the day-to-day world. These experiences need to be complete in that they include the whole activity, because without the overview of the distance senses the deafblind child will not connect the parts to the whole. This fact is sometimes misunderstood by those whose expertise is with individuals who are intellectually challenged, because of their frequent use of task analysis. The only possible way a deafblind child can form whole concepts is from having whole experiences.

From the point of view of cognitive development this 'whole/whole' approach is absolutely necessary. In order to quantify and delineate the stages one will observe in applying this approach McInnes and Treffry have outlined the 'Interaction Sequence' (1982, 20–3).

Stages of Interaction

In *Deaf-Blind Infants and Children* McInnes and Treffry stated that 'Until the child gains confidence through experience, we can anticipate that specific stages will occur in each new interaction with the environment' (1982, 36). These stages are as follows:

1. resist the interaction
2. tolerate the interaction with the intervenor
3. cooperate passively with the intervenor
4. enjoy the activity because of the intervenor
5. respond cooperatively with the intervenor
6. lead the intervenor through the activity once the initial communication has been given
7. imitate the action of the intervenor upon request
8. initiate the action independently.

The authors have provided an exhaustive explanation of each of the stages of their model. It is highly recommended that readers acquaint themselves with that source. It is sufficient for our purposes to recognize these stages as indicative of a process of exploration and learning that is grounded in social connectedness. (See chapter 2 for a discussion of Instructional Intervention and the integration of this sequence with the Presentation Sequence and the Interaction Sequence.) The emotional bond between the teacher and the deafblind student is utilized to draw the child into experiences that he or she would otherwise not perceive or explore. As familiarity with that experience increases, the student is able and motivated to engage in the activity with decreasing levels of direction and support. In the final stage, the student will have facility within the experience and may choose to engage in the activity with a minimum of interventional support to provide auditory and visual input and feedback.

These stages of interaction have been used as an effective guideline in helping deafblind students to establish new skills. We can underline the validity of these stages by examining our own experiences when faced with particularly difficult new skills. Consider the individual who has never skied before. For many the first stage is enough to keep them far enough from a ski slope that the issue of attempting the skill never arises. For those who move forward in the sequence there will likely be a reluctant moment at the top of the slope when the presence of a friend is the critical difference between continuing and returning to the safety of the chalet.

We need not complete this comparison to make our point. The relationship between our lifesphere and the landscape is for the most part determined by our sense of security as social beings. Even in the case of what might be regarded as independent exploration, the way has usually been paved through a cognitive survey of the landscape through written or first-hand accounts by others.

In many ways we might understand these stages of interaction as descriptors of a pedagogical technique that is necessary when an individual does not have access to sensory information from a distance. The deafblind child, unable to observe visually and unable to establish concepts about an interaction from auditory information, or from conversational information, must physically and motorically experience the interaction in order to have even the beginning of a conceptual appreciation of that interaction.

The gentle coaxing implied within the interactive sequence is clearly and fundamentally necessary in order to introduce new experiences to the deafblind student. This coaxing is not the verbal cajoling that we might see in the pedagogy of other populations. Without doubt it must be physical manipulation through the hand-over-hand method. There are inherent difficulties within this method that must be explored.

The first problem that arises in using the hand-over-hand method is related to the current tendency towards a litigious public that creates an atmosphere of fear among educators towards all kinds of physical interaction with their students. While this should not be an issue, it undoubtedly is a very real concern for many professionals in the field. For this reason it is necessary to state emphatically that the protocol relating to physical contact with students as developed by many professional associations and indeed by administrative bodies must be re-evaluated in programs serving deafblind populations.

The second problem inherent in the hand-over-hand method is much more difficult to address. There is a fine line between establishing awareness of the environment and coercively manipulating a child through an experience that they may be unable to assimilate into their lifesphere. McInnes and Treffry recognized this problem, as indicated by their cautioning, 'When the child resists an activity or new experience, do not insist. Switch to a related activity which he enjoys and return to the new activity when the tension is gone. The child must be relaxed and secure when the new activity is introduced' (1982, 32–7). This problem is one of judgment. As professionals working with deafblind children, we would expect the child to resist any new experience, but we are told to

TABLE 6.1

Stage of interaction	Subjective state
Resists	Fear
Tolerate	Trust
Cooperates	Perceptual attention
Enjoys	Cognitive awareness
Responds cooperatively	Re-cognition (Memory)
Leads	Confidence
Imitates	Mastery
Initiates	Creativity

'not insist.' This is clearly an area of practice in which teaching must be regarded as an art rather than as a science. Judicious decisions must be made regarding the relationship between the child's resistance and what is an appropriate degree of insistence. We might bring into this equation additional factors, such as mood, restfulness, health issues, and the strength of the emotional bond we have with the child. The deafblind child is always just one step away from retreating into an internal world of self-stimulation. Whenever decisions are made inappropriately to 'insist,' we may be successful in actually manipulating the child through an activity while losing the child's attention or even awareness of the landscape we wish to introduce.

An approach that may be helpful in this endeavour is to consider the subjective state of the child during each of the stages of interaction. The attempt must be made to determine what emotional experience is present within the child as we take him or her through the process of introduction to new experiences.

Table 6.1 offers a framework within which we may begin to establish a deafblind child's *emotional readiness* for movement through the stages of interaction. It is meant to guide the intervenor in gauging what is an appropriate activity in view of the child's emotional ability to integrate the content of an experience into his or her lifesphere. Whenever it is observed that the child has not moved to the corresponding subjective state within any particular stage of interaction, the question must be raised about the readiness of the child for that movement.

Every child must be cared for in terms of health, hygiene, and safety. The deafblind child of necessity will be exposed to experiences that are not reflective of the table. These experiences are care oriented and as such do not require the child's implicit permission as it is occurring within the interaction sequence. I have previously emphasized the appropriateness of the maxim 'Do with, not for,' but here a word of caution is in order. 'Do with, not for' has been used to justify expectations within lifeskills routines that fall under the category of care. There is no doubt that techniques that increase the child's awareness of care sequences, including touch and concrete cues, are important to the child's overall security and anticipational abilities; in this area as in others, however, it is necessary to determine the child's emotional readiness to take on responsibility for specific motor tasks within those sequences. Failing to do so may result in the child's acquisition of rote motoric skills that do not fit into a conceptual context of his or her lifesphere. We must take care to establish perceptual awareness as a priority in all interactions with the deafblind child. This focusing of the attention outward to the world is always the choice of the child and thus should be enticed but not coerced.

Management of Emotions

As our deafblind children grow and establish skills in all of the developmental areas, they will experience increasingly complex emotions. The simple responses to comfort/discomfort that are 'read' for the child by their principal caregiver will give way to the emerging emotions that relate to the external world. The child will move from the early feeling of 'want that,' to feelings of jealousy (control of the locus of security), frustration, happiness, anger, and on through the range of human emotions. This movement likely will not proceed smoothly, even with good intervention and educational planning.

Much of what we experience as emotion is learned from our observations of others. Subtle facial expressions, body language, and vocal tone impart feeling content to our everyday language. The deafblind child does not have these observations ready at hand, in contrast to the hearing/seeing child. The deafblind child must experience first hand each potential emotion in a variety of situations before he or she will be able to identify emotions arising from within. Well-trained teachers and Intervenors will assist the child to name and to respond appropriately to emotional content as it arises during the natural course of daily life. They will also inform the child of emotional displays by other individuals within the child's lifesphere.

Helping the deafblind child to manage emotions and behaviour should be done pro-actively through the type of clarification and informing that is suggested above. Unfortunately, the wealth of observational material needed and the intensity of emotional situations make this a difficult task. Additionally, the deafblind child will likely experience delayed language development. This delay not only will make the proposed teaching more difficult but will also cause frustrations in the child, since wants, needs, and interests cannot be adequately expressed.

Recreation

All of us need to have pleasurable experiences that we find interesting and engaging. Ideally, this is true of our vocations (although often it is not), but most definitely it must be true of our recreational pursuits. The world of the deafblind person is by definition a world devoid of the visual and auditory stimuli that dominate our culture (television, radio, etc.). The deafblind person is isolated in a most profound way. Not only media sources but social groups in general contribute to this isolation. Intervention can only report and inform about social dynamics; it can not reproduce the experience.

Parents of deafblind children readily indicate how difficult it is to find toys that can capture their child's interest. As stated earlier, breaking into the deafblind child's world and successfully establishing attention to the external world is often a project in itself. We must recognize that sensory deprivation will inevitably challenge even the brightest minds and in most cases will lead to a life in which long periods of boredom must be endured. These perceptual 'downtimes' will be adjusted to in different ways, depending upon the options available to each individual. As teachers we must attempt to establish recreational skills that can provide as wide a variety and as deep an interest as the student is able to manage. If we consider the interaction sequence as outlined above, we see that at the fourth stage the child begins to enjoy the activity. Enjoyment at this stage is not specifically related to the activity; rather, it is a result of the pre-existing bond with the intervenor. As the child moves further through the sequence, this enjoyment gradually becomes centred in the child as an intrinsic pleasure relating to performance of the activity. This shift is not fully realized until the child reaches the initiates/creativity stage. As teachers we must recognize the importance of reaching this stage in order to provide students with the experience of self-directed pleasurable experiences. We must not, however, confuse this stage with independence or with a cessation of the need for intervention. Intervention will continue to be necessary in order to provide feedback about efforts made, to provide any new information that might be relevant, or to facilitate social aspects of the activity.

Each individual will expand his/her lifesphere according to a combination of different factors. Personal security, exposure to opportunities at an appropriate stage of readiness, and personal preferences will determine what is assimilated into a lifesphere. We must not allow ourselves to presuppose what any individual may find to be a useful pastime. We may, however, continue to offer exposure to what we feel may eventually be valued by the individual.

Having addressed the issue of the need for recreational opportunities, we must take one step further and consider that for some deafblind individuals at their particular stage of development the option chosen may be self-stimulation of one kind or another. Although long-term planning may help the individual to broaden the options available to him/her, in the short term we must be willing to respect the decision the individual has made. This stance is essential if we are to avoid the pitfalls of labelling the self-stimulatory behaviour as a problem to be eliminated. We must consider the number of self-stimulatory behaviours that are prevalent in our culture (nail-biting, head-scratching, etc.) and see that the actions of the deafblind person are part of the same continuum. Unless a behaviour is injurious to himself or another, or unless the behaviour is so bizarre that it effectively isolates the individual from social contact, we should not attempt to extinguish that behaviour. Undoubtedly, it is preferable to provide suitable stimulation at an early age in order that self-stimulatory behaviours do not either develop or become ingrained habits. Unfortunately early identification and appropriate intervention are the exception rather than the rule, and as professionals in the field we rarely, if ever, encounter the proverbial blank slate among our referrals. The deafblind child who presents with established self-stimulatory behaviours should be provided with opportunities to develop alternative recreational skills through a planned program using techniques as outlined above in 'stages of interaction' and applied with consideration of the child's subjective emotional readiness.

Behaviour Management

A text of the present type is often consulted only when a specific problem presents itself that is of such a confounding nature that it sends teachers scurrying to the professional library in hopes of a sure fix. Behaviour management problems are of such a nature. It is seldom, however, that there are simple solutions to behavioural difficulties; hence the term 'behaviour management.'

Behaviour must always been seen in a context. Factors that are constituent of that context may be environmental, interpersonal, medical, psychological, cognitive, familial, or communicative. In order to address a behavioural concern, one must establish the relevant contextual factors. This process might be likened to an investigation by a detective. Many avenues must be explored before a working hypothesis can be formulated.

There are still a few behaviour therapists that feel that the stimulus-response approach is sufficient to understand human activity. Fortunately, the majority of behaviour management specialists now recognize the importance of contextual factors as behavioural determinants. Deafblind educators have long recognized the problems that result from an inability to communicate and to anticipate change. Emotional reactions are to be expected when an individual is unable to communicate thoughts and wishes because their functional language skills lag behind cognitive abilities. Likewise, when an individual is unable to anticipate physical changes to the environment or to discern meaning behind movement through space, upsets will occur. Many of the techniques explained in other sections of this text came about through the recognition that deafblind individuals have needs in regards to obtaining information that ordinarily would be acquired as a matter of course through the distance senses. A discussion of behaviour management in regard to the deafblind must begin with the admonishment that unless the basic components of a program suitable to the deafblind population are in place, one should expect difficulties. In such a case the problem lies not in the child but in the program, and all efforts to 'correct' the child's behaviour will be counter to the best interests of the child.

In spite of excellent programs, behavioural problems do arise. The following model is meant to provide a framework through which individual problems can be addressed. Success is not guaranteed, or perhaps even possible, but if the model is applied with empathy, perseverance, and creativity, many difficulties may be dealt with effectively to the benefit of the deafblind individual.

This model has five stages. The stages form a chronology of actions. Each action is appropriate to its specific point in the chronology. Deviation from the chronology should be avoided, especially in the light of emotions that are often highly charged in the individuals who are dealing with the day-to-day problem behaviour. In order to effect lasting change in the behaviour, it is very important that a team approach be maintained by all those involved.

Figure 6.1 will assist the reader to see the relationship between the five stages of the model presented and various subsections of enquiry or actions within each stage.

Stage 1: Identification

The behaviour in question must be targeted clearly. General terms, such as 'aggression,' should be avoided in favour of more specific descriptors. The identification should state what the behaviour is, when it occurs, where it occurs, and who is present when it occurs. If there are several behaviours that appear to form a complex pattern, it is advisable when planning strategies to target the most serious behaviour of the group and to recognize the others as extensions of the key behaviour. If the behaviours are indeed connected, strategies that are effective in ameliorating the targeted behaviour will likely have a positive effect on the entire complex.

Stage 2: Analysis

The heart of behavioural management lies in successful analysis of why the

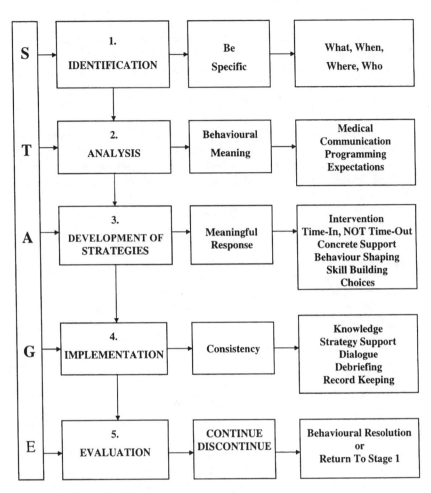

Figure 6.1   Behaviour Management

individual is acting in the particular fashion that he is. In stating this we have indicated a fundamental premise to our approach. We are stating in no uncertain terms that behaviour is meaningful. This does not indicate that some behaviour is meaningful; rather, *ALL behaviour is meaningful.*

The significance of indicating that behaviour has meaning is that we begin from the position of trying to understand the behaviour and avoid the pitfall of starting from a judgmental presupposition. Unfortunate as it seems, there is often a tendency for careworkers of all kinds to dismiss the idea that there is a meaningful context to behaviour. We hear the phrase 'just a behaviour' and the summarization of an individual's actions as being the result of his or her being a 'bad' person. These judgments and the accompanying attitudes will be very detrimental to efforts towards effectively assisting the individual displaying the behaviour.

When we state that behaviour is meaningful, we are also saying that behaviour is communicative. This is because we as humans are able to see meanings both in our own actions and in the actions of others. We have already indicated the contribution made by this ability in mothers to the development of infants through the 'reading' of their gross sounds and movements. We may interpret actions as indicative of their underlying meaning. This is the task we undertake during behaviour analysis.

In order effectively to analyse a behaviour as to its meaning content, we must gather information about the behaviour. When does it occur? What occurs prior to the behaviour? Afterwards? How often does the behaviour occur? Daily? Weekly? Are there routine activities that are in a time relation to the behaviour? Does it occur in a specific location? Is this location near or on a route that would be travelled in going to another location? All of the questions that need to be asked cannot be listed. Each situation brings about its own set of enquiries. There are, however, categories of questions that, although not exhaustive of the possibilities, can act as guidelines.

Category 1: Medical

The first consideration must be medical. Many behaviours may be indicative of discomfort or of an imbalance. Deafblind individuals may not have the functional language to indicate that they are experiencing pain. In a study of one group of deafblind children it was found that a majority of the children who displayed self-injurious behaviours (head-banging) were suffering from middle-ear infections. Many medical conditions have the potential to cause such an effect. A short list might include glaucoma, bowel problems, arthritis, migraines, or sinus problems. A doctor must make these determinations, but the medical professional often must rely on the people who work with the individual on a day-to-day basis to provide information to assist in the diagnosis.

Category 2: Communication

Congenitally deafblind individuals for the most part learn communication skills from first-hand experiences. Vocabulary that names these experiences and creates an ability to refer to the experience at a temporal and spatial distance provides for the possibility of concept development beyond the immediate sensory memory. Each concept must be developed through carefully planned activities that reveal ever widening aspects of the particular experience. This process inevitably leads to conceptual gaps in understanding because of the difficulty in planning for every relevant aspect of the experience being addressed. It is well understood by teachers of the deafblind that students regularly have difficulty transferring skills from the setting in which the skill was acquired to a new setting. As well, generalization from the specific experiences of the deafblind individual to a wider context that would reflect common social knowledge is especially problematic. These aspects of the acquisition of language by deafblind individuals have the potential to create the misunderstandings and miscommunications that often underlie behaviour problems. Some of the possible areas of language that may give rise to behavioural problems are as follows.

Miscues

Rudimentary language systems that rely on objects or routines carry with them the danger of inadvertent exposures. In such a case the student who understands a bib as a signal that eating will follow may find it difficult to distinguish the bib from something used to protect clothing during a painting activity. The student may be perceived as not enjoying the painting activity when, in fact his or her expectations have been frustrated.

Routines

In the absence of representative symbolic language, the sequence within which familiar routines occur takes on greater significance. Most of us with well-established language systems do take comfort in the familiarity of routines. For the deafblind individual who has not established complex language, the sequence of activities, the routes travelled, or even simple things such as the clothes worn can produce anticipation of an impending event. The individual's response may range from excitement followed by disappointment if the anticipated event is a personal favourite or to fear and irritability if the event has a negative associated memory.

Incomplete Concepts

The hearing/seeing child may decide after enjoying Christmas for the first time that the next day should bring about a repeat performance of the presents and so on and will have to be carefully told that he will have to wait until next year. The child likely will not have a concept of one year, but through repeated conversations and experiences, she will eventually integrate the concept of year with the concept of Christmas such that her expectations can match the reality of the calendar. The deafblind child also will learn a concept first and then modifications to the concept through subsequent experiences. The process of teaching these conceptual modifications can also provide the basis for confusion in the child's world and can lead to emotional responses that must be managed carefully.

Mislabelled or Misunderstood Emotions

All of us must struggle to identify our feelings. The congenitally deafblind individual does not have the opportunities to observe emotions in others or to experience the wealth of children's literature, media sources, nursery rhymes, and so on that help children to think about feelings. As previously mentioned, awareness and identification of emotional states must be built through the deafblind individual's immediate experiences. This process has the potential to foster interactions that require very thoughtful management by intervenors. Along the way the child may have difficulty in sorting out the content of his or her emotions as well as the socially appropriate responses to those emotions. Teachers must be able to guide this process and educate peripheral personnel such that the possible interactions are seen as belonging to this learning style, not simply as a deviation of behavioural norms requiring disciplinary or remedial action.

Emerging Interests

As the deafblind student gains skills and awareness of environmental options, a new activity can capture his or her interest. Difficulties in communicating this new interest can lead to interesting behaviours. One student began to approach people in public places and make a motion that resembled the sign for light. Upon reflection we were able to understand this behaviour as the student's way of indicating he was interested in cameras. When opportunities were provided for the student to use a camera the behaviour ceased.

All of the preceding examples and explanations are meant to give insight into the nature of possible communication-based behavioural difficulties. The list is not exhaustive, and each child's development will take its own course; teachers must be creative in their attempts to analyse their students' behaviour patterns.

Category 3: Appropriate Programming

The point has been amply made that deafblind students must be emotionally and cognitively ready for the content of their daily program. In addition to the content of programs, teachers must carefully monitor the pace of their activities. Too much or too little stimulation can lead to acting out on the part of their deafblind students. As a general rule, activities that require the student to use residual vision and hearing for extended periods of time can be expected to produce fatigue. As well, periods of intense activity of any kind may leave the child needing a little time to withdraw into his or her own idiosyncratic self-stimulation behaviours. As previously mentioned, these behaviours have a regulatory function that allow children to cope with the confused sensory impressions that are a constant in their lives.

Category 4: Consistency of Expectations

The deafblind child will likely have several Intervenors. Everyone that the child interacts with is in some sense intervening by providing additional environmental information. As the deafblind child develops, the circle of people who share interactions with the child grows. With more Intervenors, there is an increased possibility of mixed messages or inconsistent messages about what is expected. While different settings may allow for subtle differences in expectations, the child must be given consistent messages from the Intervenors at home, school, and other settings.

The foregoing categories of potential problem sources is a beginning. There are undoubtedly other categories not mentioned, such as changes in family construction or dynamics. Each situation must be looked at anew if the underlying problem is to be discovered and an appropriate response planned.

Stage 3: Development of Strategies

Appropriate strategies for dealing with behavioural problems among the deafblind are as varied as the triggering situations mentioned in the previous section. Fortunately, if good detective work has been done during the analysis stage, the appropriate strategy will be defined by the content or context of the behaviour itself. The behaviour must be understood in its meaning to the child. This aspect cannot be overemphasized. Prescriptive lists of strategies linked to specific behaviours would be counter-productive. There are, however, some comments that can be made about strategies in general.

Intervention

Although intervention is much more than a strategy for managing behaviour, whenever problems do develop, it may be useful to consider possible adjustments to the level of intervention being provided to the student. A change in either the quantity or the quality of the intervention might be needed.

An example of when intervention changes were an appropriate strategy, while a more mainstream approach would have possibly exacerbated the situation, is that of a child who would bang her head on the floor when frustrated. The therapists involved, who were not trained as deafblind specialists, felt that the appropriate strategy was to put a helmet on the child. This act, of course, answered the therapists' need to ensure the child's safety, but it did not look at the child's need as indicated by the behaviour. Instead, intervention was provided in a more constant fashion, so that the child's safety was protected through the physical efforts of the intervenor. This approach allowed the child to experience comforting tactile care in the form of holding, rocking, and massage during those periods of upset and provided opportunities of reducing the child's frustration by anticipating outbursts and using redirection techniques before incidents occurred.

Time-in, Not Time-out

Time-out is used quite effectively with seeing/hearing children. The premise, of course, is that the child will want the activity and/or the attention of the teacher and will modify the behaviour in order to regain both. This strategy works well if the child can see and hear the wonderful things that are being missed. The deafblind child may very well have no ongoing awareness of what is being missed and may have less than a passing interest in either the content or the social context of the activity.

Social disapproval and withholding of participation can be used effectively in some circumstances if the methods are reoriented in the light of the child's loss of distance senses. The child must remain aware of the ongoing activity. The child needs to maintain proximity to the intervenor such that a dialogue can be maintained in which the joys of the activity are extolled while the child is reminded of the expected behaviour for re-involvement. This dialogue may take many forms, depending on the communicative/cognitive level of the child and the degree of functional residual vision and hearing that the child displays.

Concrete Support

Many behavioural difficulties can be addressed through the use of concrete materials that clarify the student's world. Calendar systems that enable the child to anticipate activity sequences are often very effective. (Calendar, in this sense, is any cue or symbol system that provides the deafblind student with a method of anticipating personally significant events. See chapter 12.) These systems give the child a means of establishing rudimentary time concepts relating to the duration of non-favourite activities and to the required 'wait' until favourite activities resume. A more detailed description of calendar use can be found in chapter 4, 'Communication,' and chapter 12, 'Community-Based Adult Programs.'

Other concrete supports, such as achievement or reward charts, can help the child to understand clearly both expectations and consequences. It is sometimes useful to incorporate these types of system to focus the child's attention on compliance with a physical object rather than with a specific person. This technique can help to avoid the pitfalls of power struggles between the child and the teacher.

Experience booklets that assist in providing communication options are both a necessary tool of daily programming and a remedial strategy to clarify the child's wishes and interests.

Behaviour Shaping

Many behaviours identified as problems are not inappropriate in themselves; rather, they are a problem because of the time, location, or context in which they occur. These behaviours can be managed by establishing circumstances in which the child may be given permission to engage in the action.

An example of the above strategy is the child who was constantly destroying blankets and clothing by pulling threads. When this child was given a box of assorted materials and encouraged to pull threads to her heart's content, the destructive results of her hobby were eliminated. The term 'hobby' is used very intentionally to emphasize that this was a recreational activity for the child. When the behaviour was shaped to occur in programmed downtimes, the play aspect of pulling threads was a source of relaxation and comfort to her. In addition, shopping expeditions for new and interesting textiles became a motivating focus for development of cognitive and communication skills.

Skill Building

Establishing skills before problems develop is the optimal way to manage behaviour. Behaviours of all kinds are learned. When a need is satisfied, the behaviour that prompted the satisfaction will be repeated. As teachers of the deafblind, we must walk a thin line between encouraging behaviours that communicate needs and discouraging behaviours that socially isolate or threaten the child's well-being. Reading a child, in the sense of interpreting behaviour, is the foundation of all language and social development. By knowing when to respond, when to ignore, and when to redirect; we are forming the child's concepts about the effectiveness of emerging behaviours. Whenever possible, we must attempt to anticipate the child's next developmental need and provide the means for the child both to communicate and to satisfy that need.

Under the heading 'Skill Building,' a mention must be made regarding the need for deafblind children to have a method of relaxation. Relaxation goes beyond the contentment of engaging in a favourite activity. Relaxation is a physical response characterized by soft muscle tone. Deafblind children need to learn tactile acceptance of comforting touch from another. We must remember the previously mentioned difficulties of infant/parent bonding and the frequency of tactile defensiveness in deafblind children. Each child will have unique experiences in this regard, but a major portion of a deafblind person's social life will be tactile. Just as colour and sound fill the lives of others, deafblind individuals need a spectrum of tactile sensations. Being able to relax in the comfort of a caregiver's touch is a necessary starting point in building this spectrum.

Choices

Issues of control underlie many situations in which behaviour has become a problem. All people must have choices in regard to their daily experience. The scope of options available to us change and widen as we progress through childhood, adolescence, and adult life. Teachers of the deafblind need to recognize this developmental process in the lives of their students and provide appropriate choices to them. There are no yardsticks to establish what constitutes a reasonable level of control at any given stage of development, but within individual programs consideration must be given to the child's need to experience expanding opportunities to express him/herself through meaningful choice making.

Stage 4: Implementation

Once a strategy is devised, it is important that the planned approach be implemented effectively. There is a single key to this stage of the model: consistency. Through team meetings and dialogue, everyone who interacts with the student must have knowledge of the strategy. More important, all of those people must agree to support the strategy. Although this approach sounds like common sense, it is often at this stage that the model breaks down. Team members can be affected by the emotional content of their interactions with students and can begin to feel the pull of personal agendas. During the period of implementation, open dialogue must be encouraged and opportunities provided to resolve any conflicts that develop. As well, in cases of severe problems, such as aggressive behaviours, provision should be made for debriefing after episodes of reoccurrence.

During implementation, records that monitor the ongoing results of the strategy are accumulated. The form and content of these records will vary according to the problem addressed. A general caution is required here. Statistics and time studies are unlikely to be sufficient unless they are accompanied by additional notes indicating contextual information about reoccurrences. It is the context in which the behaviour occurs that may reveal the meaning of the behaviour. This information will be important when the strategy is evaluated.

Stage 5: Evaluation

The implementation stage will have a timetable for duration and criteria for success. At the appropriate time a decision must be made as to whether the strategy is working. At this point questions should be raised regarding continuation, modification, or discontinuation of the strategy. If it is decided that the strategy was not effective, the process must start again at Stage 1, using whatever new information has become available during the initial attempt.

Final Thoughts

It is my sincere hope that the model of behaviour management offered here is found to be of some help in assisting young deafblind individuals to resolve their difficulties. We must remember that behavioural problems are social in nature and that we cannot separate the child's problem from the social context of which we are a part. The child's behaviour reflects as much about our inability to discover the meaning of his/her world as it does about the child's inability to understand the world at large.

Summary

1. The preconditions of social-emotional adjustment are:
   • the ability to form emotional bonds
   • an awareness of self
   • an awareness of environmental choices
   • the ability to manage emotions and behaviour.
2. Establishing an emotional bond is the first step in social development.
3. The security of an emotional bond allows us to explore the environment.
4. Social-emotional development is characterized by pendulum movements of

our attention between our locus of security and new aspects of our environment.

5. Deafblind infants must be provided compensatory sensory information to promote attachment to their mother and to avoid the development of patterns of startle reactions.

6. Self-stimulatory behaviours are adaptive in nature and assist the deafblind child to cope with incomplete or confused sensory information.

7. The deafblind child needs to experience control through resonance activities.

8. The deafblind child gains experience in the environment through hand-over-hand guided exploration.

9. The deafblind child progresses through stages of awareness and competence within each new activity (see Interaction Sequence).

10. The interaction sequence must be applied with sensitivity to the child's subjective state and emotional readiness.

11. Deafblind children must learn about emotions from direct experience.

12. Unless appropriate techniques are utilized within an educational setting, the deafblind child can be expected to display behaviour problems.

13. Behaviour management should begin with an attempt to understand the meaning of the targeted behaviour to the child.

14. Confusion in communication and concept development often underlie behavioural difficulties.

REFERENCES

Bowlby, John (1969) *Attachment and Loss*. New York: Basic Books
McInnes, J.M., and J.A. Treffry (1982, 1993, 1997) *Deaf-Blind Infants and Children: A Developmental Guide*. Toronto: University of Toronto Press
Nafstad, Anne (1992) *Space of Interaction*. Publication No. 9. Dronninglund, Denmark: Nordic Staff Training Centre for Deafblind Services
Stillman, Robert D., and Christy W. Battle (1984) *Developing Prelanguage Communication in the Severely Handicapped: An Interpretation of the Van Dijk Method*. New York: Thieme-Stratton

7

Social/Sex Education for Children and Youth Who Are Deafblind

TOM MILLER

Introduction

'I am convinced that it is not a question of IF our child should have sex, but WHEN and WHERE. And we must accept the fact that sexuality education cannot be too early – but it can be too late' (Betty Pendler, special needs parent and advocate). This quote points to the ongoing controversy in social/sex education among families of children with and without disabilities. It is a topic that is both personal and highly public and that throughout the history of both regular and special education has been viewed as a subject of top priority and then subsequently ignored. It is a topic overlain with emotion and a diversity of personal and cultural values and, especially in the area of disability education, ignored until a crisis or problem erupts.

In the early 1970s there was a great deal of awareness and activity regarding the social/sexual rights of people with disabilities. A variety of curriculums, articles, workshops, and policies were developed to address the needs of both students and adults with single or multiple disabilities. Unfortunately, owing to a variety of factors, the intensity of these efforts gradually waned and social/sex education for the disabled continues to this day to be a severely underdeveloped component of both school and community living programs. All too often, social/sex 'education' occurs only on an informal and reactive level, that is, as a response to a crisis. My purpose in this chapter will be to offer a concrete and 'proactive' approach to addressing the social/sexual issues of children and young adults with deafblindness.

Problem Overview

Why does the child or young adult with deafblindness often make significant strides in the structured activities of self-help skills or prevocational training and then demonstrate such severe social deficits, such as lack of initiative, inability to structure his/her own free time, poor decision-making skills, or inability to form social relationships? What are some of the factors that lie at the root of this issue? This lack of social-emotional development seems to stem from the interplay of many factors, which cannot be truly isolated from one another. The purpose of this overview, however, will be to reflect upon some of the causes of this social lag and to illustrate the role of both staff and parents in remediation of social/sexual learning deficits.

Social/sex education for the deafblind, indeed for all children and youth, is a lifelong learning task that needs to be addressed from infancy onward. The basic premise of this chapter is that the child or young adult who is deafblind, at any level of functioning, has both social/sexual rights and responsibilities and that both staff and parents have a responsibility to educate and to create environments that allow these individuals to develop to their fullest potential. The information that will be presented covers a broad range of functioning levels and has been used successfully with children and young adults who are deafblind. The approaches and information also recognize the diversity of cultural and ethical opinions on social/sex education, but experience with their use has again shown them to be adaptable to a diverse set of values and across a wide range of individuals. Since there has been very little written in the area of social/sex education for persons who are deafblind, in this chapter a compilation is included of some of the successful interventions used with children and youth with deafblindness over the past fifteen years. These approaches have been adapted from literature related to individuals both with and without disabilities. In reading this chapter, please maintain an open mind and begin to consider how and when, not if, the topic of social/sex education is critical to the full development of children and young adults who are deafblind with and without additional disabilities. An outline of topics that will be covered follows.

Some Aspects to Consider in Social/Sex Education for Individuals with Disabilities

1. Ourselves and Society
2. The Individual with Deafblindness
3. Content of the Social/Sex Education Program
4. Techniques for Social/Sex Education Training

Ourselves and Society

In order to understand issues in social/sex education for children and young adults who are deafblind, we need to look briefly at the topic of sex education in general. The primary issue is dealing with the topic of 'sexuality,' not only for the disabled. Social/sex education is a controversial topic for each of us and for society in general. We have simply to pick up the newspapers, watch television or videos, or listen to music on the radio, and we are bombarded with images of social expectations and sexual images of who we are supposed to be, or at least what certain segments of society believe we should be. In the light of these images and the issues of curriculums within public schools, stereotypes, and misconceptions, it is apparent that a great deal of social confusion exists within the field of social/sex education as to what should be taught, who is to teach it, and how it should be taught. In general, unfortunately, among children and youth with and without disabilities social/sex education, if it occurs at all, occurs in a 'reactive' mode. All too often the result is non-teaching or ignoring the topic until it becomes a crisis, often prefaced by the adults in the situation with a giant 'OH NO!!!.' The crisis is generally handled in a negative manner through suspension, punishment, or the 'just say no' approach, with little emphasis on constructive learning or enabling the child to understand and problem solve more effectively in the future. As adults and caregivers, however, particularly in the area of social/sex education, we have to begin to realize that ignoring or not addressing this issue creates a situation where children and youth with or without disabilities are left to fumble along to interpret and to form values and impressions relative to social/sexual lifestyles and relationships without guidance or input.

Although in dealing with social/sexual issues we can never totally overcome the feeling of 'oh no,' we can approach the topic of sexuality for the disabled in a proactive manner, that is, by trying consciously to teach and address social/ sexual issues throughout the individual's life span. Utilizing a proactive approach places an emphasis on education and intervention that views social/ sexual experiences for children and youth with or without disabilities as 'opportunities' for learning, as signs of growing up, and as a stepping-stone to further development of decision-making skills to the best of the individual's abilities.

We can never totally solve the dilemmas of society regarding this topic, but we need to decide upon the actions that we, as adults and caregivers, will take in dealing with the subject of social/sex education for children and youth who are deafblind. Essential to our decisions is development of a level of self-knowledge and awareness about our own feelings and attitudes towards social/sexual topics both for ourselves and for the disabled. Beyond a greater emphasis on developmental play and social tasks during early childhood, the first step in social/sex education of children and youth who are deafblind is staff/parent attitude and values clarification and education. Given the confusion that exists concerning social/sex education among individuals without disabilities, the exploration by staff and parents of both personal social/sexual values and an ability to deal with this topic becomes of primary importance. Through workshops and by making resources available that deal with attitudinal and informational topics regarding social/sexual development and people with disabilities, both parents and staff can be aided in identifying and clarifying personal values. This initial step will enable us to initiate conversation among ourselves and/or with the individual with disabilities and to begin to develop or access resources to foster the social/sexual development of children or clients. Self-reflection will enable us first to see how we acquired our own social/sexual knowledge and behaviours and then to apply this experience to, or perhaps correct, the way children and youth who are deafblind learn these behaviours and put them into practice.

A key issue that makes this topic difficult for us can be found in reflection upon our own lives. For example, the following exercise uses three basic questions to help us to explore some of our personal feelings and/or beliefs regarding sexuality.

- Where did you learn about sex?
- What messages did you receive about it from those sources?
- What feelings did those messages create?

When this exercise is used with staff and caregivers, consistent trends or patterns in responses occur. Respondents most often report learning about sex from friends, magazines, television, radio, and books, with only a handful stating that schools or parents were their primary sources of information. If, as we shall see later, the child or young adult who is deafblind has no access to such incidental learning, how much more incumbent does it become for us as adults and caregivers to bring such learning to them? Without our intervention, how would the child or youth who is deafblind manage access to appropriate social/sexual knowledge when even the most common ways in which we acquired information are often inaccessible to them?

In addition, the messages and feelings about sex reported by workshop participants most often have a negative connotation. Confusion, guilt, anxiety, not something to talk about, and private are the most frequent responses, with few participants mentioning the positive aspects of intimacy and relationships. These attitudes and feelings, though common, should not stop us from trying to approach the topic of social/sex education, but rather, they should encourage us to look for both more accurate knowledge and ways to share appropriate information with children and youth who are deafblind.

In order to begin to provide social/sexual education to children and young adults who are deafblind, we can use the above exercises to help us to reflect upon our attitudes towards sexuality, our level of accurate knowledge regarding sexuality, and, even more important, our attitudes, feelings, and beliefs regarding sexuality for people with disabilities. We need to examine our feelings regarding the rights and responsibilities of individuals who are deafblind in the areas of sexual expression, privacy, access to information and services, the ability to choose relationships and living arrangements, and, in general, to make decisions that affect their social/sexual lives, which allows them to develop to their *fullest potential* (Gordon 1974).

Do we hold any of the myths regarding sexuality and the disabled, for example, that they are asexual, oversexed, dependent and childlike, a threat to others in the community? Do we react to the idea of sexuality and the need for social/sex education for the disabled with disbelief; revulsion; avoidance; suppression; or active encouragement (Chipouras et al. 1979)?

The first step towards a social/sex education program for people who are deafblind is the realization that the person with a disability, whether it is blindness, deafness, cerebral palsy, or multiple handicaps, does not by virtue or his/her disability cease to be a social/sexual being. It is coming to the realization through self-reflection and seeking out accurate information that it is most often our misconceptions about sexuality and disability that not only hinders our ability to view the disabled as social/sexual beings but, even more, stifle their development of appropriate social/sexual expression, self-concept, and the motivation to live as independently as possible (ibid.). It is achieving the realization that just as our own social/sexual attitudes and behaviours are shaped or distorted by our daily interaction with others, the media, and experiences, the person with disabilities, no matter the type or degree of infirmity, is daily being moulded and affected as to his/her social/sexual development by the social attitudes and interactions with the people in his/her social situation. Finally, it is achieving the realization that the loss of incidental learning through the senses of vision and hearing for deafblind individuals makes it even more imperative for us to intervene and interpret life experiences and to provide access to information to allow them to achieve social/sexual independence to their fullest potential.

The development of a social/sex education program for the deafblind begins with the belief that children and youth who are deafblind have the same basic social/sexual rights and responsibilities as we do. It begins with expanding the definition of 'sex' beyond the 'act' to the realization that sex is 'who we are,' that our maleness and femaleness are an integral part of all our day-to-day interactions and instruction with children and youth who are deafblind.

The definition of sexuality needs to take into account the integration of its physical, emotional, intellectual and social aspects (Chipouras 1979). Sexuality refers not only to body parts or the 'physical aspects of sexual expression,' but to the total person, the individual, and the full range of his/her social values, social relationships, and awareness and performance of social responsibilities. In teaching social/sex education , we need to adhere to this broader definition of sexuality. Social/sexual development is not limited to the home or classroom, but is totally integrated into our daily existence. Our world is a social world, and living on any level, no matter how basic, of necessity involves relating to oneself and to others. In all our work, socialization, and interests, sexuality is an expression of one's personality and is evident in every aspect of one's interactions.

Through self-reflection and acceptance of this broader definition, we further realize that social/sex education is not a static process. Unlike a skill, such as hand washing, which you teach and then say knowledge is achieved, our social/ sexual expression is relative to age, living situation, social groups, and so on, and changes in learning and/or life circumstances for the individual with deaf-blindness will lead to the need, or better an opportunity, to teach a higher-level social skill or to make a needed adaptation.

In the next section we shall look more specifically at the impact of deafblind-ness on social/sexual learning and further refine our roles and responsibilities in this essential area of deafblind education.

The Individual with Deafblindness

Since social/sexual development is an ongoing process, it is necessary to con-sider some of the early childhood factors that might hinder the progression of social/sexual learning for the individual who is deafblind with or without addi-tional disabilities. Unlike a child without disabilities, who is able, beginning at birth, to receive and respond to physical, verbal, and social stimulation from his environment and those around him, the child who is deafblind begins life in a state of sensory deprivation. The nature and extent of the child's impairment of near and far senses imposes upon him/her varying degrees of social isolation. For the child who is deafblind, the loss of auditory social language and full visual interaction with the environment creates severe limits on the child's early mobility, directed exploration of his world, and, most important, vicarious social learning input.

The child who is deafblind very often lacks contact with other children, and frequently both parents and staff are confused as to how best to stimulate or interact with the child beyond basic needs fulfillment. Basic developmental interaction patterns, such as meaningfully playing with or seeking out objects, playing with parents, imitative play, and cooperative play with others, are therefore often limited experiences for the child. Sensory impairments decrease exposure to the repeated social/sexual experiences that sighted children and youth visually experience throughout their day. Opportunities to observe parent-to-parent hugs or affection, use of simple phrases of politeness, expressions of emotion, flirtatious behaviours and/or body language cues, verbal innuendoes, moments shared between best friends, variations in styles of dress, and so on, all taken for granted by individuals with vision and hearing, are too often inaccessible to the child who is deafblind, leading to a cumulative deprivation in the area of social/sexual learning. As a result, the child who is deafblind often builds his/her own world and finds satisfaction in self-stimulating behaviours.

What happens when this socially and emotionally underdeveloped person enters adolescence? The adolescent who is deafblind must not only puzzle out the physical changes of this period, but must also deal with its new social demands. Because of physical growth and often adequate development in other areas of learning, the adolescent who is deafblind is suddenly confronted with attempts by others to adapt his or her social behaviours to age-appropriate guidelines within specific contexts (e.g., work or home). Some behaviours, for example, hugging or being physical with staff, are no longer viewed as cute or appropriate and become instead 'problem' behaviours in need of modification. During this period, the individual with deafblindness often remains in a state of social isolation relative to peer interaction. Because of the unique modes of communication used by learners who are deafblind or the limited ability to acquire language, an inability to express feelings and emotions may exist and often results in frustration and acting-out behaviours. The school or work site, with their emphasis on structure, may foster further frustration and/or continued compliance or rigidity, without offering opportunities for making choices or moving towards greater personal growth. Even the student's leisure time may continue to be so programmed that opportunities for spontaneous social interaction and initiative may be hindered. Finally, a lack of role models within the living situation and/or a lack of awareness on the part of staff or parents as to how to observe and foster social and sexual development may further impede movement towards social-emotional maturity.

In addition, the lack of basic concepts, such as body-parts labels, appropriate/inappropriate touch, how to say no assertively, dealing with strangers, and social/sexual decision-making skills places the individual who is deafblind at significant risk for physical and/or sexual abuse.

Development of these social/sexual skills and behaviours is essential for integration into society and for enabling children and youth who are deafblind to achieve and develop social relationships to their fullest potential. Our role as parents and professionals becomes one of mediator or facilitator. We need to help to bring the realities of social/sexual experiences into focus for the individual who is deafblind and to expose and interpret the multitude of social/sexual cues that are lost given decreased sensory awareness. Ideally, our role will be one of partnership, where school and parents alike work together to develop the social/sexual skills *essential* to the lifetime success of children and youth who are deafblind at every level of functioning. Accomplishing this role requires openness and a willingness to work together to look at the realities of life that children and youth who are deafblind will face in the *real world* and to identify the resources and/or how each of us will personally bring them this essential knowledge. Since social/sex education is really an ongoing process that occurs whenever staff or parents and students interact, the implementation of a social/sex education program requires each of us to identify, particularly in the area of sexuality issues, our level of comfort with various topics and to develop our own skills or to seek out appropriate knowledge, resources, and/or individuals to teach these essential life tasks.

Within social/sexual learning situations, a model developed by Annon (1974) offers a decision-making hierarchy to enable each of us to determine our level of comfort with a topic and to seek additional personal or professional resources as needed. The model provides a progression from simple permission giving to providing limited information and specific suggestions, and/or to seeking intensive therapeutic intervention. It offers an opportunity for staff and parents to work together in defining their respective roles in dealing with social/sexual issues in the lives of children and youth who are deafblind and realize that it is acceptable to seek help and not to have all the answers about how to intervene in or facilitate each child's or young adult's social/sexual development. After a discussion of some of the content areas of a social/sex education program, we will look in greater depth at techniques we can use to define and achieve our role of mediator or facilitator in working with children and youth who are deafblind.

Content: What and When to Teach

Social/sex education is more than just the facts: it is a way of life. Social/sex education is an intimate part of our daily life with the child, adolescent, or young adult who is deafblind, whatever the level of functioning. The social/sexual life tasks are the same for individuals who are deafblind as they are for individuals without disabilities, but owing to an array of developmental and experiential issues, the rate and type of access to information will vary. The saying 'There are two things we can give our children, the first is roots and the other is wings' (Anonymous) offers an analogy for what we are trying to teach the child or adolescent who is deafblind in developing social/sexual knowledge and skills.

The content of what we teach in social/sex education needs to be seen as fully integrated into all the life skills that our children learn from birth onward. The roots of social/sexual development for children and youth who are deafblind lie in the development of self-esteem, communication, choice and decision-making skills, control, and forming a network of supports and relationships. The wings of social/sexual development are the content areas of social/sexual skills and knowledge needed to enable them to participate as fully as possible in life.

Before reviewing some of these content areas of knowledge for different age levels, let us look briefly at one of the key developmental tasks of early childhood relative to social/sexual development. This key area is the development of self-esteem, which according to Dorothy Briggs is 'the mainspring that slates every child for success or failure as a human being' (1975, 3). In reviewing the tasks of self-esteem development for children ages birth through young adulthood, it is important to remember that children with disabilities also need to go through these life tasks, but as we noted earlier, their rate of development may vary with the degree of their disabilities. Our role as facilitators or mediators, however, requires that we keep these tasks in focus and realize that all of the skills, such as self-help, communication, play, fine motor, and mobility, which we so conscientiously put into our individualized education plans, have as their ultimate goal the development of self-esteem and social/sexual independence.

Because, as we noted earlier, so much of the development of social skills and self-esteem were acquired incidentally during our early childhood years and adolescence, we need both to recognize the ways we are currently nurturing their development and to look at ways we can do better. During the early childhood period (birth to six years), as parents, professionals, and caregivers, through our touch and handling we communicate to deaf-blind individuals the concept of '*I am lovable*' and form the basis for later life attachments. '*I exist*' or '*I am separate from you*' comes as we structure the world of the child who is deafblind to allow him/her greater freedom, choice-making, and the ability to control events in the environment through communication and action. The simple goals that we often set of choosing a snack or toy are important precursors to the later larger decisions in life. The sense of '*I can*' comes with increased independence and mastery over their environment (Briggs 1975, 3–4, 124–38).

In the middle years (ages six to twelve), the child enters a period of achievement and improved competence, when he/she begins to move towards greater interaction with peers and adult models other than parents, thus developing the sense of '*I am worthwhile*' (Briggs 1975, 4, 139–72). We need to consider how the living and school situations are offering opportunities to expand these children's sense of growing independence and movement into the world.

The young adult or adolescent years (ages thirteen to twenty) mark a period of definition of the self, discovering and clarifying who one is in relation to one's sexual orientation, one's readiness for an occupation, and improving one's self-confidence. These issues often continue to evolve into the adult years, where one expands one's sense of self-awareness and ability to give as well as receive, and increases one's sense of self-respect (Briggs 1975, 153–76).

The social/sexual challenges or issues for the adolescent and young adult who are deafblind are the same as for individuals without disabilities, but their ability to grow in these areas is often more limited by their social environments and learning opportunities than is that of their peers. Many of us, as both parents and caregivers, are faced with the challenge of creating age-appropriate learning situations in areas such as friendships or dating, while we ourselves still wrestle with these issues in our personal lives. We are challenged as to how to communicate social/sexual cues, which are often non-verbal for us, into language and/or concepts understandable to the person who is deafblind. Later, in a discussion of techniques, we shall see that the limitations of teaching and expressing these concepts are most often a function of our need to be creative and socially engineer learning opportunities for children and young adults with deafblindness.

Although it is an artificial separation, the 'wings' of a social/sex education program for learners who are deafblind parallels in content what each of us needed to learn in early childhood and young adulthood. Since within the space of this chapter a detailed explanation of each of the curriculum content areas cannot be given, the reader is encouraged to utilize the curricula and resource materials cited in the references in order to grasp the full range and scope of resources available.

Social/Sex Education Core Curriculum

- *Understanding oneself: self awareness* – body parts, body language, feelings, self-control, physical development, gender
- *Understanding bodily functions* – toileting, grooming, hygiene, menstruation
- *Understanding individual differences* – uniqueness, puberty, body image, positive self-concept
- *Understanding the need to respect self and others* – privacy, self-image, assertiveness
- *Understanding relationships with others* – family, friends, strangers, dates, decision-making skills, avoiding abuse and exploitation

- *Understanding adult lifestyles* – single, married, gay, parenting, group home
- *Understanding medical aspects of sexuality* – conception, birth control, AIDS, sexually transmitted diseases, prevention
- *Understanding sexuality terms (signs)* – body parts, actions

In reviewing this list, it might be easy to say that these topics apply only to higher-functioning children and youth who are deafblind, but access to this knowledge to the highest degree of their potential is a basic right of all individuals who are deafblind. The lack of social/sexual development all too often is the result of waiting to expose the child or young adult who is deafblind to these essential life concepts when we feel that they are ready to learn them. If, as stated earlier, even persons without disabilities often do not have full access to knowledge in these core areas, how can we expect progress among children and young adults who are deafblind if we do not attempt to supply them with such information? Although, for the more severely disabled, exposure to signs and information will differ in degree from the level of social/sexual knowledge provided to the higher-functioning child or young adult who is deafblind, staff awareness of the individual's right to factual knowledge is essential.

In the life of all children these tasks are not begun at arbitrary ages, but are developmental from birth; children with deafblindness, however, require constant efforts to make conscious learning that is taken for granted in the sighted world. For example, a child is not suddenly given the names and labels for emotions at age three. His/her parents have been providing that information since birth, and it has constantly been reinforced by visual and auditory images and interactions both with peers and through various media. For the child who because of deafblindness has had limited opportunities for incidental learning, we must consciously provide this input using accessible modes of communication and tactile input. This task isn't easy, but once again the difficulty lies not with the child so much as with our beginning to make social/sexual learning a conscious part of our day-to-day interactions with our children.

How often in the day-to-day existence of a child who is deafblind do we use signs for *all* their body parts or do we refer to them as boys or girls? If input will later equal output in terms of learning and language, then it seems essential that we use language in the area of social/sexual learning with greater frequency to develop truly the child's sense of self. The individual education plan (Personal Plan) of each child and youth who is deafblind must incorporate goals related to the present level of social/sexual development and challenge the attainment of greater independence and skills.

Often we neglect to deal with social/sexual issues, stating that the person who is deafblind is not ready to be exposed to or learn a specific topic, but in this area, as in other areas of learning, children will not internalize and/or act upon that which they do not understand. We need to be careful that in our waiting for moments of readiness we are not simply avoiding the topic of social/ sexual education. For example, holding off presenting sign or language input relative to sexual body parts or gender until one feels the child is ready runs the risk of *never* inputting that knowledge and/or missing prime teachable moments. As is the case with all learning, our challenge is not to underestimate the ability of the child who is deafblind to accomplish these tasks; rather, we should provide ongoing opportunities to refine and/or develop these skills. Roots can be healthy only if given enough sustenance and room to grow. The child who is deafblind can accomplish these tasks only if given opportunities to practise and rehearse the social/sexual skills we all too often take for granted in our own lives.

Adolescence is inevitable; we cannot stop the processes of physical development, but we can hope that the social/sexual knowledge we have shared with children who are deafblind will better prepare them for it. The tasks of adolescence for the individual who is deafblind will be the same as they are for all teens, but the rate at which and how the information is presented may vary, along with the opportunities to practise and master the social/sexual skills of this period. The significant issues that physiological changes create may vary, depending upon the extent of additional emotional and physical disabilities. For example, for the adolescent who is deafblind with additional disabilities, the physical changes and mood swings of adolescence may be expressed by acting out or masturbation at inappropriate times and places. For the more cognitively able individual who is deafblind, the key issues might be meeting and maintaining friendships or dating. The content of this adolescent/young adult period, which continues into adulthood, is once again the content that each of us needed and continues to need to learn in our social/sexual dealings with one another. It is the content of self-development and self-care and the tasks of relating to others socially and sexually.

Our task is to act as a support or sounding board to enable the child or young adult who is deafblind to balance their needs and to master the social/sexual tasks of this period to the level of their fullest potential.

Techniques

What techniques can we most effectively use to teach the person who is deafblind these essential life tasks given their wide range of functioning levels and living situations? This is where the actual teaching of social/sexual skills to

children and young adults who are deafblind has often run into its greatest difficulty. We can usually convince ourselves that we need to address the topic, but
when we look at the individual who is deafblind, we shake our heads and wonder where to begin. The key point, however, is not where to begin, but how and
when most effectively to deliver or facilitate social/sexual learning for the deafblind individual.

Children and adolescents who are deafblind are so diverse in terms of their
levels of functioning, living situations, and levels of social supports, that no one
answer can be given as to how or when to teach them. Since each child, youth,
or adult brings to each situation his/her own unique personality, level of skills,
and learning style, their needs and intervention strategies must be considered
from an individual perspective. Rosalyn Kramer Monat has outlined the factors
that affect individuals with multiple disabilities ability to exercise their social/
sexual rights and responsibilities in the following manner:

• COGNITIVE LEVEL: that is, the degree of impairment (e.g.: mild, moderate, severe, profound)
• ADAPTIVE SKILLS: that is, self-concept, social attitudes, peers, parents,
  staff, laws, and so on
• ENVIRONMENT: that is, living situation – independent, group home, family home, residential facility, and so on (adapted from Monat 1982)

Each of these factors would affect both the type of approach used in communicating social/sexual rights and responsibilities to the individual and the
degree to which he/she will effectively be able to exercise those rights. For
example, at the lower end of the developmental and living spectrum, the intervention approach may be more behaviourally oriented and/or concentrate
more on staff behaviour regarding client rights to privacy and age-appropriate
physical handling. At the higher end of the spectrum, more formal instruction
and education coupled with providing the individual with the freedom and
opportunity to exercise his/her rights and responsibilities would be the method
of intervention. Figure 7.1 (Miller, 1994) attempts to outline graphically the
internal/external factors in decision-making for planning social/sex education
interventions.

An effective intervention must achieve a balance in the often conflicting
forces of the physical development of the person who is deafblind, his/her functional levels of language, cognitive, and social/emotional development, his/her
living situation, and the additional environmental factors of social, parental,
cultural, and staff expectations. The level and method of intervention should to
be viewed as a continuum; variations in approach should be based upon the

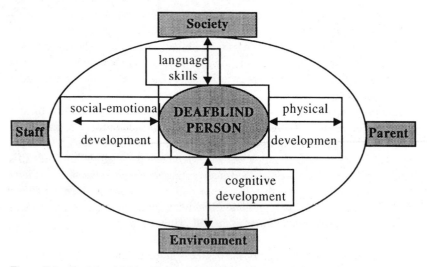

Figure 7.1   Decision-Making Factors in Planning Social/Sex Education

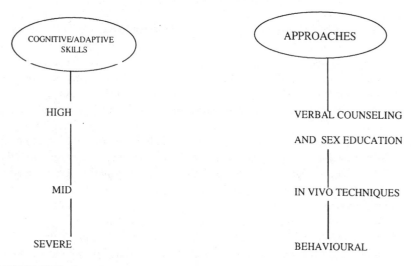

LIVING SITUATION: home; dorm; institution; community group home; own apartment

Figure 7.2   Educational Approach Based on Skills

child/young adult's level of adaptive and cognitive skills and his/her present-future living situations. See figure 7.2.

When all of the following techniques are utilized, the emphasis needs to be upon 'action.' We all learn by 'doing' and the learning of *functional* social/ sexual skills can be 'a lot of fun.' The key feature of a method for instructing children, adolescents, or adults with deafblindness (with or without additional disabilities) in social/sexual skill development is using an approach that is both adaptable to their wide range of functioning levels and that raises staff confidence and comfort in dealing with these issues. One such approach, which has been used successfully with severely challenged to high-functioning students has been developed by Jean Edwards and S. Wapnick in their two curricula, *Being Me* (Edwards 1979) and *Feeling Free* (1982). A brief summary of their approach follows.

The key concepts proposed by Edwards and Wapnick (1982) offer a method of defining social/sexual behaviours and tasks by the four workable categories of: 'Appropriate/Inappropriate' and 'Public/Private.'

'Appropriate/inappropriate' refers not to when a situation is right or wrong, but to whether or not the behaviour matches the situation. In many instances, it is a commonsensical decision (e.g., choosing whether or not it is appropriate to wear sandals in the snow), while in other instances it is tied to societal expectations or judgments (e.g., how we meet or greet strangers as opposed to our more intimate greetings with family members).

The second set of categories, 'public/private,' is defined as follows: 'Public' refers to any place where people can or may see you 'Private' refers to any place where there is little or no chance of being seen (e.g., bathroom or bedroom with doors and curtains closed). These terms also stress age-appropriate behaviours and encourage decision-making skills by children and youth who are deafblind with or without additional disabilities. Finally, these categories are adaptable to planning interventions for a wide range of functioning levels, and they contribute to relaxing attitudes dealing with social/sexual situations.

Although discussions around cultural sensitivity should occur and be taken into account when decisions are being made on how to define certain behaviours within situations (e.g., home vs. school), in our experience these terms can be used to define the majority of social/sexual behaviours and can serve as a jumping-off point to develop intervention plans and social/sex education lesson plans. For example, whether in the home or in the residence, it is inappropriate for an adolescent who is deafblind to masturbate in public. A learning sequence can be developed based upon the individual's level of functioning to teach the appropriate time and place to masturbate in each living situation. Or, at the higher end of the developmental spectrum, education regarding social/sexual rights and responsibilities for making decisions about sexual intercourse and the use of safe sex can be taught using interactive techniques and models.

Although the Edwards and Wapnick curricula (1979; 1982) provide us with a concrete framework to define many topics of social/sexual learning in the home, school, group home, or other community living situations, a variety of techniques or approaches should be used to put a curriculum into action.

The approaches that I shall overview have one overriding concept: as staff and caregivers we need both *to seize the moment* and *sometimes to create the moment* to optimize social/sexual learning opportunities for the child or young adult who is deafblind, whatever his/her level of developmental functioning or degree of independence.

The following are some techniques that have been useful in developing concepts of social/sexual rights and responsibilities among children and youth who are deafblind.

Role Playing

Role playing can be utilized across the full spectrum of functioning levels. For example, to prepare a child within the severe to moderate range for the onset of menstruation, since many children who are deafblind within this functional range have difficulty dealing with changes in their routine, the child should be introduced to the wearing of a sanitary pad on a monthly basis.

Role playing situations (e.g., on an actual mobility lesson), where staff who are unfamiliar approach the student to try to persuade him or her to come with them, can be used to teach children and young adults in the mid- to high-functioning range about self-protection techniques and how to deal with strangers.

Activities, such as dancing, eating in a restaurant, or dating, can also be rehearsed through role playing with follow-up practice opportunities in real-life situations. Finally, role playing and/or reverse role playing, where the staff or caregivers act out the child's behaviours, can be used to 'debrief' or review social/sexual situations, such as workplace or community behaviours, after community experiences have occurred.

In Vivo Counselling/Teaching

In vivo counselling/teaching uses moments of opportunity for social/sexual learning that occur throughout the day. Especially for children and young adults who may not be able to learn out of context, in this technique the appropriate behaviour and language are replayed or demonstrated within the actual situation. For example, if a child consistently leaves the bathroom and returns to class with his pants undone, staff would not adjust the child's clothing in the hallway or classroom area, but rather would return to the bathroom to illustrate the appropriate time, place, and behaviour to do up one's pants. In the case of another student, who consistently lifted up her shirt in public to adjust her bra, staff and family members intervened by taking the student to a restroom or other private area and rehearsing and teaching the appropriate language and behaviours for a private activity.

Photos, Slides, Pictures, Drawings

Photos, slides, pictures, and drawings can be utilized in both fostering language and choice making around both public/private and appropriate/inappropriate social/sexual behaviours. These media, whether hand-drawn pictures, self-produced slides or photos, or commercially available slides or photos (see Edwards and Wapnick 1979, 1982; *Stanfield Publishing Catalogue* 1997; *Special Education Curriculum* 1979), allow the child or young adult who is deafblind both time and multiple opportunities to review images of social/sexual situations and expressions of emotion or feelings and/or to learn basic body parts or gender concepts. For example, language experience stories or the Van Dijk method of conversational signing, magazine pictures, or actual photos of the child or adolescent who is deafblind within certain situations could be used to offer language about feelings or behaviours within those situations.

Video

Video offers the opportunity to replay actual social/sexual situations to reinforce both positive behaviours and to offer options or learning opportunities for dealing with inappropriate behaviours. For example, while a group of adolescents who were deafblind were being videotaped in the work activity centre, a female student was observed periodically reaching under the table to rub the thigh of a male student sitting next to her. Both students had been involved in a social/sex education program and exposed to the concepts of public/private and appropriate/inappropriate (Edwards and Wapnick 1978, 1982). The videotape was replayed individually with the students to review and provide language around the topics of public and private behaviour in the workplace, where such behaviour might be more appropriate, and public and private body parts and the right of the person to refuse or allow such touch.

Models

Although it is best for children and youth who are deafblind to be given the names/signs for their sexual body parts during normally occurring opportunities from an early age (e.g., bathing), lifelike models of sexual body parts (Jackson Pelvic Models) and/or anatomically correct dolls (e.g., Teach-a- Bodies; Victoria House Dolls) can be utilized as instructional and intervention aids. Concepts such as safe sex, sexual intercourse, menstruation, apprpopriate/ inappropriate touch, and the birth cycle can be taught through these models. The case study that follows this technique overview illustrates one such use for these models.

Books, Audiotapes

Although there still needs to be an increase in the number of books that are Brailled or recorded in the area of social/sexual education for use by children and young adults who are deafblind, this medium is often overlooked for mid- to high-functioning students. An audio tape such as *Your Changing Body* (Allen 1974) offers time for guided self-exploration; it can build both language and concept skills and offer a base for instruction in bodily changes and development. Books on tape or in Braille can also offer a common jumping-off point for parents, staff, and the child or young adult to share information on social/sexual topics.

Peer Support Groups

Peer support groups offer an opportunity for children and youth who are deafblind to explore social/sexual issues within a safe context. Such groups offer an opportunity for discussion and/or role playing to enable children and youth who are deafblind to be exposed to, practice or review strategies for dealing with social/ sexual issues in their lives. Teen weekends sponsored by schools for the blind, deaf, or deafblind or community based organizations for the deafblind could be utilized to provide an opportunity for career and social/sexual education.

Pulling It All Together

Let us spend a moment to pull all of this information together to develop an action plan to raise our awareness of how we might begin to foster more effectively the development of these essential life skills among deaf-blind individuals at all ages. A planning sheet, as shown in figure 7.3, will enable both staff and parents to begin to approach and work through social/sexual situations from a common framework. This framework clarifies each individual's level of comfort and ability to deal with social/sexual situations and to participate in the definition of workable outcomes. The questions are ones that easily can be internalized, so that the development of social/sexual knowledge or reactions to

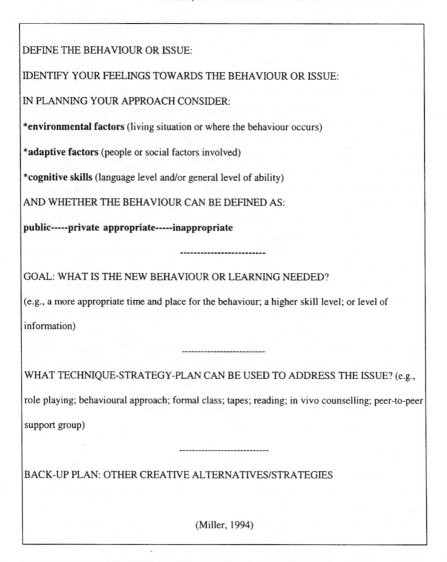

DEFINE THE BEHAVIOUR OR ISSUE:

IDENTIFY YOUR FEELINGS TOWARDS THE BEHAVIOUR OR ISSUE:

IN PLANNING YOUR APPROACH CONSIDER:

environmental factors (living situation or where the behaviour occurs)

adaptive factors (people or social factors involved)

cognitive skills (language level and/or general level of ability)

AND WHETHER THE BEHAVIOUR CAN BE DEFINED AS:

public-----private appropriate-----inappropriate

GOAL: WHAT IS THE NEW BEHAVIOUR OR LEARNING NEEDED?

(e.g., a more appropriate time and place for the behaviour; a higher skill level; or level of

information)

WHAT TECHNIQUE-STRATEGY-PLAN CAN BE USED TO ADDRESS THE ISSUE? (e.g.,

role playing; behavioural approach; formal class; tapes; reading; in vivo counselling; peer-to-peer

support group)

BACK-UP PLAN: OTHER CREATIVE ALTERNATIVES/STRATEGIES

(Miller, 1994)

Figure 7.3   Social/Sex Education Program Development Sheet

social/sexual situations for children and youth who are deafblind at any age can become as automatic a part of our home or school curricula as the activities of daily living.

Using the case example given in figure 7.4 (pp. 222–3), we can decide how we might wish to handle the behaviour in a given situation to foster both optimal social/sexual learning and understanding for this particular student to his fullest ability. The student TP in this case was a sixteen-year-old male at a residential school. The student demonstrated a mid- to high-functioning scatter of skills. In terms of language development, by using a combination of signs and pictures the student was able to pick up new concepts and learn new behaviours. The behaviour identified was occurring at both home and school and was of concern within both settings. The family felt comfortable with the fact that the staff and school were trying to develop a workable program to address the behaviour. The following offers a brief illustration of how the Social/Sex Education Program Development Sheet was utilized. After ruling out potential physical reasons and medical issues (e.g., medication) for this student's inability to achieve ejaculation, staff were asked to fill in the sheet prior to a staff meeting, and their perspectives were shared and discussed to arrive at the following plan.

In TP's case the above intervention resulted in more appropriate behaviour relative to time and place for social/sexual activity. The planning sheet offered staff and the family a common ground for beginning to address the issue and creatively working together to enhance TP's quality-of- life opportunities. Once again, for further content areas or examples of role-play topics, the reader is referred to the resource list at the end of this section.

Policy Development: Moving Ahead

Social/sex education for children and youth who are deafblind needs to occur as a home-school partnership. At present, all too often both parties at best defer to the other or at worst do not address the issue until some developmental crisis ensues. The school and parents need to work together to develop a vital atmosphere that offers optimal opportunities for the social/sexual development of each student as a unique individual personality. As is the case in all areas of learning for the deafblind, perhaps even more so in the realm of social/sex education, the need to balance staff expertise with parental cultural and/or other beliefs and with the uniqueness of each individual child or young adult who is deafblind is essential if optimal growth is to occur in this area. Schools, group homes, residential facilities, and agencies who provide services to children, youth, and adults who are deafblind should develop policies that clearly outline individual rights and staff and client responsibilities in the area of social/sex education and behaviours. Inservices and training for both parents and staff should be offered to communicate clearly that the goal of the school or agency, as they are in all other areas of learning, is to enable the individual who is deafblind to achieve the fullest possible level of social/sexual independence.

A clearly defined policy, developed wherever possible with the input and review of staff, parents, and consumers, should outline not only the philosophy of the school or agency, but even more important, the roles and responsibilities of the child, youth, or adult who is deafblind and the staff to enhance social/sexual learning. Since policies will vary with individual settings, for examples of useful policies the reader is referred to Gail Brown's *Human Sexuality Handbook* (1994), Pat Allen and LeeAnn Lipke's *Your Changing Body* (1974), and J. Edwards and S. Wapnick's *Being Me* (1979).

Summary

This chapter has offered a brief overview of some of the critical areas in the development of social/sex education programs for children and youth who are deafblind. As outlined in the key points below, the challenge both to improve and to enrich the lives of children and youth who are deafblind in the area of social/sexual development belongs to each of us, and the rewards for the implementation of effective programs will be fuller and more effective lives for all.

1. Social/sex education continues to be a controversial and generally ignored part of curricula and training materials for children and youth who are deafblind.
2. A pro-active approach needs to be implemented in teaching social/sexual skills to children and youth who are deafblind.
3. The first step in developing and implementing a social/sex education program for children and youth who are deafblind is to clarify our own personal values and attitudes towards sexuality and sexuality for the disabled.
4. Children and youth who are deafblind do not cease to be social/sexual beings because of their disabilities, and they possess the same social/sexual rights and responsibilities as persons without disabilities.
5. Deafblindness can severely limit access to both incidental and direct social/sexual learning and opportunities.
6. The role of parents and staff is to mediate, facilitate, clarify, and provide opportunities for social/sexual learning for children and youth who are deafblind.
7. The content of a social/sex education program for children and youth who are deafblind is intricately related to all facets of deafblind education, but

DEFINE THE BEHAVIOUR OR ISSUE: TP

The issue centres on the development of appropriate self-stimulation (masturbation) to avoid current practices of self-injury. TP across the day pulls at his scrotum. Although he achieves erection, he does not seem to ejaculate. Behaviour is fairly constant and occurs in public areas.

IDENTIFY YOUR FEELINGS TOWARDS THE BEHAVIOUR OR ISSUE:

Parents and staff are interested and willing to attempt intervention and feel comfortable in addressing the behaviour.

IN PLANNING YOUR APPROACH CONSIDER:

*environmental factors (living situation or where the behaviour occurs)
The dormitory area will be used as intervention site to stress the private nature of the behaviour.

*adaptive factors (people or social factors involved)
Staff and family will be encouraged to use consistent sign and place interventions in both home and school settings.

*cognitive skills (language level and/or general level of ability)
TP can read print and responds to both signs and pictures. It is the feeling of the team that he could transfer use of models to self.

AND WHETHER THE BEHAVIOUR CAN BE DEFINED AS:

public-----private appropriate-----inappropriate

Figure 7.4   Case Example: Social/Sex Education Program Development Sheet

GOAL: WHAT IS THE NEW BEHAVIOUR OR LEARNING NEEDED?

(e.g., a more appropriate time and place for the behaviour; a higher skill level; or level of information)

Goal is to encourage behaviour and limit it to an appropriate place, that is, a private space such as his bedroom.

WHAT TECHNIQUE-STRATEGY-PLAN CAN BE USED TO ADDRESS THE ISSUE? (e.g., role playing; behavioural approach; formal class; tapes; reading; in vivo counselling; peer-to-peer support group)

The strategy will entail the use of the Jim Jackson sex education models along with KY-Jelly. The team identified 1:00 p.m. as an appropriate time to offer TP private time and space. The sign for private time will be used along with a Polaroid of the Jackson model and jelly to allow TP a way to express his need for private time. The model will be presented to TP along with the Polaroid and the sign for private time. The model will be used to indicate to TP that it is the same as his penis, and using K-Y Jelly, stroking behaviour will be demonstrated on the model. TP will then be instructed that he can do the same. The student will be fully clothed throughout instruction and will be left in his room for private time to see if he will translate modelling to his own body without further intervention. Two staff members will carry out training protocol.

BACK-UP PLAN: OTHER CREATIVE ALTERNATIVES/STRATEGIES

To be determined after a trial period with initial intervention. Possibly, it will entail additional ways to instruct TP on body parts and their functioning.

Figure 7.4   (*concluded*)

particular attention needs to be given to increasing self-esteem and access to social/sexual learning opportunities.

8. As parents and staff, our role is to seize and create optimal moments for social/sex education within the real-life experiences of children and youth who are deafblind.

9. In program planning and implementation we should consider the functioning level of children and youth who are deafblind, their present and future living situation, and the utilization of appropriate communicative and interactive techniques.

10. Schools and community agencies serving children and youth who are deafblind should develop policy statements that facilitate opportunities for persons who are deafblind to access their social/sexual rights and responsibilities to their fullest potential.

Appendix I
Fifteen Facts of Deaf-Blind Sexuality Education
by J. Neff

1. It should be remembered that SEX is something we ARE, not something we DO.

2. We must recognize that deaf-blind children, adolescents and adults, like all others, are sexual beings with sexually related needs.

3. Be aware that it is never TOO EARLY to begin the purposeful sexuality education of any child, especially that of a deaf-blind child.

4. Sexuality education should be considered a learning experience that will enrich a child's life, giving him/her more understanding of themselves, their family, and society ... in short, a positive approach.

5. The sense of TOUCH is the most valuable learning tool that can be employed in teaching the complex concepts of sexuality.

6. Immediately upon entering a program, a child should be evaluated in order to determine the extent of self-awareness and sexual understanding. A program to meet the child's needs should be incorporated into the total course of study/care.

7. Never assume anything!

8. Just as an adult must manage many aspects of a low functioning deaf-blind child's life, so be it with his/her sexuality.

9. Each aspect of a child's sexuality must be considered a matter of 'HOW' and 'WHEN' it can best be approached rather than a matter of 'IF' it needs to be dealt with.

10. To effectively handle a child's sexuality, one must first be comfortable with his/her own sexuality.

11. Attention must consistently be given to the deaf-blind individual's social, emotional, and cultural understanding and development as well as to their communication development.

12. Be aware of mannerisms and activities that either carry sexual connotations or are indicative of one's particular sex membership which are assimilated through the use of one's vision and/or hearing.

13. Knowledge is never as dangerous as ignorance.

14. Be aware that an individual's image of himself is a basic part of their sexuality.

15. Gender identity is of prime importance to everyone, especially the deaf-blind individual.

(Reprinted with permission of author Jan Neff)

RESOURCES AND REFERENCES

Allen, Pat, and LeeAnn Lipke (1974) *Your Changing Body*. Audio tape. Chicago: Perennial Education

Annon, Jack S. (1974) *The Behavioural Treatment of Sexual Problems*, Vols 1 and 2. Honolulu: Enabling Systems

Bell, Ruth (1980) *Changing Bodies, Changing Lives*. New York: Random House

Briggs, Dorothy (1975) *Your Child's Self-Esteem*. New York: Doubleday

Brown, Gail T. (1994) *Human Sexuality Handbook: Guiding People Toward Positive Expressions of Sexuality*. Springfield, MA: Association for Community Living

Chipouras, S., D. Cornelius, et al. (1974) *Who Cares? A Handbook of Sex Education and Counseling Services*. Washington, DC: George Washington University

Dechesne, B.H.H., C. Pons, and A.M.C.M. Schellen, eds (1986) *Sexuality and Handicap*. Springfield, IL: Charles C. Thomas

Edwards, J., and S. Wapnick (1979) *Being Me*. Ednick Communications, Box 3612, Portland, OR 97208

– (1982) *Feeling Free*. Ednick Communications, Box 3612, Portland, OR 97208

Frank, Roger, and Jean Edwards (1988) *Building Self-Esteem in Persons with Developmental Disabilities*. Ednick Communications, Box 3612, Portland, OR 97208

Gordon, S. (1974) *Sexual Rights for the People ... Who Happen To Be Handicapped*. Syracuse, NY: Center on Human Policy Development, Syracuse University

Greenberg, Polly (1991) *Character Development: Encouraging Self-Esteem and Self-Discipline in Infants, Toddlers and Two-Year-Olds*. Washington, DC: National Association for the Education of Young Children

Griffiths, Dorothy M., Vernon L. Quinsey, and David Hingsburger (1989) *Changing Inappropriate Sexual Behavior*. Baltimore, MD: Paul H. Brookes

Hargie, Owen, Christine Saunders, and David Dickson (1987) *Social Skills in Interpersonal Communication*. London: Croom Helm

Jackson Pelvic Models, 33 Richdale Avenue, Cambridge, MA 02140; (617) 864–9063

Katchadourian, H.A., and D.T. Lunde (1975) *Fundamentals of Human Sexuality*. New York: Holt, Rinehart and Winston

Kolodny, R., J. Masters, and V. Johnson (1979) *Textbook of Sexual Medicine*. Boston: Little, Brown

Kroll, Ken, and Erica Levy Klein (1995) *Enabling Romance*. Bethesda, MD: Woodbine House

Marshall, Hermione (1989) 'The Development of Self-Concept,' *Young Children*, 44–51

McGinnis, Ellen, and Arnold Goldstein (1990) *Skillstreaming in Early Childhood*. Champaign, IL: Research Press Company

Miller, T. 'Social/Sex Education for the Deafblind.' Keynote Presentation: Fourth Canadian Conference on Deafblindness, Fredericton, NB, 1994

Monat, Rosalyn Kramer (1982) *Sexuality and the Mentally Retarded*. San Diego, CA: College-Hill Press

Monat-Haller, Rosalyn Kramer (1992) *Understanding and Expressing Sexuality*. Baltimore, MD: Paul H. Brookes

O'Day, Bonnie (1983) *Preventing Sexual Abuse of Persons with Disabilities*. St Paul, MN: Minnesota Program or Victims of Sexual Assault

Pomeroy, Wardell B. (1981) *Boys and Sex*. New York: Dell

– *Girls and Sex*. New York: Dell

Project MORE (1978) *Developing Responsible Sexuality*. Hubbard, IL

Ratner, Marilyn, and Susan Chamlin (1987) *Straight Talk*. New York: Viking Penguin

Santa Clara County Social Skills Curriculum (1990) Developed under SCORE Regionalization Project. To order contact B.J. McCallum, 1296 Maripose Ave., San Jose, CA 95126, at (408) 971–1353

Special Education Curriculum on Sexual Exploitation (1979) Comprehensive Health Education Foundation, 208 Pacific Highway S., Seattle, WA 98188

Teach-a-Bodies Instructional Dolls. P.O. Box 101444, Ft Worth, TX 76185; (817) 923-2380

Tymchuk, Alexander J. (1985) *Effective Decision Making*, Ednick Communications, Box 3612, Portland, OR 97208

Victoria House Dolls. P.O. Box 663, Forestville, CA 95436; (707) 887-1516

Zilbergeld, Bernie (1978) *Male Sexuality*. New York: Bantam

Zimbardo, Phillip (1978) *Shyness*. Boston, MA: Addison-Wesley

8

A Family Viewpoint

NORMAN BROWN and GINI CLOKE

Introduction

In reading this chapter, you must bear two things in mind. First, our experience is drawn from living in England, and, although it has been heart-warming to find from international contacts that parents' basic concerns and experiences are the same regardless of background or culture, we are aware that there are differences among cultures that affect family function and support. While we have tried to remain aware of possible differences and to emphasize what may be universal, the reader must remember that we are sharing thoughts and experiences that should not be taken as necessarily or always true. You must bring your own self to their interpretation. Secondly, we have decided not to attempt a scholarly exposition with many referenced authorities, since that would demand a book rather than a chapter and would limit what we want to say. The only references given are to key texts that have seminal significance. We are therefore offering our own distillation of experience and what we have drawn from others in the hope that you will gain from what is written here as much as we have gained from others we have met. You may find few answers, but it is often helpful simply to know that you are not alone in what you feel and are experiencing.

In writing, we refer mainly to 'parents' and 'professionals,' using the latter word to cover anyone who is paid for providing a service. We hope that this broad generalization will not offend too many readers. It certainly makes the writing easier. In lumping together all professionals we have also lumped together all parents. We have drawn no distinctions among birth parents, step-parents, foster parents, and adoptive parents, because we find more similarities than differences among them and are confident the reader will easily identify what does not apply to particular circumstances. In writing, we also found ourselves referring to our 'children' even when we were speaking of adults. We therefore decided to keep that approach, reflecting the truth that our offspring remain conceptually our children, regardless of age, and also to avoid tortuous language. The reader is urged to consider the truth of our observations rather than to think they are specific to particular ages; we shall point out when age is significant.

We have both been privileged, although we did not at first realize this, not only in having in our families deafblind sons, Gini's Ian and Norman's Stephen, but in having been for many years members of and having worked for Sense (the National Deafblind and Rubella Association in the United Kingdom) which has brought us rich contact with many families in our own country and around the world. We must thank them all, along with our partners and daughters, for what we are now trying to share with you. Some readers will recognize here what has appeared in previous articles and presentations by each of the authors, but we hope there is sufficient that is still thought provoking for everyone.

In this chapter we shall start with broad and general issues, moving to more specific matters before finishing with some recommendations that you may consider making a part of your own work.

Special but Ordinary

The first question to be answered is 'Are there elements concerned with having in the family a child who is deafblind that are so special that they require consideration in a separate chapter?' Are not all parental reactions shared and common? Can we not join in with others or simply share the services provided for other families where there is a disability? In many particulars we can so share, because we are as normal, and therefore as individual, as anyone else, but there are specific issues that cannot be ignored.

There are special elements for the family with a child born deafblind, because there are special elements for a child born deafblind, and they result from factors that make deafblindness a unique disability. Because vision and hearing are the major avenues of learning as well as the main communication receivers for most of us, the deafblind child has massive problems in making sense of the world and in relating to it and everything in it. And among the things in it are us. We parents are the ones with the first and continuing responsibility to bring the world to the child and the child to the world in an understandable way, and we cannot do that if we have not first brought ourselves to the child and the child to us in a loving and empowering way.

Therefore, one very special element for the parents of a child born deafblind is the result of impaired communication between infant and prime caregiver.

Here we are not speaking of communication in terms of formal language but in terms of basic social interaction. In the development of an infant, the infant is the main instigator. All parents worry about their responsibility for the development of their children, especially their first child; yet research shows that, of the interactions between a baby and a mother, the baby is responsible for initiating and continuing two-thirds of the interactions and the mother is responsible for only one-third. In that very early, loving, bonding, secure, and confidence-building interaction, it is normally the baby who leads the way. Parents are the great responders. This is probably just as well, since most of us embark upon parenthood with no previous training, and it may account for the fact that so many parents do a reasonably good job. If we wish to oversimplify, but with more than a grain of truth, we could claim that a parent is an adult who has been educated by a baby.

What happens if the baby is unable to lead? Or, more exactly, what happens if the signals the baby is giving out and receiving are not those we recognize or expect? Our 'education' is sadly lacking and the infant's development is hindered because we cannot join effectively in that developmental journey.

The Importance of Emotional Engagement

Increasingly, consideration is being given to the inferences of the Bonding and Attachment Theory (Ainsworth 1978; Bowlby 1982) for all development and to the place of real personal relationship in the massive need that deafblind children have for security, reassurance, and interaction (McInnes and Treffry 1982; Wyman 1986; Nafstad ,1989; Van Dijk 1991). Such considerations are discussed more fully in chapters 3, 4, and 6 of this book.

Many congenitally and early adventitiously deafblind children and adults display some of the characteristics of deprived children (Fox 1983), not because they were deliberately deprived but because the lack of or the impairment of their own proactive and reactive behaviour, sometimes compounded by actual separation through hospitalization, interfered with the early emotion-stabilizing, language-developing, and cognition-enhancing interaction with their primary care-givers. What may be necessary is the satisfaction of that primary need before there can be progress through even the first stage of development. But here we have to consider not only the effect on the child, who is in fact attempting to use everything available to him or her. What may be the effect upon parents who have so much love to give and yet have a child who displays some of the characteristics of a deprived child? It may not be realized that congenital deafblindness can lead to this state if the dual impairment is not compensated, or if there is enforced absence because of special treatment or hospitalization.

Sadly, confusions can also result from following 'good' but mistaken advice, or from having no advice at all. Parents are likely to add any apparent failures to their own threatening load of guilt and perceived inadequacy.

It is hard to keep giving if you seem to be getting little or nothing back, if your presence does not seem to be recognized or enjoyed, or if your advances appear to be rejected. You may easily slip into a state of being grateful to leave matters, and babies, alone if they are not bothering you, because you have more than enough on your plate already. It is not unusual for parents to speak of having to persuade their child to accept cuddles and physical contact, as if the child needed to be taught how to receive and give love. Luckily, the loving persistence of parents brings results, and the evidence provided by children who have benefited from good early intervention shows that nothing is inevitable.

Within deafblind theory, the principle of attending to such possibilities is increasingly stressed. It is vitally important for the emotional and mental health of all the family, including the deafblind child, to help rather than hinder the early building of relationships in the puzzling world into which the arrival of a deafblind baby plunges everyone.

This is not to say that nothing else matters, or that there should be no working on developmental programs that parents can begin following with their child. It is a caution to keep a balance. Recognition of the vital importance of early intervention may lead to a distortion of parent-child interaction if we are not careful to keep a balance. Hogg and Sebba (1986) are not alone in noting that parents of children perceived as disabled tend to adopt a more directive than interactive role with such children, and Van Dijk (1991) is aware also of the dangers of unconsciously encouraging such a tendency, while encouraging parents to institute teaching programs, mentioning the conclusion of Rogers (1988) that gentle support of a parent's spontaneous interactions with his or her disabled child seems to be more effective than emphasizing situations in which the mother has to carry out teaching tasks or therapy.

Enough now of the references, but this point underlies everything we wish to say, both to fellow parents and to involved professionals and friends. While recent study of congenital deafblindness prompts us to look at earlier and earlier stages of normal development for our starting point and our concepts, all study underlines the vital importance of building a good relationship as the necessary precursor to any successful developmental work. To put it more simply, underneath all the perceived or feared problems, my child is a child, and the best early intervention you can give is to help me respond better to what my child is trying to instigate or convey. The earlier you can do that the better, for then I and my child can get on with growing in harmony. Work among congenitally deafblind adults who have not had good intervention reveals the same truth, that responding appropriately and lovingly is a better starting-point than imposing a program.

Of course it would be unfair to leave everything to the deafblind child, and we parents need all the help we can get in taking up our responsibility for helping our child to move on. Nevertheless, communication in its ever widening sense will remain the greatest challenge, and the inability to involve our children in discussion of what is happening to them will be the greatest heartache. We shall become very sensitive to behavioural expression that tells us our child's current and past situations, but we shall be reduced to inspired guesswork when contemplating the future.

We can already see that there are special elements for families with a child who is deafblind. They are not elements that make such parents different from other parents; they are elements that present special challenges to perfectly ordinary parents.

Emotional Reality

In this chapter, we are being forced to address generalities – a daunting task in the face of such a diverse group of individuals and families. Yet there are some broad patterns that we think will give a basis for discussion.

An individual's emotional state plays the major role in governing energy and performance. Parents have to face their demanding but uncertain future without 'time out' to absorb what has happened and to prepare for it. Sometimes, in fact, we deal with our feelings by ignoring them or by swamping them in attention to necessary action. Rather than grieving and then getting on with things, we have to grieve as we go. All the emotions we experience are normal reactions, shared in varying degree by all, and they do look and feel very like the emotions associated with a bereavement or any major loss.

It was common, in fact, a few years ago to read that parents of disabled children mourned for the child they did not have. The authors do not find that to be so in their own experience or in the experience of the many such parents they have met. What is found is a necessary grieving – not for the children we did not have but for what has happened to the children we did have – and that is a very different thing. The emotional processes may be the same, but the outcomes and positive spin-offs can be quite different. The confusion and anger that in true mourning for someone who has died will have no positive outcome for the person mourned can be channelled into a driving force that produces real benefit for the disabled child whose limitations are grieved over. Reactions to the news of a child's disability seem to show a common pattern: first, the immediate shock, anger, and disbelief leading to, secondly, grieving and a feeling of isolation, an isolation that is sometimes even sought; thirdly, there is a process of adaptation characterized by information-seeking before the fourth and life-long process of adjustment begins.

You will have observed that not only have we chosen to say 'grieving' rather than 'mourning,' which is the term you may encounter in the research, but we have chosen 'adjustment' rather than 'acceptance' for the last stage. Acceptance is another concept about which we have reservations. We have never really 'accepted' what happened to our sons; it does not seem acceptable at all. However, we did adjust – time and time again. There were certainly key times of try-ing to face reality and 'accept' what was the reality at that time, but the exercise has had to be repeated at each of life's major milestones and sometimes in between. When sisters have made significant steps to independence – learning to ride a bicycle, changing to senior school, finding the first boyfriend – the comparison of progress and possibilities could not be avoided. Yet the spiral of adjustment continued with many little 'acceptances' along the way until com-parisons became meaningless and fell away, making the adjustments a little easier each time.

Earlier, we used the term 'necessary grieving,' because it does seem neces-sary to acknowledge those emotions some people may suppress as negative. Much of life involves coming to terms with things that can be good and bad at the same time. The pressure to be positive and to get on with life can cause us to bury other real and legitimate feelings, but there is a time limit on doing so. We know of two parents, admired and acknowledged as successful and competent, who suddenly and unexpectedly broke down completely. Subsequent treatment led to the realization that they had not allowed the grieving process, and it had lain hidden until time and a relatively minor upset produced a catastrophic out-pouring.

For most parents, the grieving and adjusting merge to become what could be called a coping force, or active coping. The loving anger can drive us on in seeking the best provision. We can solidify it into endurance to keep us going when our strength has failed. We can share it with others when that magical link of likemindedness is forged. But underneath everything there is an unremitting normality at work, and underneath all the questions is one we never dare voice: 'What about me?' It is a question that involved professionals will have to ask for us, because our emotional state will have as much effect on their work as will the emotional state of our child.

Newly involved professionals should consider the stage of adjustment that they have entered at. The reason their far-sighted plan is rejected may not be that it is bad, and it may not be that it will never be accepted. The cause of rejection could be that the parent is not yet ready emotionally to accept it at that time.

Emotion and Reason

It is fair to add that a newly involved professional may have to inherit the legacy of previously involved professionals. Some things seem never to be forgotten. For example, parents will remember vividly how the news was broken or how they learned about their child's disability. If the trauma was particularly negative, the subject may continue creeping into conversations even when the 'child' is a mature adult. This leads to two considerations. First, how should distressing news be broken? Secondly, a professional's greatest difficulty may be getting around the hurt and suspicion engendered by previous professionals' insensitivity in order to work cooperatively with a family.

As far as breaking distressing news is concerned, it would seem that it is definitely better to break it than to withhold it. The agonies of not knowing are far greater than the agonies of knowing. The former leaves you with absolutely nothing positive to do. What is very apparent, however, is that what is spoken is often very different from what is heard, especially when the emotions are engaged. It is remarkable how many parents are sure they were told that their child would be a vegetable in comparison with how many doctors swear they have never said such a thing to anyone. We shall not go deeper into this topic except to say that increasingly we see the value of either having a friend or supporter present when such news is broken or ensuring that what is said is noted down or is followed up by a written record for parents to question and digest in the necessary time. This process may have to happen more than once. Even when initial diagnosis is attempted, the truth usually unfolds slowly, with further revelations coming when you have scarcely recovered from the last. Introduction to a supportive network of other parents is invaluable at such times and should always be an adjunct to diagnosis.

The benefit of having a supporter alongside can be enormous in all crucial meetings throughout life. It can alter the balance of power when parents are faced with large numbers of high-status people, because it concentrates the mind of any professional if independent witnesses are present. It also frees the parent to be human, that is, an emotional being. With no support, a parent has to become his or her own professional, struggling to be objective and reasonable when the heart is leaping and lunging as each comment brings a surge of memories and anxieties with it. Both authors have played a support role for other parents. We were able to note the comments, marshal the arguments, ensure the parents' concerns were heard, take the reasoned route, while the parents, free of the burden of objectivity, could more vividly and spontaneously react. It is an effective combination and is much more likely to produce results than is a meeting from which unsupported parents emerge distressed, unsatisfied, and with the feeling of having been outmanoeuvred in some way.

Some professionals may hate the approach recommended here, claiming that emotion should play no part in their professional discussion. Yet it is, in fact, their own emotion – fear – that dictates such a course. It is strange that professionals who claim to know how to deal with emotionally disturbed children cannot cope with emotionally normal adults. In the best meetings, time is always allowed for parents to express their feelings, because not until feelings have been released can the reasoning begin.

Parent couples, themselves, can be forced to adopt the two roles, one the emotional and the other the reasoning partner, but doing so can emphasize roles between wives and husbands and in fact distort both.

Aiding Adjustment

As far as dealing with the news is concerned, what seems to be most requested is, first, full information, secondly, someone to talk to, and thirdly, practical advice. Giving 'full information' requires the giver to think about what that means. It entails taking into consideration the timing of the telling, the environment for the telling, the language of the telling, and the recording of the telling. Otherwise, the opportunities of the occasion will be lost. It is no good giving me life-changing news in circumstances that suit you; you must give it in circumstances that enable me to take something positive from it.

The 'someone to talk to' need not be the news-giver, although the best news-givers always allow future contact for answering those questions that do not form for a day or two. The best person to talk to may be another parent, though not any parent. Parents still nursing their own distress and finding it difficult to respond to another's except by recounting their own bitter experiences may not be the best people to meet a family with a new baby. The choice of a parent who has been through what you are facing and has emerged with love and hope intact, however, cannot be bettered. In very early days, it may be too soon for a parent with a baby to meet a congenitally deafblind adult, which is why we are speaking here of parents rather than families. Family mutuality will come later.

Caution has to be exercised over encouraging parents to join with families whose children are not deafblind. This may seem an overly divisive and negative statement, but deafblindness so impairs awareness of others, of how to react, relate, and communicate and, very much, how to play in the accepted sense, that experiences with other children and other families where seeing and/ or hearing is no problem can leave the parents of a deafblind child constantly explaining, constantly excusing, and ultimately demoralized and depressed as the most apparent differences in their deafblind child are expressed. The natural tendency for like to seek like becomes an imperative where parents of deafblind children are concerned. Parents can and do join in with family groups facing different disabilities, but only if their own needs are being met elsewhere. For many families the only chance of regular physical meeting is within a context of other disabilities, and therefore, for families with a deafblind child, distance-spanning contact with similar families by letter, telephone, or newsletter has always been a life-saver. Introducing the family to a national or international deafblind organization should be a part of every professional's good practice.

The request for 'practical advice' reflects that huge desire to have something to do in the face of feelings of complete powerlessness. It means that the 'person to talk to' is often an early Intervenor, visiting teacher, or adviser, who can answer a little of all three requests, being able to explain what diagnostic terms may mean, who has practical advice to give and who has a sympathy that comes from genuine affection for children or adults who are deafblind. Even where parents are in contact with other parents, they always appreciate and seek out someone who has professional knowledge as well as a liking for their child.

Parents sing the praises of those who saw their child as a child, were good listeners, had some practical suggestions and explanations, and who helped the parents to put them into operation in an enjoyable way. In the face of early chaos, it is wonderful to meet someone who can give us back our child and bring back some fun into interaction.

Mutual Respect and Recognition

It can be difficult sometimes to work out exactly what is the best approach to take, especially when both parents and professionals feel their own competence threatened by the others' supposed expertise. Perhaps a useful starting point could be to consider what each has that the other wants. Such thinking may help both parties to work out how best to cooperate.

What does the parent have that the professional needs? Certainly vast areas of knowledge. If only the right questions are asked and the right listening is done, parents carry in their memories a voluminous case history of their child that cannot be found anywhere else. Parents will also have great understanding of things specific to their child and the child's condition that otherwise may be totally puzzling or totally missed. This may extend from the meaning of particular behaviours in particular circumstances to the most successful approaches in all circumstances. In this context it is appropriate to remind everyone that taking a parent's comments seriously has been proved to be more likely to lead to correct answers than an insistence on only objective investigation. Not only do deafblind children perform poorly with strangers or in situations strange to them, but it is too easy to dismiss a parent's comments as neurotic or as wishful thinking when, in fact, they are the result of years of watchfulness. It is strange to think that a professional judgment will be confidently made after half a dozen observations, while a parent's judgment, based on thousands of observations in a myriad of different contexts, is ignored. Unconscious observation is one of a parent's greatest allies, although it is often dismissed as groundless intuition.

The parent also will have the child's trust and recognition. Although it is to be hoped that involved professionals will win such acknowledgment, it should never be at the expense of the parent, and it may be a long time before the parent can leave the working team. There will be many elements that work only if the parents are involved, at least initially. There are also many things that a child will attempt only if asked by a parent. Without extrinsic motivation to tempt a child into new experiences, the motivation provided by a trusted and liked person is the most powerful. This truth remains constant and becomes important when involved professionals themselves become trusted and liked and they gain this world-expanding power. Initially, however, rather than interacting with the child, they may have to guide the most trusted person to do so, and that may be difficult for some professionals to accept.

Behind the parents is, of course, the whole family and the family home. There, the child or young adult will have learned a way of relating and communicating and a particular form of dependence and will have developed certain priorities and routines, preferred tastes and evocative smells, and a steadily increasing store of memories, all of which can be used by a discerning professional to enrich programs and expand experience, even when the child is not in the parental home. Striking a somewhat subversive note, parents will also have freedom from professional codes of conduct and a concentration on one child only. This freedom can make them powerful agents in effecting change in policy and provision where a professional feels constrained. They can therefore be powerful allies. There have been many occasions when parents and their friends have spearheaded reforming movements at local or national levels in ways not open to professionals but using the information freely given by professionals.

What do professionals have that the parent wants? Parents will certainly hope that a professional has a broader perspective than they have been able to gain, relevant skills, relevant training, and a knowledge at least of sources of information and expertise. Parents will also benefit from a professional's degree of detachment. Although there may be murmurs that professionals can walk away from the situation and they cannot, parents recognize that that kind of respite is vital not only to a professional's sanity but also to the success of any sustained program for the child. We cannot have everyone on twenty-four-hour duty.

Both authors have benefited from the fact that professionals have kept working and planning when for a time both were too exhausted to do either. Parents will also hope that professionals have the power to change things, or at least will help in effecting change. It is very important, therefore, for professionals to consider the limits of their own powers before promising or appearing to make promises to parents. Raised expectations that are then dashed can have a devastating effect on a family.

Coordination of Input

Being clearer in one's role and willing to state limitations as well as strengths is a healthy beginning, but having a good partner is only part of the jigsaw for most parents. Just how many partners are there? Can there be too many partners? Is it possible in fact to have too much help? The problem is coordination and harmonizing. The aware professional may be daunted by the number of other professionals with whom contact and cooperation must be maintained, but the overall role of coordination usually falls to the parents. For a while, in Sense, there was an unofficial inquiry among the parents to see exactly how many involved professionals a child could have at any one time. The record was held by a Scottish family, which had thirty-two people actively involved in the child's life. What kind of family life can you generate if thirty-two people command your attention and attendance? There are not even enough days in a month to give a day to each. Your home may not seem your own, subject as it becomes to repeated invasion. How do you take in and apply all the advice that is given? The blessing of having a key figure who will be the main point of contact and coordination cannot be overstated, although usually the best we can achieve is to have a key figure for each major area of service – education, social, and medical. It is surprising how often little is done, even at a microlevel, to coordinate and conserve resources. Multiple visits to different centres for different reasons can be stressful but are nowhere nearly as annoying as multiple visits to the same centre for different reasons. We find it hard to believe that more than one activity cannot be arranged for the same day among specialists. We also find it hard to accept that, among a population noted to be at risk from anesthesia, necessary operations or investigations requiring anesthesia cannot be coordinated.

The Specialist in Deafblindness

What cannot be bettered is the early involvement of a specialist in congenital deafblindness, where many of the multiple effects are understood, where little needs to be explained and by whom much can be done. Correct assessment is the only foundation for appropriate programs, and one cannot arrive at a correct assessment by cobbling together a number of separate assessments from different specialties. There may be a team approach, but a deafblind specialist must be on (preferably leading) the team. In a multidisciplinary situation, the presence of a specialist in deafblindness is essential, and increasingly, professionals who are trying to work in a multidisciplinary context are expressing their need for a knowledgeable coordinating person.

Problems of coordination can be accompanied by those of perceived status, hinted at earlier. A psychologist once told us that the fear parents had of professionals was as nothing compared with the fear professionals had of parents. This misplaced sense of status and power can lead to worries and even dislikes that totally cloud all issues upon meeting and can even encourage avoidance of meeting. Status problems can exist among professionals themselves, where actual position in a hierarchy can be confused with value of opinion, so that the advice followed is that of the most powerful person rather than that of the most knowledgeable.

To leave coordination to the parents is not therefore the best practice. However much is learned by workers in the field of deafblindness, for the family it is usually the first time anything like it has been encountered. Unless the family members are fortunate enough to know someone who has experience in this area, it is likely that everyone they meet will also be faced with a first-time unknown situation and will, like the parents, dip into such experience as they do have to guess at what might be appropriate for a deafblind child. Parents may find themselves either completely abandoned or taking ineffective action 'on the best advice.' Some parents have even given up their children 'on the best advice.' Others have tortured themselves and the whole family in an attempt to force so-called normal development on a child with unique needs. It must be recognized that a unique disability requires a unique professionalism.

Family Environment

Stephen's sister was instrumental in making Sense forsake the concept of 'parents' for one of 'family' (by standing up at an international conference and proposing it!), and by so doing she opened the way to a much wider acknowledgment of the influence of social circles of extended family, friends, neighbours and society at large with all their subtle interrelatedness. We have space to share only a few thoughts on this topic here.

Although it is certainly true that the arrival of a child who is markedly different alters the whole world, not just the family, there are considerations that become concentrated within the immediate family. One consideration is that the family does not become totally as one in the face of great challenge, although the members may learn to operate as such. The members remain individuals and have to make their own journeys of personal discovery and development, often rearranging their relationships within the family along the way.

The arrival of any child has an effect on the dynamics and possibilities within a family. The arrival of a disabled child will greatly increase those normal pressures. Even if no other children are present, the relationship of the parental partners will be affected. That relationship will certainly be robbed of time and almost certainly will be robbed of focus – and here we do not refer to the ability to focus but to what is focused upon. Society will accept that the overriding concern of the family must be the disabled child, and the family may come to believe the same or to feel that there is no choice in the matter. Unfortunately, society will also believe that the overriding concern will of itself remove the family from all other concerns, especially those that take up the majority of other people's time and attention, such as personal relationship problems. If the family comes to share that belief, the result can be the neglect of such issues or even the substitution of the child's problems for them, until what has been neglected erupts with destructive force. There have been some families where the removal of a child's problem resulted in the family's putting another one in its place, because the family did not operate without one. There have also been occasions when the removal of a child's problem resulted in family break-up, a possibility that can become particularly acute when a child enters an adult residential placement and the parents are faced with reassessing their own identities, relationships, and future. Even where there is no such threat to family function, there is no law that says all members of a family must feel the same – or feel the same at the same time. Family members may well be at different stages of adjustment. As a generality, we tend to expect fathers to take longer to adjust than mothers, which may reflect the closeness mothers usually have to the child minute by minute, but it may also reflect the difference in expectations and upbringing between men and women in our society.

What is remarkable in families with a disabled child, in fact, is not how often the parents' own relationships are weakened but is how often they are not. Parents are more likely to become a powerful team than the opposite, but there should be no assumptions. This is the point where the reader must exercise the greatest caution. The authors' experience is of families in a Western culture, where a history of families' having to move around the country to pursue employment has broken the old pattern of living among lifelong friends and relatives. Many parents now have to rely on what is sometimes called the nuclear family, meaning only parents and children, living many miles from members of the extended family. Such a small family unit can therefore find itself without the friendly support of relatives or long-term neighbours, who are a normal part of the life of families in other lands or cultures. For families who have moved to a different country, this situation will, of course, be greatly magnified. In writing of what we have learned in the United Kingdom, therefore, we may be writing of things that seem strange to readers with other experiences. Always remember that your experience is more relevant to you than ours is to you.

In essence, we are saying that whatever the size of the family unit, if you are dealing with a deafblind child, you are dealing with a whole family. All the 'normal' pressures and characteristics of family life will be present and will affect what can be done with and for the deafblind child. Sometimes it is necessary to realize that what is offered as a problem with the child may be a problem in the parental relationship. The great mistake will be to think that the child is the cause of the problem. The authors do not believe that a disabled child causes cracks in marriages. The increased pressure may open out any cracks that are there, or may divert us from repairing them, but we cannot pass responsibility for causing break-up to the child. An even greater mistake would be for an Intervenor to take on the role of marriage counsellor in a desperate attempt to help. The results can be catastrophic. This is another reason for being clear about roles and responsibilities – and limits. There are, however, some helpful or preventative measures that can be taken.

Mothers and Fathers

Much of the work with any disabled child tends to be mother orientated. Traditionally, in Western culture this was simply because involved professionals worked when the father was also working, so that any visit to the home found only the mother there. In any case it was understandable to give most to the person with the main burden of care, usually the mother. However much a mother tried to pass on to a father what had been heard and shown, not as much got across as had been absorbed by the mother. Also, the child would often seem to respond more readily to the mother, who had had more time and contact to build the interactive relationship, while the father's attempts to do the same seemed far less successful. This can lead to a father's feeling inadequate and to his backing off to concentrate on other roles, such as the advocate, breadwinner and supporter, emphasizing what is already a role tendency and leaving, in fact, even more of the burden of caring on the mother. Both partners may then feel overburdened and guilty for different reasons, and there is potential for friction.

Any potentially divisive effect can increase as the child grows. When a child is small, it is easier to find baby sitters who will allow the parents to go out together, but as the child grows and is perceived as less appealing and more challenging, it is harder. Some parents rarely go out together without their child. One goes out only if the other remains to look after the child. Maybe unconsciously, the marriage becomes a serious business, focused on stress and problems. The only time one is free and relaxed is when one is not with one's partner. This state is not healthy for a relationship.

Fortunately, it is becoming rarer to find professionals who are not alive to this situation, who will not take pains to involve both father and mother in what they and the child are engaged in, and who see different forms of respite as vital for the family's health. One of the best services organizations around the world offer is a holiday program for deafblind children and adults. Some even offer holidays for the brothers and sisters. Others add holidays for the whole family. Increasingly, also, conferences offer holiday or family-camp facilities as part of their conference provision. Such initiatives help enormously in allowing families to feel like families, where sometimes they can be enjoying themselves together and at other times they can be enjoying themselves apart. The vital element is that for a while they are free of the responsibility of care and can even dare to be carefree.

It is still common, however, to consider families as a unit and to assume that they have one attitude and approach. Although the father may take the role of spokesperson at any meeting, his wife, in fact, may not always be represented by what he says. A child may be subject at home to two very different regimes according to who is caring for him or her at the moment. Father may be convinced that a more directive and disciplined approach is for the best, while mother may feel that a regime that proceeds gently and removes pressure gets the best results. If neither agrees with the regime followed by a school, the child will be subject to three different management systems, which can be expected to produce confusion and some self-defensive strategy of withdrawal or action. It is therefore important to seek opportunities and environments where all family members and involved professionals can exchange thoughts and feelings freely, if not always honestly.

Honesty

Being honest is not as easy as it sounds. It may be salutary for the reader to reflect for a moment on just how honest are thoughts expressed in different contexts. When last were you completely honest, and with whom? Often we are most honest with people who do not matter to us.

With all the pressures I as a parent see my partner under, do you think I am going to unburden myself to her, to him? That would not be fair, would it? I must keep silent and put on a brave face; for when my deeper thoughts do occasionally burst out they cause panic. Even with concerned and understanding professionals I can rarely be completely honest. How will my honesty affect their decisions about my child? How will they interpret what I am asking for? What will they think of me? As adult services have appeared, the authors have noted another barrier to honesty. Parents have become so concerned for the staff who have now taken over the responsibility and stress of caring that they will not voice concerns that might stress or distress staff further. One answer seems to be to have a parent liaison person who can be approached with concerns and can ensure that they are addressed without the agonies of what seems like a formal complaint. Both authors have had such a role at different times.

Time and a growing relationship will ameliorate many of these difficulties among parents and professionals, but sharing thoughts and feelings with other families is often the best therapy. It is an immense relief when mothers meet mothers, siblings meet siblings, and fathers meet fathers and can unburden themselves to others who recognize the same fears and feelings without being directly involved. The release that comes from expressing horrible thoughts to someone who knows that does not mean you do not love, because they have known the same, is surely one of the most wonderful aspects of families meeting one another with time to talk. It always leads on to clearer minds and the confidence to be more honest with professionals.

Brothers and Sisters

In many homes, the siblings, the brothers and sisters, are the great allies and the great truth-tellers. Tortured by consciousness of the time and priority that has to be channelled towards the needs of their deafblind child, many parents feel it is their other children who are the handicapped ones. Here is another rich source of guilt and grief. We can make the mistake so often made when considering our deafblind child; our consciousness of what the child is missing makes us feel that the child is also conscious of loss. If a child has no experience for comparison, nothing is loss; all is possibility.

Overall, the experience of families concerning the brothers and sisters of deafblind children is remarkably positive. With few exceptions, the siblings have not emerged as damaged and resentful beings; quite the opposite, in fact. Although their development is greatly influenced by the experience, it seems to foster a deeper and more aware personality rather than the reverse. This is not to say that there are no problems along the way, but to say that the likelihood is for positive rather than negative outcomes in the long run.

There seem to be three periods to bear in mind, and here we are oversimplifying. When we are young everything is normal. It is only when others point out differences that we may feel our circumstances are odd. So the golden rule with young brothers and sisters seems to be: if they have no problem, do not give them one. Young children are more accepting than older ones, and this applies to our young children's young friends as well. As long as he or she is not too big, our deafblind child is more likely to be fascinating than frightening and will be absorbed happily into their world.

Certainly any professional involved with the family must acknowledge the brothers' and sisters' presence and value. Involving them in what is being done with the deafblind child will pay dividends all round. They are very perceptive and motivating in the deafblind child's life. What is very helpful for younger siblings is to arrange times for them to play together with other siblings of deafblind individuals whenever there are family conferences or gatherings. To find they are not alone in their experiences of life is very healthy, and great friendships can begin.

When they are approaching adolescence, brothers' or sisters' personal pressures and concerns are normally so overwhelming that issues arising from a deafblind sibling are of secondary importance or cannot be taken on board among all the others. This can be a period when brothers and sisters seem to draw away for a time. The urge for acceptance by one's peers is often so strong that anything that affects that acceptance assumes massive importance. It is difficult to be positive about your deafblind brother or sister when you cannot even be positive about your shape, hair, or clothes in the face of peer-group offensives. Having a deafblind brother or sister is just one more difference among the many you are struggling with as you begin the change from child to young adult. Some teachers have helped to turn what could be a cause of isolation into one of admiration by getting brothers and sisters to give their classmates a presentation about deafblindness and their experiences or by deliberately raising the subject themselves to allow positive input. But overall, adolescence does not seem to be a good period for heavy intervention.

Enormous benefit has been found when brothers and sisters reach an age when they are naturally thinking about and analysing their life experience. Here, the greatest benefit seems to come, as it does with parents, not from talking with psychologists or therapists but in talking freely with one another. Sense's experience has been that to facilitate meetings among older brothers and sisters of deafblind individuals, with no one else present, has led to such a liberating exchange of feelings, fears and, yes, perceived guilt, that the results have been instant and long lasting, giving them their own informal support network and strengthening relationships. Fears that dangerous emotions might arise needing professional help have proved groundless. Fellow siblings have proved just as able to deal with matters as fellow parents are, especially if older ones are present. Little organization is required. It seems that once true feelings have been unburdened in like-minded and like-feeling company, there is little need to repeat the exercise, except to help others. At one time it was thought that maybe a brothers' and sisters' group was as necessary as a parents' group, but it appears not to be so. Siblings of deafblind individuals are not so burdened, and once the first unburdening has happened, they prefer meeting occasionally socially rather than formally. For brothers, such meetings can be invaluable, especially in cultures where males do not easily speak about their feelings. We know of one man whose first transforming admission to fellow siblings of his true feelings about his deafblind sister did not happen until he was thirty years old. Until that time he had carried his burden alone, only to find after thirty years that it should not have been a burden at all. Siblings are often those who point out to parents by behaviour or words when certain facts must be faced and decisions taken. It cannot be overestimated how much they contribute to the sanity and survival of parents. How much we over-involve them or shut them out in an attempt not to burden them or overlook their rightful place is a complex mixture of personality, belief, and background, but they are golden threads in the unfolding tapestry of families' lives.

The Extended Family

When considering the wider family, we again have to be cautious. Some families have found that they have received more support from people outside the family than from those within it. While grandparents in particular can be a tower of strength when children are small, it seems that relatives of the parents often hurt too much to be effective helpers. Relatives also go through their own confusion of emotions upon learning of the arrival of a deafblind child. There can be a natural grieving coupled with a fear of comparison with their own unaffected families. We even know of a family with a deafblind child who were not invited to visit for fear of the parents' being distressed among normally sighted and hearing nieces and nephews. In fact, the exact opposite was true. Grandparents have to grapple with a double grief. They grieve not only for their deafblind grandchild but for their own child, the parent. More consideration needs to be given to the extended family to avoid having what should be positive support become a confused distancing.

Social Changes

Similar, although less, emotional confusion affects friends and colleagues of parents. Most families find that the arrival of a deafblind child alters the pattern and content of circles of friends and acquaintances. There is not space here to explore this topic fully, and any attempts by parents to affect changes are limited by the capacities and choices of people over whom they have no claims or controls. It is necessary, however, to realize that the arrival of a deafblind child will alter a family's entire world, social as well as emotional and physical. Such families enter one of society's minorities and may even feel they have no place in society at all, except as supplicants for service.

It would be grossly unfair to give the impression that all people flee. The challenge of responding or not responding to a deafblind individual brings forward wonderful people as much as it deters others. There are many communities where a deafblind individual and his or her family are warmly included and where friends of the family have provided the most practical support of anyone. Such inclusion tends to happen more frequently in small and stable communities rather than in larger towns or cities, but even in cities there are unexpected meetings with kindness and openness from ordinary people that gladden the heart.

Single Parents

For single parents, singleness is the main problem. It is very hard to be the centre of someone else's universe, realizing that everything depends upon oneself. Not a thing must be forgotten, every eventuality must be foreseen and planned for, and there is no room for flexibility. All parents must feel this during the periods when they are in sole charge, but for the single parent this is a constant state. There is no point even in screaming for help if there is no one to hear. Life must be reduced to limits within which one can cope. Respite or a supportive network becomes vital rather than desirable.

For involved professionals, working with a single parent can have particular delights and hazards. Certainly there may be a closer and more smoothly working relationship, where focus on the child is shared without distraction. An involved professional may also find a much greater openness on the part of the parent in sharing personal feelings, because the parent may have only the professional to share such things with. The danger may lie in the parent's seeing the professional as a real friend and looking for more than child-centred support and more involvement than should be given. This reaction is quite understandable and may be inadvertently encouraged by an inexperienced professional seeking to foster a good relationship with a child's parent. But isolated parents can be very emotionally vulnerable and judgments may become clouded on both sides. A professional can never become a substitute marital partner. The price is too high for all concerned. Similar dangers can, of course, arise among professionals and married couples, if the parents have become emotionally detached from one another.

Nor can a professional afford to become part of any power-play over a child between parents who are separated, or who are using the child as a weapon against one another. Whatever the temptation to side with one or the other, the major allegiance has to be to the child, and continued involvement must be judged upon benefit to the child.

Personal Identity

What so easily can be lost in caring for a deafblind child is a sense of one's own personal identity. One becomes Stephen's father or Ian's mother, not only to all the world but also to oneself. It is not easy to keep up outside interests, and ordinary social occasions can reduce us to silence. We cannot swap opinions on the latest films, plays, and books, because we have seen none, and, although people may express the opinion that we must be saints, they will not want to hear too much of how our days are spent. After a time, not being saints, we may become bores. Better, perhaps, not to be there. We hardly dare add that sometimes the change in our views and priorities makes the concerns of others seem trivial and equally boring.

It is possible that we may indeed become obsessed with our child. Family members still in employment will have an escape, although the freedom to pursue a career will be severely limited by comparison with others who have no such limits on their time and finances. If both partners have been forced out of employment into full-time caring, as can happen if there are no services able or willing to take on their adult or challenging child, it will be very difficult to escape the whirlpool that sucks one down to total absorption in the child, and no one to feed on but one's partner. Such a situation is not only a closed circuit, it is claustrophobic.

Changes over Time

The needs of the family change with time, usually as the child changes, but it is possible to see three stages, or rather three shifts of concern, that are very common. The stages roughly follow those of a child's education and affect not only the changing needs of the child but the changing demands and expectations of society as a child grows. These stages correspond to the pre-school, school, and post-school periods.

As we have already mentioned, the pre-school years are a time of searching and adjusting. The search is for information, for diagnosis, for treatment, and later for rights and the best placement. It is a time when the greatest task may be that of coordination and simplification in the face of a multitude of professionals and professional visits, and the greatest help, therefore, is early contact with a sympathetic specialist in deafblindness.

At school age, once the great hurdle of finding an appropriate placement has been jumped, there is, from the parents' point of view, a welcome transfer of focus to the teacher. Suddenly the number of involved professionals shrinks, because many of the necessary services are arranged by or through the school. Now the greatest worry may become the finding and maintaining of respite, especially during the long school holidays. If the child is in a day placement, these periods of respite, which are usually seen as periods of refreshment for the parents to enable them to continue their caring role, may have their greatest function in preparing both child and parent for the necessary distancing that is a prelude to independence when the child becomes an adult. The old saying used to be that your school-days were the happiest days of your life. For parents of a deafblind child, their child's school-days seem the happiest days of the parents' lives. It is a time when, for a while, there is certainty of provision, a clarity of law over what will be provided, a definite program for the child, and a smaller number of people involved. It can be a time when parents seem to back off or take a rest, but really they are entering a new period of adjustment.

Two families we know of in Latin America and one in the United States will smile at mention of taking a rest. Not only did they not take a rest, they actually founded and ran the schools that their children attended. Parents in other countries may be more inclined to weep, knowing they have no appropriate provision at all. But again, we are forced to speak of what we know. We are omitting the struggles and advocacy many parents face, even in our own country, before their children, in fact, get the recognition and access to provision that they need.

Advice to Education Services

When you are considering our willingness to cooperate, also consider our ability to cooperate. We shall have some ability that is innate and some that will develop with time.

You may wish to spare a thought for our emotional and other resources at a particular time and what we might need to help us cooperate more effectively. Simply providing the opportunity for caregivers to participate is not enough; they must be enabled to participate effectively.

Help us to respond and initiate more effectively, and teach us what we want to know rather than only what you think we need to know. Let us know what you are doing with our child, how you are doing it and why, so that we can back you up wholeheartedly.

In honest appraisal with us of difference in environment, pace, interests, and pressures between where you work and where we live, let us work out together what are priorities, what needs to be consistent, what needs to be transferred between settings, and what can be transferred. We may then arrive at what is to be normal in our child's life.

When the time is ripe, let us consider together the long-term expectation and whether there is a long-term plan. We need to know who is working in harmony.

Give us a named person for our main link and invite us to meetings that are not simply in response to crises, or we shall always arrive geared for defence or attack.

Give us comprehensive information in a language we can understand, help us to see the significance in it, and give us time to chew it over and respond. Consultation without information is liable to become an empty exercise. Think of Effectiveness rather than Efficiency. The time to listen, the time to talk and the time to decide may not be the same. Time is so important; we have so little to spare, you are pressured for results, yet our child travels slowly. If we can all learn from the child, perhaps we can get time on our side.

Transition

As the time for leaving school approaches, fear returns in full measure. Now the worry is over post-school provision, over the need for continuing education, for a life-placement plan. Here, again, we have to pause. In some countries a child will have a right to a place in a supported group home. In others there may be not a right but at least a possibility. In yet others, the very thought of any child moving from the parental home is anathema, because the family home is also the extended family's home and encompasses the family's occupation, in which everyone has a part to play. In western countries, where 'nuclear' families bear the burden alone, it can become impossible to continue caring for a congenitally deafblind young adult in the parental home. There is also an acceptance in such countries that deafblind persons as well as other family members have a right to independent living and development. It is of such a social context that we speak and to which we shall return later.

Priorities

Expectations can cause conflict if they are not clear. If, as a parent, I feel that any service offered is merely filling the time until my child will be returned to my care, I shall be far less motivated to cooperate with that service than if I feel we are all working towards something else. There is a radical difference between programs in countries where supported group-home living is the expectation and those where there is no planned future. Even while programs are running, there are different priorities that need to be faced. At the very least we have to question one another about them. Here we can consider cultural diversion as well as personal difference. We realize that there can be no common worldwide practice. Take a small illustration: while half of the world is struggling to teach deafblind children to eat with a knife and fork, the other half is struggling to teach them to eat with their fingers. The motivation in both halves is the same – to have the child acceptable in social gatherings.

At the personal level, also, the same motivation can lead to different outcomes. School staff may have spotted that use of hearing aids encourages a child to make noises in response to stimulation and, seeing the possibility of training residual hearing, insist that hearing aids must be worn at all times. A parent may have spotted that the use of hearing aids encourages a child to make noises that alarm the public and therefore quietly dispenses with hearing aids so that the child remains silent and acceptable in public. It would be a brave parent who admitted this action to teachers. Here, we have the teacher's priority of using every available opportunity to train residual hearing clashing with the parent's priority of having a child who is socially acceptable.

What is going to be accepted as normal? What are the priorities? What weight have the rights of the caregivers versus the rights of the person cared for? In essence, where does my responsibility lie – and does it change as a child grows older? Such thoughts underline the power, and therefore the responsibility, exercised by the person actually in contact with the deafblind individual.

The examples of different priorities mentioned above contain an element of choice, but sometimes parents have priorities that override others. Most parents will try very hard to continue in the home what is being attempted in the school. But homes are not schools, and everything that happens in them has to be done by family members; there are no back-up staff and no off-duty hours. The demands of getting the washing, shopping, cooking, and caring done within the time available will often entail cutting the time needed to allow a deafblind child to complete a task. Parents will guiltily find themselves doing things for rather than with their child, hoping the teacher will never find out.

It is vital that professionals consider carefully what is essential in a consistent program and what is possible. Otherwise parents may retreat to silence rather than share honestly what they see as their shortcomings. Here, again, the strength of a good family-child relationship should not be forgotten. One of the authors remembers vividly being reprimanded by a very irate teacher upon taking his son back to school after the holidays and feeling forced to confess to not having been able to follow through any of the programs sent home with his son. The teacher was not angered by the missing of programs but by the parent's distress over it. In no uncertain terms it was pointed out that teachers teach and parents parent, that it was obvious that the boy was loved and that was why he was so open to interaction and learning, that fears of unalterable regression were groundless, and that the parent was never to get into such a state again. Shaken but mightily relieved, the parent was able to enter a more productive phase of honest negotiation with the school with priorities reaffirmed: in the home, loving is more important than teaching, although it is not enough on its own.

Readers who have programs that utilize paid intervention for the preschool and school-age child can quietly congratulate themselves that their Intervenor system is one safeguard against the dangers mentioned here, but readers in other countries without that blessing will still be with us and must be supported by a realistic, comprehensive program for their child that can be implemented within their family resources of time, energy, and overall priorities.

The concept of the Personal Program easily can be misunderstood. The twenty-four-hour, 365-days-a-year programming insisted upon by McInnes and Treffry (1982) may mistakenly be seen as a constant regimentation of the infant, child, or adult with deafblindness, rather than what McInnes and Treffry were, in fact, insisting upon: a total approach that is designed to recognize and to use effectively the contributions that educational programs, therapeutic programs, community programs and the family can make to overall development. Such a program should never take control away from parents. It should never appear to require that parents' and siblings' interactions with the deafblind member of the family be at a level beyond what the family feels it can realistically support.

As explained in chapters 1 and 2, no professional should ever allow a program to be suggested that is beyond the resources of a family or that merely duplicates school-based activities. If poor programming does allow this to happen and there is failure to recognize the changeable priorities and pressures that parents experience, then any sense of cooperation and choice will be lost over time. Parents may mistakenly try very hard to continue in the home what is being attempted in the school rather than having a clear understanding of how their own special contribution can be made within their own family context.

Confidence

One of the most significant occurrences during all these possible changes is not the growth or destruction of competence but the growth or destruction of confidence. Confidence also changes over time, and involved professionals can build or destroy it. It is very easy to de-skill someone.

During the child's first years, parents develop an expertise and knowledge that few can match. They are often the ones who carry out successful programs and who provide the knowledgeable centre of the network serving their child. This preschool expertise can be severely tested when their child starts school. Now there is a professional teacher in charge. Their child's programs are carefully designed, monitored, and instituted when they are not around. Suddenly, they are moved from centre stage and are expected to carry on the school program instead of being the instigators of routines that others have to follow. The philosophy and approach of the school concerning parental involvement will be crucial at this stage. Certainly there will be traumas of adjustment, which can be damaging, but they can also be reassuring and liberating if handled well. Communication will be a vital element for the parents as well as for the child.

In your communication with us, remember to give us what is missed in our experience, the things that normally a child would tell a parent. We miss out on the gossip and the tale-telling and the recounting of good and funny things more than we do news of what has gone wrong or is worrying. Obviously you will not gossip and tale-tell, but do not neglect the chat. We love to share in the smiles and understanding that a child's chatter and reporting would normally stimulate.

Another great confidence-breaker can be simply the increasing size of the child. It is difficult to view one's own increasing incompetence with calmness, especially if one has the reputation of skilful management, but if there has not been preparation for a management strategy that does not depend in the last instance upon physical strength, a growing child can quickly become unmanageable and will, in fact, come to rule the home. This is perhaps a reminder that, although we emphasize responding to the child, that does not mean always letting the child have his or her own way. Always remembering the child is a child means accepting our responsibility to guide and train acceptable behaviour. If we do not do it, how is the growing child to learn how to behave? There are instances, unfortunately, where a growing child really has become unmanageable and beyond the strength of a mother to contain. In some instances this situation has led to fathers' giving up their jobs to be at home full time, and in the case of single parents it has led to a child's having to go into full-time residence away from home. It is very important to obviate either of these situations if at all possible, so that any moves are for positive, not negative, reasons, and careful cooperation with families is required to make sure we are all looking ahead in what we do.

Puberty can cause problems for all of us, even when we know what is happening to us and why. For a deafblind child, and therefore for the parents, it can be a confusing and frightening time. The changes, along with growth spurts, increasing strength, and possible changes in behaviour patterns, put added strain on parents' ability to cope at home. This stress can lead to a rapid loss in confidence and competence.

In all cases there will be physical changes or degeneration that demand adjustments, but one of the things for which we rarely prepare is success. As our child becomes capable of more and desires more, we have to provide more of both time and of experiences for the child, often being asked for more input when we are growing weary and less resilient. If we parents seem ungrateful for all your efforts and are still asking for help, especially after school and in the holidays, remember that your successes demand more from us and we do not grow younger.

It is easy to overlook the effect of long-term stress. A certain amount of stress is good for us, keeping us alive and alert, but if it continues too long, there comes a point where the effects are damaging. Although the authors cannot prove it, it seems that twelve years is some kind of limit. Because this age coincides with puberty in the child and often a change to secondary schooling, it is hard to say what is due to what, but the authors have found the twelve-year mark a significant one in terms of peak distress. We are speaking here of exhaustion rather than depression. It is easy to mistake weariness for depression, but this is a case where medication will not help; rather, help is the best medication.

One duty professionals have is that of preparation. Readiness – for taking a break, for accepting additional help, for separation, for independence – is important for nearly all our families. Yet we are never really emotionally prepared, nor can we be. The most we can do is to take a risk on the best advice and cope with the consequences.

Post-School Separation

Well before the time for leaving school approaches it is necessary to consider the options available, and parents may appear reluctant to do so. If it is complicated and stressful to find a suitable school for our children when there is a statutory requirement for education to be provided, the problems associated with finding an appropriate long-term placement can be overwhelming. Luckily, planning for such a transition is part of the education policy in some countries and a right to a group home exists in others, but even there, the period when a child becomes officially an adult is one of the most traumatic parents will face.

Along with the months of meetings and discussions, assessments and financial considerations, parents will also be trying desperately to come to terms with their conflicting emotions about their vulnerable and possibly difficult young person's moving away from home.

Each of the professionals they meet during this process will have come into contact with a small facet of the parents' life and will have encountered a few of their emotions and attitudes. But they should be aware that they have seen only a part of the whole and that their words and actions at this critical stage can have more effect than they could guess. It is impossible to imagine what it must be like for our children as they go through all the traumas of growing up, but often they seem to be ready to move on before we are. One sometimes gets the feeling that deafblind children in the senior classes of schools are bored. School-based life is no longer challenging or interesting enough, especially if many of the tasks they are required to do are the same ones they were doing when they were five years old. School-leaving age is, after all, arbitrary, and it pays little attention to individual needs. As a generality, despite the necessary period of adjustment and relationship-building, our children usually handle the transition to an adult placement better than we parents do.

Letting Go

When our other children leave home, there is a gradual separation to prepare us. They develop their own lives, start staying out late, spend more time with friends than with us, increasingly make their own decisions, often in defiance of us, and slowly move towards living independently. Parents and growing children also talk, discuss, argue, and plan as they start to lead separate lives.

For most of our deafblind children none of this is true. There is often no way of explaining that they are leaving home in three months' time, next week, tomorrow – possibly forever. Maybe we can take them to visit their new home, show them their room, introduce them to the people they will be living with, and so on, but there is no way of preparing them for the enormous upheaval about to happen. Even when preparatory work is done, many young people seem to think their first arrival in their new home is for a holiday, and it is only as time passes without the expected return to home that the truth begins to dawn.

Strangely, it seems that the more stressful and difficult it has been for the parents to look after a young adult at home and the more anxious they are to find a suitable placement, the more intense and yet unexpected are the feelings when the time for separation actually comes. The enormous relief at not having to bear the responsibility any longer can quickly be replaced by a terrible feeling of having failed as parents. However rational and logical one is, it can still be extremely hard to overcome such acute feelings and to face the daunting prospect of filling the huge hole that has suddenly appeared in life where the caring used to be and the realization that a new identity has to be found.

Professionals who care for and work with a young adult need to be aware of the possible turmoil and anguish that parents may be suffering. There is potential for conflict and a misunderstanding of seemingly irrational parental reactions as the struggle to let go continues. Some parents may appear to vanish for a while. Others may criticize the smallest detail, constantly visiting unexpectedly, telephoning, or complaining. We have even known parents who have contemplated suicide. Thankfully, we can also report that in every case except one the parents came through this stage and found a new life for themselves as they witnessed the new life for their child. The one exception was a parent who could not cope with the separation and removed the child from the group home he had entered. All the others now bore anyone who will listen with repeated praise for how well their child and the staff are doing.

The process is really another bereavement, and for many parents it seems to be the most powerful loss they encounter. So, to readers involved in adult residential work, we would say: please be patient with us if we cause worry and confusion among staff, keep the contact and information flowing, and remember that we shall come through it. Remember that the one witness whose testimony we shall accept is our own child. If you concentrate on our child's well-being, all eventually will work out.

Thankfully, not all transitions are so painful. Much will be influenced by what has happened before. Important factors are whether a child is moving on from a background of a day placement or a residential placement and from a traditional family setting or a single-parent family and whether that background has been basically happy or merely bearable.

If the child is moving on from a day placement, home life will have been, for the parents, one of high stress and adrenaline. As we have mentioned before, there will be a huge gap when the child goes away, and possibly a loss of personal identity when the main caregiver is no longer 'parent.' There will be a period of re-learning for parent as well as for child, and worry and constant oversight (which may be seen as interference) is possible while trust and acceptable communication develops.

If the child is moving on from a residential school, he or she will still be seen as having lived at home but there will be differences. Parents will have learned to trust others for longer periods, ideally, and will be used to times when their child is away. They will have had a mixture of their own life and periods of

caregiving. There may be a carrying over of expectations from previous placements that may have to be challenged, but the notion of shared responsibility
should have been established.

The child from a hospital (institutional) placement is seen as not living at
home. Parents will already have gone through a bereavement process and may
feel particularly inadequate and guilty, especially when they are first in contact
with other parents who have managed to keep on caring for their child in the
family home. The impossibility of adequate staffing in any hospital setting will
have required a containment policy for the child (by medication and/or 'training'), which the parents will have had to accommodate or ignore. Their child
may have become institutionalized, with minimal home contact. The authors
know of parents who arrived at a large mental handicap hospital to visit their
child but could not face what they would find inside the walls and returned
home. For one mother this became a pattern: travelling to the hospital, grieving
outside, then going home. Once her child entered a group home the family pattern changed to one of regularly and joyfully visiting their child. There are
always chances of a new relationship when good services arrive.

An adult placement greatly increases fears and raises new issues with as yet
no clear answers. Sexuality and risk-taking among the relationships and activities of adult services cause particular worries, as do questions of control and
intimate personal care. All is overlaid with the realization that in law (in most
countries) parents have no rights over an adult child. Are parents truly sharing
now or are they handing over control? Are any conflicts actually over practical
matters or is there a conflict of love?

Rather than adjusting to our child's independence in the accepted sense, we
are adjusting to our child's changed dependence. We are learning what it is to
see our child turn to others for emotional as well as practical support. The
authors no longer think of independence as the acquisition of skills that enable
independent action, although we revel in their acquisition. We think of independence as emotional independence, which is built from growing confidence
in good experiences with people, and which enables a person to form new
relationships and to move from childlike dependence upon one person to
admittedly dependent but increasingly adult relationships with more and different people. Most of our children will not progress to adult living where
they can be left to fend for themselves; they will always need supportive environments, which do not have to be in the parental home. They can still move
on to their own homes, and the critical element will be not their practical
skills but their acceptance by others, helped by their ability to relate successfully to others.

A Final Word

In writing this chapter we have been forced not only to exclude much, but to mention more negative things than we hope would plague any parent or professional. It is hard to avoid presenting a picture of overwhelming threat, yet we and other parents have learnt so much, have met such love and such lovely people, and have experienced such heights of delight among the difficulties that we grieve at not being able to share those aspects also with you. That is why we wrote at the beginning that we had been privileged in having in our families deafblind sons. We are what we are because of the experience. We have not been able to do justice to ethnic, cultural, or religious differences or even the basic ones of personality, but we hope you will forgive us for that omission. We in our turn will not forget, now that we are in calmer water, that parents in our footsteps may not yet be able to say what we have said. We hope this chapter will help them and their families along the way.

Ten Commandments

How are we to summarize what has gone before? Let us give you, instead of a summary, a lighthearted but serious set of commandments to consider. Speaking as a parent to a professional:

*1. Thou shalt make sure I am talking with someone who knows
what he or she is talking about.*
Because my child is deafblind, that someone must understand congenital deafblindness. If you admit your ignorance but put me in contact with someone who does understand, I shall think highly of you. If you admit your ignorance but do nothing, I shall not think highly of you. If you pretend you know and I find out later that you do not, I shall find it hard to forgive you.

2. Thou shalt not forget I know what I am talking about.
I do not know everything, which is why I have come to you, but that does not mean I know nothing. Let us put our heads together like thinkers, not like rams.

*3. Thou shalt seek to find someone who has experienced
what I am experiencing.*
Help me to find such people, even if it is only by giving me an address of an organization that might know of them.

4. Thou shalt be practical.
I want practical and realistic advice. A pat on the head and reassurance that I am doing all that can be done is not acceptable. I already know that I am not doing all that can be done.

5. Thou shalt support rather than direct me.
I want to express my love. Help me to do that effectively. I need information and advice rather than counselling and commands. I shall need counselling only if I carry the mistaken belief that somehow I am responsible for my child's impairments.

6. Thou shalt include me in everything to do with my child.
I want to be involved. Give me the necessary information, inclusion in planning, a part in decisions and programs, and the confidence to participate effectively.

7. Thou shalt not train my child without training me.
I want to learn. I want to be ahead of my child in everything my child has to learn, so that I can draw my child on to greater things in the right way.

8. Thou shalt accept my humanity.
I want to be allowed to be human. I cannot be wholly professional where my child is concerned, but I can be the most brilliant amateur you have ever seen. Do not worry if sometimes I weep as I go. Be prepared to cope with my highs and lows as you do with those of my child.

9. Thou shalt accept thine own humanity.
Always keep an open mind and have an eye to yourself and your own personal luggage. You are too valuable to my child to burn out, hide, or escape into pretence. My child is teaching me the glories of human failure and triumph. Join us.

10. Thou shalt not tell me thou understandeth; thou shalt show me.
If you want a more sensible summary of the situation, look up the section on parents in John and Jacquelyn McInnes's statement of their philosophy in *Deafblind Education* (1996).

Actual Bereavement

Although this is a book dealing with the lives of congenitally deafblind individuals, we feel we cannot end without a brief note that we hope will not be relevant to all readers but will become part of the experience of many professionals. It concerns the death of the person with whom we have engaged.

Speaking as a parent, in losing my child I may for a while lose my whole world. If the only people with whom I felt understood and to whom I could talk freely were the professionals who cared for and about my child, I may lose them all when my child is no longer around and they have no service to deliver.

To whom, then, can I talk? Who will help me through the mourning by listening and by reminiscing about the one who is lost? I would appreciate it if you would stay in touch for a while and allow me to be around occasionally until I can manage on my own in this new world in which I have to learn to live.

I shall have to deal not only with the 'normal' progress through bereavement but also with some strangely conflicting reactions. Although feeling the ache of loss, I shall also recognize the removal of pressure, which may stir the guilty suspicion that I am relieved rather than grieving. In fact some people may mention such relief in an attempt to comfort me. Even other parents may find their shared grief troubled with such thoughts; for many will at one time or another have wondered whether it would not have been better for their child to die rather than that life should continue with such uncertainty and pain. It may well be that I withdraw from all contact, in the belief that no one really understands my twisting and confusing emotions. At such a time it is a real blessing if someone is around who really knew my child and the love that was generated.

Two other thoughts rise. One of the authors, Norman, had to face the final and real 'acceptance' when Stephen was twenty. The bad times had passed. It looked as if the good times were coming. Yet Norman had to allow Stephen to go, to say thank you to him and for him, and to turn to new challenges. 'What enabled me to do that,' says Norman, 'was the certainty that Stephen knew I loved him and also that I knew he loved me. I found that thought of ultimate comfort and have often worried over families where the youthfulness of the child or the severity of the disability has prompted parents to say that they are unsure whether their child knows he or she is loved or even loves them.' This is an area that early Intervenors need to work on – looking for and pointing out evidence the child gives of recognition of love.

A second point is also important. Professionals may find themselves coping with repeated bereavement, especially among young children with complex disabilities, or in adult placements. This is an area where professionals, if they are to remain open, engaged, and motivated, may need more support than parents. It may seem strange, but we as parents urge such professionals to look to one another and to their own support systems, and we hope that some of us can be included in such support, which helps us all to retain humanity, not to become scarred, numb, or destroyed.

Summary

1. There are special considerations for families with a deafblind child that revolve around the building of relationships and the emergence of communication.

2. The best early intervention is to help parents to develop their relationship with their child by recognizing and responding to the infant's expressions and attempted interactions.

3. It should never be forgotten that the child who is deafblind is a child, who has the same need for love, security, reassurance and interaction as any child.

4. On the arrival of their deafblind infant, parents have to face the future without time to prepare, and life becomes a spiral of continual adjustment rather than a process leading to acceptance.

5. Reaction to an infant's disability shows a common pattern of shock, anger, and disbelief, leading to grieving and feelings of isolation, before adaptation and information seeking lead to ongoing adjustment.

6. Professionals must allow for a parent's emotional state and stage of adjustment.

7. The reception by the family of the current professional will be greatly influenced by the sum of the knowledge, skills, attitudes, and empathy of all previous professionals encountered.

8. There is great benefit in allowing parents to having a supporter at all crucial meetings.

9. Families with a deafblind child need contact with other families with deafblind children.

10. Parents have a vast store of knowledge and other advantages concerning their child that the professional should respect, utilize, and in some cases help the parents to organize to aid understanding.

11. Professionals should evidence a broader perspective, relevant skills, training, knowledge, and a degree of detachment, which can aid the family of the deafblind individual.

12. Involvement of a specialist in deafblindness is essential for the design and delivery of any effective program for a deafblind individual.

13. When a professional is dealing with a deafblind child, that professional is dealing with a whole family, and each family member is an individual.

14. The arrival of a deafblind child alters family dynamics, social circles, and future possibilities.

15. A disabled child is not a root cause of family breakdown.

16. If one is not careful, caring for a deafblind child can result in loss of personal identity.

17. It is part of the professional's responsibility to involve both parents in all aspects of professional support.
18. Siblings involvement may pass through stages but outcomes are usually positive.
19. The needs of families change over time.
20. Differing priorities among parents, educators, and other professionals should be acknowledged and addressed.
21. The recurring challenge faced by parents is not lack of competence, but rather lack of confidence. Attention needs to be paid to confidence building and the humanity of all involved.
22. Planning for adult life should begin well before the child leaves school.
23. Special allowance must be made for the emotional trauma surrounding a deafblind young adult's entry into adulthood and possible permanent move away from the parental home.
24. There are Ten Commandments that should guide all professionals in their work with parents.

REFERENCES

Ainsworth, M.D.S., M.C. Blehar, E. Waters, and S. Wall (1978) *Patterns of Attachment: A Psychological Study of the Strange Situation*. Hillsdale, NJ: Lawrence Erlbaum

Bowlby, J. (1982) *Attachment and Loss*, Vol. 1: *Attachment*. New York: Basic Books

Fox, A.M. (1983)   The Effects of Combined Vision and Hearing Loss on the Attainment of Developmental Milestones. *Proceedings of the First Canadian Conference on the Education and Development of Deaf-Blind Infants and Children*. Toronto: Ontario Ministry of Education

Hogg, J., and J. Sebba (1986) *Profound Retardation and Multiple Impairment*. Vol. 1: *Development and Learning*. London: Croom Helm

McInnes, J.M., and J.A. McInnes (1996) A Philosophy behind Education.   *Deafblind Education* 18 (July–December), 11–13

McInnes, J.M., and J.A. Treffry (1982) *Deaf-Blind Infants and Children: A Developmental Guide*. Toronto: University of Toronto Press

Nafstad, A.V. (1989) *Space of Interaction. An Attempt to Understand How Congenital Deafblindness Affects Psychological Development*. Publication No. 9. Dronninglund, Denmark: Nordic Staff Training Centre for Deafblind Services

Van Dijk, J. (1991) *Persons Handicapped by Rubella: Victors and Victims – A Follow-up Study*. Lisse: Swets and Zeitlinger

Wyman, R. (1986) *Multiply Handicapped Children*. London: Souvenir Press

9

The Preschool Years

JOHN M. McINNES

Introduction

Some professionals have difficulty with the term 'consultant.' They would like a term such as 'home visitor' or 'specialist in deafblind education and development' to be used. The author sees the first as being too limiting. The consultant is in the home and the school to consult, that is, to share, ask for and give advice, demonstrate, and talk things over. The consultant comes with some specialized knowledge, but is visiting the home, school, or community to do much more than 'tell.' If the term 'consultant' causes you concern please read the section on the consultant's role in chapter 16. For those seeking detailed suggestions on programming for and working with infants and children who are deafblind, they may be found in *Deaf-Blind Infants and Children* (McInnes and Treffry 1982), which is devoted solely to that topic, as well as in chapter 4, 'Communication.'

In chapters 1 to 8 several important points have been established that, when taken together, indicate the necessity for early identification and immediate action to begin to ameliorate the problems faced by an infant or young child challenged by deafblindness and the problems faced by his or her family. They may be summarized as follows:

1. Deafblindness is a unique, low-incidence disability.
2. An approach designed specifically to meet the special needs of the infant or young child who is deafblind must begin at once if the possibility of deafblindness is suspected.
3. Having a Personal Plan for the infant or child from the time of identification does not indicate the creation of a highly organized or regimented

implementation of a program. Initially, stress will be on bonding and communication in activities that take place during normal family routines.

4. It is important to use specialized methods and techniques when working with infants and children with deafblindness in areas such as Communication (chapter 4), Cognitive Development (chapter 5), Social Development (chapters 6 and 7), and Motor Development.[1]

5. If they are to provide suitable support, both nuclear and extended families as well as community professionals must be given accurate information concerning deafblindness, the present level of functioning and the future development of the infant or child, and the resources available.

6. Unlike the situation associated with many other disabilities, there usually is no pool of community knowledge where parents and community professionals can find accurate information.

7. The use of standardized tests and scales to provide an accurate assessment of the child's level of functioning is inappropriate (chapter 5).

8. An overall approach (chapter 2) focusing on the integration of medical treatment follow-up, therapeutic and developmental programs, communication development, sensory stimulation, sensory integration, and life-skills programs will be best developed by a specialist in the area of deafblindness in cooperation with parents and community professionals.

9. The family, community professionals, and others who work with the infant or child must be shown how to use appropriate intervention techniques.

10. The family have specific expectations of professionals who provide support for their child.

11. Individuals who make decisions concerning appropriate levels of support for both the child and the family must be educated to understand the needs of the deafblind child and the stress placed on the family.

Overview

Developing support for the infant or child with deafblindness will follow a specific series of steps:

1. Identification and referral
2. Initial evaluation
3. Initiating parental consultation
4. Personal Plan development and implementation
5. Ongoing formative evaluation
6. Education and training for parents, family, and professionals
7. Introduction of Intervenor(s) to the home and other settings

8. Identification and utilization of community preschool services
9. Preparation for entrance into formal educational programs.

Identification and Referral

Identification

From reading chapters 4 to 8 one can understand the importance of early identification and subsequent appropriate handling, interactive communication, and programming. Despite this understanding, however, problems will arise from two sources. An infant's vision loss and hearing loss may not be identified at the same time. Increasing numbers of deafblind infants are born with one or more additional disabilities. Good medical practice dictates that severe medical problems are addressed in an appropriate order, utilizing the most effective medical and therapeutic techniques. While the severity of physical problems may take precedence, the importance of identifying and approaching the infant as having deafblindness and of providing appropriate stimulation during periods of hospitalization cannot be overlooked.

When the problems caused in the areas of communication, cognitive-conceptual, and social-emotional development are taken into account, the disability of deafblindness is the denial of appropriate interaction with the environment and thus the denial of the motivation to initiate activities leading to development and the opportunity to learn. As the medical specialists who studied the Nordic definition of deafblindness stressed (chapter 1), when deafblindness is suspected, the infant or child should be treated as deafblind until it is proved that the identification is inappropriate. There can be no excuse to deny the infant an appropriate level of stimulation because he or she is hospitalized.

Referral

Experience has shown that members of the medical profession, including family physicians, medical specialists, and staff of children's hospitals, have proved very willing to call upon specialists in the field of deafblindness if they are aware of their existence. Specialists in the field of preschool services to infants and children with auditory impairment or visual impairment are also willing to refer infants and children if they are aware of the need for, and the existence of, services for infants and children who are deafblind. It is the responsibility of the consultants in the field of deafblindness and the centres from which they work to inform these groups about their existence and services. If it is suspected that he or she may have both a visual and a hearing loss, no infant or child is too disabled not to require services specifically designed to meet the needs of the person who is deafblind. Parents will occasionally initiate contact with a centre, but, as has been pointed out previously, the lack of a broad pool of community knowledge makes this the least likely source of referrals.

Initial Evaluation

When an infant or child is referred, an initial evaluation should be set up within the following fourteen days. If the referral was by telephone, the centre should have a procedure in place to ensure that the call is either taken by, or returned by, someone knowledgeable in the field of deafblind infants and children within twenty-four hours. There is no valid excuse for not meeting these two time lines. This is not the time to leave the parents without support.

The Process

On the basis of extensive experience, the first recommendation is to avoid the term evaluation and all it implies when discussing an impending first visit to the home and after you arrive. Rather, the consultant should talk about 'getting to know the infant or child and the family.' With the above said, the author has also found there are four basic pillars upon which the success of an initial evaluation will rest.

1. The evaluation should take place in the infant or child's most secure setting, usually the home.
2. The evaluation should be carried out by a team of two, an observer and an interacter.
3. A parent, or the parents, should be present, together with any other family members or professionals whom the parents wish to have present.
4. The team should encourage the parents to share their observations and should listen to what a parent says his or her child can do (see chapter eight).

The last point upsets many professionals. It has been our experience that, almost without exception, if a parent says 'my child can ...' and he or she does not do it during the initial visit, the infant or child will do it at some time during the next one or two follow-up visits. The parents' emotional bond, and thus ability to motivate the infant or child to give a desired response, is far stronger than that of team members, no matter how talented they feel they are in working with such infants or children.

Initial Evaluation Location

The initial evaluation should take place in the infant or child's most secure set-ting, usually the home. If you are going to have a successful interaction with the infant or child, you want to do everything possible to ensure both the parents' and the child's comfort and relaxation. When the home is used, the child is sur-rounded by a familiar environment and normal routines have suffered the least disruption.

In addition, when the initial interaction takes place in the home, the parent has not had to cope with a child who has

- parents who are nervous for days before the visit to an evaluation centre, anticipating their child's failure because of their knowledge of how their child acts in new situations or when they go to doctors' offices or hospitals
- been disturbed by travelling long distances in a car, or worse, by public trans-portation; and who anticipates 'hurts' because most long trips result in visits to doctors' clinics or hospitals
- been 'sleeping' in a strange bed and is out of sorts or even unmanageable
- been upset by being bombarded with unfamiliar smells, tactile experiences, and people
- been asked to eat strange food, or his or her food in unfamiliar surroundings.

Sometimes it is thought to minimize these problems by having the child and parent come and stay in accommodations at the clinic or near by. The reality is that parents often tell us that doing so may make the problem worse, because most of the above conditions are present, and, in addition, the parent accompa-nying the child is left to provide twenty-four-hour support without relief. Most deafblind infants and children do not adapt to new environments either over night or within a few days. The implication that they will do so flies in the face of all that we know about these infants and children. Put simply, the deafblind child and his family usually do not function as well in a strange environment or when routines are disrupted. Later, when recognition and bonding has been established between the consultant and the child, and the parent's trust is such that he or she is not apprehensive, the infant or child may be successfully brought to a clinic if it is thought necessary.

Initial Evaluation Interaction

Professionals who evaluate children become expert in forming a relationship with the child that brings forth the child's best efforts. Most professionals can establish such a relationship in a short period of time – except with a deafblind child. The positive relationship that may take minutes to establish with other children can take hours to establish with the deafblind infant or child, particularly during the first visit. For this reason time should be taken initially, and periodically, to observe the parent interacting with the child. The relationship will certainly be further affected if the individual interacting with the child has to stop to record significant happenings or to answer questions. Initial evaluations may take from three to five hours. The actual time allotted must be flexible. Even after observing the parent, the member of the team interacting with the child may require many attempts to establish true communication and to begin to see a child that 'can.' Occasionally, it may be necessary for the team to come back for a second or even a third visit to effectively get to know (evaluate) the child's level of functioning, particularly if the responses received from the child differ markedly from those described by the parent.

The Team

It is for the above reasons that the author advocates the use of a team approach. It has been found that a team of two professionals, both of whom have extensive training and experience performing initial evaluations, is the most cost-effective, efficient, and supportive way to perform such evaluations. The team members take the roles of interactor and recorder. It is often wise to wait until the team has met the child before the decision as to who will fill which role is made. The deafblind infant or child may begin to interact more positively with one team member than the other.

Using the team approach frees the interacter to concentrate on forming that very necessary relationship with the infant or child. This leaves the recorder available to answer questions and record significant interactions while the interaction is taking place. *The Developmental Profile for use with individuals with Congenital Deafblindness* (McInnes 1996) is a useful tool for recording such information and for making sure that no significant areas are overlooked. This tool is not a scale and is not designed to give scores. It is designed to ensure that no important area will be overlooked during the evaluation and that all significant medical and developmental information is recorded. No matter what instrument is used, well-trained team members will know the recording tool so well that its contents will be second nature to them.

Purpose of the Initial Evaluation

The purpose of this initial evaluation is to establish the following.

a) Decide if the child is deafblind. (As previously stated, if there is doubt, and regardless of additional problems, initially treat the infant or child as deafblind.)

b) Identify the present level of functioning in all areas of development.[2] What the parent tells you the child can do is equally as important as what is observed during the visit.

c) Identify areas of most likely progress in the following six months. This identification will lead to an initial set of recommendations and provide part of the basis for the writing of the first Personal Plan. (See chapter 2 concerning the contents of the first few plans.)

d) Obtain a detailed medical, therapeutic, developmental, and, if applicable, educational history. The time spent in hospital, the amount of stimulation received during that time, and the appropriateness of the developmental programs received are information that is essential if one is to understand the child's present level of functioning. The assembling of this information may take place over a number of visits. As parental trust grows, more detailed and accurate information will be forthcoming.

e) Obtain information about the child's and the family's routines. When such information about the family is missing, it is all too easy to make suggestions and design a plan that is unworkable, which only leads to feelings of frustration and guilt for the family. All of this information is essential if you are going to begin to develop an effective Personal Plan for the infant or child.

The Recorder

The recorder should be alert to all interactions initiated or repeated by the child, to any use of residual vision and hearing, communication, and all other indications of functioning level. A good team will develop a communication system between the two members that will enable the interactor to draw to the attention of the recorder communication attempts through muscle tightening, small movements, and so on, which may not be readily observable.

The recorder should carefully choose times to gather information from the parents or others. At first, most of their concentration will be on what the infant or child is doing (often with fear and concern) and on what the interactor is doing and how he or she is doing it, with thoughts of being able to repeat the techniques later. This is not the time to begin to gather information and history.

The Interactor

The interactor should begin by ensuring that the child is as relaxed and comfortable as possible. In almost every case in which the author has participated in an initial evaluation in the child's home, the child was dressed either in 'Sunday Best' or in new clothing. Both of these types of outfits may make the child uncomfortable. Thus, a good starting point to relax the child is to eliminate this potential problem. The interactor and the child remove clothing, usually hand over hand, until the child is dressed in a comfortable way. The interactor sits on the floor with the infant or child lying or sitting between the interactor's legs during this activity. Each item of clothing is placed in a particular place. It is surprising how often the child will demonstrate memory by making assisted motions to recover specific pieces of clothing hours later when the interaction is over and re-dressing is begun. When the infant or child has additional disabilities, care must be taken to ensure that nothing is done that will cause discomfort or other problems. This arrangement usually will increase the child's security and encourage freedom of movement. Parents may be apprehensive, and the recorder should explain to those present the reasons for this routine. *The interactor should always be ready to ask the parents for advice as to preferred activities or a demonstration as to how best to interact physically with his or her child, particularly when additional disabilities are present.*

Next, the interactor will usually introduce movement of the limbs and the concept of 'more' or 'stop.' In Souriau's terms (chapter 3), they are becoming communication partners. From this point on, interaction will take place guided by the infant's or child's responses. The interactor may wish to introduce new physical activities or play materials as the interaction continues, however, and should do so carefully. Major mistakes many interactors make are (a) to rush in using too many objects too quickly and (b) to think that the toys and other materials, rather than their interaction with the infant or child, will be the motivating factor. The infant's or child's experience usually lies in physical relationships and motor activities involving themselves and an adult. In using this interactive approach, much will be learned.

If the child rejects, or has had enough of a specific activity, leave it and return to it later if there is more to be learned. In our experience, it is not unusual for an infant or child who was judged to have 'a short attention span' to initiate, or accept, returning to an activity many times throughout the interaction and functioning at an increasingly higher level each time. It is often at this stage, when you have worked for hours, that a parent will say, 'He does that with me, but when I told my doctor he just looked at me.'

The emphasis throughout is on interaction and communication. As the interaction progresses, the interactor should give the infant or child a break periodically either by returning him or her to the parent or by encouraging independent investigation of the 'new things' and even the interactor's person. After the break, the infant or child is encouraged to return to activities with the interactor. If there is any reluctance, start by reintroducing an item or activity that was enjoyed prior to the break. As the final act, and a signal to the infant or child that *it's over,* co-actively retrieve and put on the clothing that was removed initially and return the infant or child to his or her parents for the last time, with an appropriate *'good bye.'*

Parental Questions

After the child's needs have been taken care of by the parent, the interactor should be prepared to discuss what he or she demonstrated and observed. Parental questions and observations concerning the interactor's work with the child should be encouraged. When this interchange is completed and the questions and comments by the team are finished, the parent(s) and other people present should be invited to ask further questions. If the recorder has done his or her job well and made note of questions raised during the interaction, he or she should raise them again at this time for further discussion. This is the most important aspect of the first visit, and it is not unusual to be invited back in the evening, 'when my husband/wife gets home' or 'when we have had time to discuss what you have told us,' to repeat answers and answer further questions. The team should avoid being too busy or too tired. Maybe for the first time the parents have found someone who understands the needs of their deafblind child. They will be eager for more information.

Initiating Parental Consultation

Under ideal circumstances, one of the team that did the initial evaluation will be the consultant assigned to the child and family. When this is not possible, one of the team should accompany the consultant who will fulfil this role on his or her first visit. Regardless of which route is taken, the initial team should set a date and time with the family for a follow-up visit before they leave, providing the child is found to be deafblind. Ideally, this will begin a long association between the family and the support centre.

An expectation of such support should gradually develop among the family members, therapists, developmental preschool specialists, and medical people involved. The expectation must never be allowed to exceed what the consultant and centre can deliver. Occasionally, one will hear a consultant say, 'That family only wants to see us once or twice a year.' There are several possible explanations for this reluctance. The family is fortunate enough to live in an area where appropriate, knowledgeable local support is available. On the other hand, it may be that the initial evaluation team did not make a good impression or did not explain clearly enough why a deafblind child has unique needs. Another possibility is that the parents or family are not at a stage in the grieving cycle where recognition of the child's problem of deafblindness is possible. Under such circumstances, if the child is deafblind and local support is not available, the centre should continue contact, merely to see how things are going and if there is anything that can be done to help. The purpose of continued contact is not to sell the service, but to remind the family that it is available and to show genuine interest in the infant or child.

The author can think of one occasion on which such contact was maintained for three years with a family before they had exhausted all other possibilities and requested support. It took a long time for the parents to accept the diagnosis, but the child made up much of the lost ground when treated as deafblind.

There are times when distance and financial constraints make home visits very difficult. The telephone, fax machines, the internet, email, and interactive communication using real-time digital cameras and computers all can help in overcoming such problems. None, however, can take the place of face-to-face visits during which the consultant is interacting with the child and demonstrating what he or she is saying.

Initially, such support should be available to the family and community once every two weeks. Later, if circumstances dictate, a longer period between visits may be contemplated. Regardless of circumstances, monthly visits are the least frequency that should be considered for the preschool child unless there is a strong deafblind support group available in the local community. There is a limit below which parents will be forced to turn to inappropriate sources for support to the detriment of their child.

Personal Plan Development and Implementation

The fully developed Personal Plan will not, in most cases, not be introduced during the first, or even the first few, six-month period(s). In the time between the initial evaluation and the development of the first Personal Plan, the consultant will

- get to know the family and community
- identify the level of resources available
- develop an ongoing emotional bond with the infant or child
- obtain a complete picture of his or her level of functioning and develop a dialogue with all family members, paraprofessionals, and professionals involved

- begin informal education and training during bi-weekly visits by demonstration and discussion
- introduce the concept of five-year goals and encourage and participate in their development.

Formative Evaluation

The author, and many others working in the field, strongly stress the need for *formative* rather than **summative evaluation**. Formative evaluation is an ongoing process, designed to identify and react to progress rather than being a fixed measurement at a specific time. A useful analogy would be that formative evaluation is represented by a video of the child, while summative evaluation is a photograph.

Each visit by the consultant will form part of the process, particularly during the first six months. He or she will gradually gain a more comprehensive picture of the child's level of functioning. At the same time, the consultant will have the opportunity to educate the parent, the family, and the professionals involved concerning the specific methods that will work with the child; to help each understand the problems presented by a loss of the use of the distance senses; and to promote an understanding of how each must adjust his or her traditional approaches to fit into and promote overall development.

The most important aspect of the ongoing consultant visits, however, is the gradual change in the parents' view of their child. An effective specialist in deafblindness will gradually change the focus from that of a disabled child who 'can't' to a view of a child with deafblindness, and maybe additional problems, who 'can.' An important part of this process lies in educating those involved to know what to look for as indicators of success. In no way should this be interpreted as proposing to give the parents false hopes.

JJ was a two-year-old child with severe disabilities. He was diagnosed as deafblind, had cerebral palsy, deformities of the spine, a general, overall weakness, and had no concept of self. The consultant worked with the physiotherapist and the family to demonstrate how therapy exercises might be incorporated into everyday routines and how communication could become a part of all activities. After six months he was beginning to recognize 'Mother' (she wore glasses), Dad (the smell of his pipe came from all his clothing), and Susan (his sister with braids). Owing to Mother's hard work, particularly during meal times when she sat him on her knee and fed him hand over hand (at least four or five tries with each food item), he began to show some occasional attempts at hand and arm control and is now beginning to show recognition of family members with expectations of certain activities. Mother had great difficulty with friends and particularly grandparents on both sides of the family because he wasn't in a high chair and they thought he should be in one. For most deafblind infants much of the interaction during the first six months will focus on the development of emotional bond(s), communication, fostering curiosity, use of residual vision and hearing, and mobility.

'When will my child walk?'
This is one of the most frequently asked questions. The simple answer is 'when it is to his or her advantage to do so.' The question you should ask yourself, however, is 'Why does my child need to learn to walk?' To answer it, you must first consider why any infant rolls over, creeps and crawls, begins to prefer a sitting position, and eventually stands and walks. The answer will be 'you,' physically interacting with the child in a variety of ways. To understand, focus on the part vision and hearing play in these accomplishments and then decide how you can compensate through interactive play for the lack of effective use of the distance senses. The child will learn to stand and walk when it is to his or her advantage unless there are extreme physical problems that prevent or make it dangerous to bear weight. It is possible that your child may not progress through the traditional stages of rolling over, creeping, crawling, sitting, standing, and finally walking. Nor should you try to motivate him or her using each stage in turn. It is not unusual for the child to go from lying, to sitting to standing because this progression will best equip him or her to play interactively with you or another person. He or she will learn to creep, crawl, and pull himself or herself up when these actions will pay off.

'Will my child talk?'
This is a very different question from 'Will my child be able to communicate?' An important and detailed answer is found in chapter 4.

'How will I promote curiosity?'
Curiosity will be promoted and developed if the initial attempts to explore the world are encouraged and participated in by people with whom the child has a bond and with whom he or she enjoys snuggling, rough-housing, and simply being with. Curiosity is one of the hardest things to encourage because of the lack of satisfaction with the results unless the deafblind infant can share the experience.

All members of the family worked very hard on getting JJ to participate actively (rather than being manipulated passively) in exercises that were disguised as games. Individuals outside the immediate family took much longer than six months to begin to recognize his progress. Most important, however, that was the family was beginning to see him as a child that 'could' (McInnes and Treffry 1982). One of the most difficult things to learn to do was to promote independence by giving JJ choices among activities, allowing him to decide that an activity was finished, and simply to be there for support rather than continued direction and manipulation.

Writing the Preschooler's Personal Plan

Once the parent's confidence has been gained and shared positive perception of the child has been developed, it is time to begin discussions leading to the setting of five-year goals (see chapter 2). It will take time to reach this point and the process should not be rushed. Until now, the bi-weekly visits and the demonstrations of what to do and how, combined with the education of both the family and the professionals involved with the child, will have provided sufficient support.

It must be realized, however, that probably only the consultant has a clear picture of where this process is going. This is not a professional secret to be guarded by the consultant. It is a projection ('vision' may be a more accurate word) that should evolve from discussions among the parents, paraprofessionals, and professionals involved with the child. It can be somewhat unsettling to some professionals the first time they are asked, 'Given the present progress and your experience in your field, how do you see (the name of the infant or child) functioning in five years?' The questions to the parent will be somewhat different. NOT 'What do you see ... doing in five years?' but rather, 'Where do you see him going to school?' 'What responsibilities do you see him having in the family?' 'What do you see him doing for fun?' 'What activities do the family like to do together?' and so on. It will probably require several sessions, maybe many sessions, to have all involved comfortable enough to answer such questions.

At the same time, the process of developing a Personal Plan will be taking place, and the consultant will be encouraging everyone to participate in assembling a history and preparing a description of the child's present level of functioning. When the history, description of the present level of functioning, and the five-year goals have been assembled and agreed upon by the team (parents, professionals, and paraprofessionals), the consultant will initiate the preparation of a set of objectives describing the success indicators that will show progress hoped for in the next six months. And as the final step, the consultant will review all the information with the family and others involved and assist them in identifying where in the existing routines individual objectives will be worked upon; suggest and demonstrate the techniques and methods that will facilitate the accomplishment of the objectives; and assist both professionals and parents to make such arrangements as are necessary to carry out new, or modify existing, routines and activities. One caveat needs repeating: no program should be suggested that so disrupts the family's routines or makes such demands on the family's time that it will not be carried out willingly. Such willingness should be composed of equal parts of the infant's or child's progress and available time. No other formula will work. The consultant who proposes or lets another propose that the family do too much is not doing his or her job. Souriau and Rodbroe emphasize that enjoyment is an essential component in communication (see chapter 4). In fact, it is an essential component in all activities.

Enjoyment is a hard thing to find if you are

- being late for work
- deprived of your friends' company to take care of your brother constantly
- scheduled so tightly that you cannot possibly utilize the appropriate approaches during therapy
- so tired and distraught that your job and/or your marriage suffers
- feeling guilty because you are not 'doing enough.'

It is the consultant's job to listen to the family, assess the family and community resources, and avoid stretching the family's resources to the breaking point.

Training for Parents, Family, and Community Professionals

Initial training for parents, family members and community professionals will take place primarily through demonstration. In the words of the poet Edgar A. Guest,

I'd rather see a sermon than hear one any day,
I'd rather one would walk with me than merely show the way.

It is not the job of the consultant to try to take the place of any of these individuals. Rather, it is his or her job to demonstrate techniques and suggest methods that will make their actions more productive.

When the parent or professional indicates that he or she is ready, a second means of increasing knowledge and confidence is for the consultant to provide the individual with the phone numbers or email addresses of others, either parents or professionals, who have had or are having similar experiences. Two points should be emphasized: (a) no such information should ever be given unless permission has been obtained in advance, and (b) initially, the selection of such contacts should be carefully made. The Deafblind List on the internet is also an excellent place for family members and members of the local support team to obtain and/or share information

Both parents and professionals have often indicated that they have benefited greatly from such contacts. These contacts have permitted them both to check the validity of the advice they are receiving and to overcome the feeling of isolation resulting from having few, if any local contacts. Consultants, particularly, should realize the importance to the family of being able to check on the advice given, and it is hoped that this book will serve such a purpose to some extent.

Workshops, training sessions, and meetings designed to address specific topics in the area of deafblindness should be available to both parents and professionals. Professionals, such as physiotherapists, and parents can be invited to address groups of both professional and lay persons, to outline the approaches that they have found successful. The most important factor is timing, particularly for parents. If timing is handled appropriately, they will increase their appreciation of the value of what they are doing, gain new insights into its importance, and increase self-esteem.

Introduction of Non-Family Intervenor(s) in the Home and Preschool Settings

In the Home

The first Intervenor will be the child's most frequent supporter. Today grandparents and even paid housekeepers often fulfil the role that was traditionally filled by mother. The next step occurs when individual family members begin to play specific roles in the child's life (see chapter 3). The largest step of all is the introduction of outside Intervenors into the home and family.

The latter step should not be attempted before the parents begin to recognize the child's progress and reach the stage where they realize that family resources, particularly those of time, are insufficient to meet the infant's or child's need for stimulation from a reactive environment. The introduction of a stranger into the home and family circle is a major event. Families will often be reluctant to take this step. The consultant should present the concept of such intervention, but it should be left to the family to initiate the request. Sometimes, the child's being supported by an Intervenor while attending nursery school will lead to parental recognition of the need for intervention in the home both during the week and on weekends.

The consultant's support of the family in obtaining intervention, training the

Intervenor to work with the specific child, and defining the role the Intervenor will play is essential. Where the Intervenor is working out of the home, it is strongly recommended that a contract be drawn up outlining the duties and responsibilities of both the family and the Intervenor. This is very important in cases where the child has additional challenges having specific requirements that must be met during the time the Intervenor is working with the child. Bureaucracies that are paying for the service often want an identified agency, such as the deafblind centre, to be in charge of, and doing the hiring, firing, and supervision of the Intervenor. Under no circumstances should the family have an Intervenor imposed upon them by an outside agency. Because of the role the Intervenor plays, the family should have a say in who is hired. The final decision may be made by someone other than the family in cases where the Intervenor is an employee of a school board or preschool agency IF the Intervenor is not going to work in the home. Even under these circumstances, the family should be included in the hiring process. An Intervenor is not a school aide. *Hiring an Intervenor without the family's approval is never defensible, for any reason, if the Intervenor is going to work in, or out of, the family's home.*

The family must have control of who is entering their house, what they are doing, and how they are doing it. The roles of the consultant and the centre are to support, educate, and train, not to dictate. A local agency may pay the Intervenor, but the family must always have the final say concerning their infant or child without the threat of loosing the support of the agency, the consultant, and the centre. It is legitimate, however, for such a funding agency to have rules governing the employment of family members.

In the Preschool Setting

After the parents, accompanied by the consultant, have visited and reviewed the available preschool programs, arrangements should be made for a return visit to the programs most favoured by the parents. During this visit a discussion with the program's director concerning the problems posed by deafblindness, the needs of the specific child, the child's Personal Plan, and how the preschool program can contribute to its fulfilment should take place. The consultant should explain his or her role in developing, implementing, and evaluating the Personal Plan and in supporting the family and the preschool program. The role of the Intervenor and the fact that it is not expected that the staff will become experts in the field of deafblindness should be also explained. The consultant should answer any questions posed by the program director or members of the staff of the preschool program.

Initially, the concept of intervention and role of the Intervenor will probably cause the most confusion and concern. It is often wise to arrange for the child and the Intervenor, accompanied by the consultant and the parent, to attend one or two sessions of the preschool program. This will give the consultant a chance to demonstrate how the child can participate in appropriate activities and do individual activities when the class is engaged in activities unsuitable for a deafblind child. Having the parent give explanations, demonstrations with their child, and answer questions will provide an opportunity for the preschool program staff to see the parent as a knowledgeable member of the team. The impression should be left that the parent and family are valuable sources of information, and that the program staff do not have to wait until the next visit by the consultant to obtain necessary information. It should also be suggested at this time that the parent should visit the program as often as weekly to ensure that the same techniques and methods are being used in both the home and the program. The frequency of the visits should be governed by the parent's ability to carry out such visits, not by either the consultant's or the preschool staff's idea of 'What should be.' The consultant should discuss this frequency with the parents and be guided by their decision prior to introducing the idea during the visit to the preschool program.

Occasionally, after the initial discussion, the consultant may suggest to the parent that other alternatives should be considered if the director or staff of the preschool program should prove

- to have entrenched views and routines that they are not prepared to modify to meet the needs of a deafblind child
- not to be prepared to have a parent or consultant in the program on a regular basis
- not to be prepared for any child in the program to have one-to-one support.

Preschool and Community Services

The introduction of the use of preschool and community services depends on

- the availability of appropriate services
- the readiness of the facility or service to accommodate the needs of the infant or child as deafblind
- the parents' recognition of the need for such services.

The final choice of the utilization of any specific preschool program must lie with the parents. In the author's experience, local preschool programs that are prepared to function as part of a larger Personal Plan are preferable to specialized community-based programs designed to meet the needs of children who are physically or mentally challenged. If the child with deafblindness has additional disabilities that are not being met, special programs may provide access to therapy that is not otherwise available, and they should be chosen for this reason only. However, no deafblind child should be saddled with expectations held by staff in programs designed for children with other challenging conditions. Unfortunately, the author has seen deafblind children placed in programs designed to meet the needs created by physical or mental disabilities and resulting employment of inappropriate methods and techniques in a non-communicating atmosphere. In each instance this approach almost inevitably led to learned helplessness and severe behaviour problems. In most cases therapy can be delivered as part of the school program or the child can leave school and go to the therapist accompanied by his or her Intervenor; thus, the lack of availability of appropriate therapy in the local school program usually can be overcome.

If a local community preschool is being considered, there must be provision for activities such as daily swimming and other out-of-class and out-of-school activities required by the comprehensive Personal Plan. Sensory stimulation boxes, play areas, and specific activities designed for other children may not be suitable for the deafblind infant or child. In fact, they may often be inappropriate because of the child's multi-sensory deprivation. The consultant can play an important role in assisting the program staff to choose those activities that are suitable and suggest alternative activities that the child and the Intervenor can do while the other children are following established routines.

One thing that is essential is that the program staff accept the presence of an Intervenor and recognize that his or her role is not one of an additional staff member to be utilized for 'the good of all children.' To this end, the consultant should continue to hold information sessions on a quarterly or half-yearly basis and provide some training for the program staff when requested. These activities should continue as long as the child is enrolled in the program.

It should be noted that once the child is enrolled in a preschool program, the consultant must visit both the home, when the child is present, and the preschool program as well as all facilities that are being utilized in the community as either part of the preschool or home-based section of the Personal Plan. Visiting only one location will inevitably lead to confusion, and even mistrust, as the consultant's suggestions are communicated from one site to the other. The consultant's demonstration of appropriate techniques in both environments, as new needs evolve, is essential.

Preparation for the School Years

As the young child approaches the age for entry to the school system, the parents, assisted by the consultant, should review the choices available. These choices may include

- a regular class in the local school
- a special class in the local school
- a special school in the local community
- a residential school serving children with another identified disability, such as hearing impairment
- a residential school with a program designed to meet the needs of the deaf-blind child.

Each of these choices will have advantages and disadvantages. The author's preference would be a regular class in the local school where support is available from a consultant who is a specialist in the field of deafblindness and who views the school's academic program as being a partial contribution to the total Personal Plan or the residential school setting that provides a specific program for children and youth who are deafblind. No choice should be seen as final, and the use of each of these two settings by one child at different ages should be expected. Unless the local community is very large, or very unusual, there will not be a class or classes for children who are deafblind or consultants specifically trained in this field.

Parents should examine each of the two choices (local school and residential school) to ensure that they will provide, or actively promote, a twenty-four-hour-a-day, 365-day-a-year program. The local school must be prepared to be flexible and to permit the deafblind child to continue to utilize community resources, such as swimming, during the school day. Deafblind children do not learn successfully by the methods used with children who face visual, hearing, or intellectual disabilities nor do they participate in the active, vigorous games that develop the cardiovascular system and muscles. Activities designed to substitute for both organized team sports and spontaneous activities of their peers must be substituted for by the use, with intervention, of swimming pools and other community facilities on a regular basis.

Parents should start looking approximately two years before they are going to seek admission to the school system (see chapter 10 for a detailed discussion). Initial approaches should be a request to visit local and area schools in which the child might enroll and a visit to any residential programs that the child might attend. These initial visits should concentrate on assessing the following features:

- the flexibility of the staff in providing individual programs
- the availability of required therapy

- if transportation is required, the availability and function of additional staff on the bus or in the car as well as the length of time such transportation will take
- the administration and school's staff attitude towards outside assistance from a consultant
- the administration's attitude towards a child's having an individual Intervenor
- the attitude towards a parent's being in the classroom frequently and for various lengths of time
- the accessibility of the facilities in terms of the child's needs.

Eliminate from the list of choices programs that appear not to be able, or that are unwilling to adjust, to meet the child's needs as deafblind. The placing of the child in a class designed to serve the needs of another disability is often suggested because of low staff-to-student ratios and/or because they already have teacher's aides in the room. Such reasoning should immediately raise doubts. The reason the class has a low number of students is because that number is all a teacher working with children who have this particular type of challenge can possibly support. The teacher is a specialist in working with this particular type of disability, and it is unrealistic to expect that she will have the time or the energy also to become a specialist in the education of the child who is deafblind. Secondly, the child with deafblindness does not need a teacher's aide who has been placed in the class to assist all children. He or she needs an Intervenor who will support him/her, not the teacher and a number of other pupils.

One principal proudly told us that his philosophy was 'All children are equally important and no one child will receive any more support than any other! No child in my school is going to receive one to one when others in the class also need support.' The author and the parents were thankful that he went into education rather than medicine, where he would have given all patients a heart transplant regardless of their needs. It is the needs of the individual deafblind child, not the philosophy of the administration, that must determine the amount and the type of support required.

When the list has been narrowed down to the best possible choices, visits by the parent accompanied by the consultant should be made to observe the programs in the classroom and the atmosphere in the school and to meet with and talk to both the teacher and the administration about the specific deafblind child and his or her particular needs. The concept of the Personal Plan approach should be introduced and discussed. Any educational system that indicates that their IEPs or IPPs will meet the deafblind child's needs should be viewed with suspicion or even rejected out of hand.

Ask about other challenged children in the school and about how their needs are being met in the classroom, at lunch time, and during recess. Observe the interaction between these children and the general school population. Is it being actively supported and encouraged by the school staff? To what extent do these children with special needs take part in the life of the school? These questions are equally valid when any of the choices listed at the beginning of this section are being considered.

Once the choice is narrowed to one or two possibilities, have the deafblind child visit the schools with his or her parents, the consultant, and, where possible, the Intervenor. These visits are important both for the information they elicit and to prepare the child for entry into this environment.

Finally, before the child actually begins to attend the school, the staff of the program under consideration should be invited to one or two team meetings. When they have had a chance to review and discuss the child's Personal Plan, they should be encouraged to indicate how specific activities and equipment in the classroom can contribute to the attainment of identified objectives. Discussions should also be held concerning activities that the deafblind child can do with his or her Intervenor when the class is engaged in activities that are inappropriate.

Entering the educational system parallels the infant's entry into this world. He or she can no more be plugged into the educational system than he or she could be expected to mirror exactly the development of the non-disabled infant or child. Just as the home and community were utilized to aid development with the support of the intervention process, so must the educational system be viewed as another array of tools and opportunities that can be utilized to promote the child's development with the aid of an Intervenor.

Additional Considerations during the Preschool Years

Requests for Support Seen as Excessive

Unless the family and their medical advisers receive a high level of ongoing support from knowledgeable professionals, they will be forced to turn to other community organizations. These other organizations often will have little or no understanding of the problems associated with the infant or child who is deafblind and may see the parents' requests for service as excessive. This is particularly true where administrators are forced to operate under general guidelines that place upper limits in terms of hours or dollars upon the degree of support that an individual family may receive. Additionally, such requests for support by the family of an infant or preschool child who is deafblind, usually for intervention hours, are often misinterpreted as unreasonable requests for parental relief or as evidence of a family that is unable or unwilling to cope and 'do their duty' in supporting the child with deafblindness. It is a rare occurrence when they represent either. This lack of appropriate support, combined with the constant need to explain, defend, and justify special services for their child, places an emotional drain upon the parents and other family members. Such constant pressure is greater than that felt by the parents of most children who are challenged, because for them a pool of community knowledge, appropriate expectations, and needed services exists; the disability faced by their children is more readily identified and understood by both professionals and the community at large.

It has been found that the use of a fully developed Personal Plan showing contributions by parents and others is often helpful in overcoming the perception that the parents are requesting excessive support. Bureaucrats and other agency members, and even extended family members, are completely unaware of the amount of time and money the parents and family are already contributing to the support of their child.

Family Failing

The family may feel that they are failing because

- there is not an appropriate level of support
- there are no community models upon which to base expectations of service
- there are no appropriate family models to turn to.

When requests for support are met with lack of understanding from other community agencies and from government agencies, the result is that the family often becomes reluctant to request adequate support out of fear that they may loose some or all of the support they have been able to obtain.

Parents repeatedly state that it is for these reasons, not the disability of the child or the extraordinary number of physical demands made on them personally that they are forced to consider giving up or to accept services that do not meet their child's needs. Even after they have stopped fighting for their child, however, they remain bitter and frustrated at seeing their child denied the life he or she might have had.

Appropriate Support for the Family

The family who are supporting an infant or child who is deafblind should have access at least twice a month to knowledgeable professionals with extensive training and experience in deafblindness and, between visits, access to a specific professional available by telephone, fax, email or through an interactive internet connection who will guarantee to return their call within twenty-four hours. Support for the family should come from one or a maximum of two such consultants at any one time. If requested by the family, this consultant should act as a case manager and be available to accompany the family, when requested to do so, to meetings with community-service groups, and medical and other professionals who are providing community-based medical, therapeutic, educational, or recreational programs and support.

When Available Resources Restrict Support

There is an optimum level of support, as described in this chapter and throughout the text. There is also a minimum below which attempts at support only cause families and community professionals frustration and resentment. When families are forced to turn to agencies and advisers who represent other fields, such as deafness or blindness, it is an indication that they are not receiving an appropriate level of support. Correspondence between the author and James Gallagher, a deafblind young man who has authored excellent internet resources, has provided the following insight into how technology can help to stretch available resources.

Alternative Approaches to Support

by James Gallagher

The technology age has come, especially for parents of deafblind children. There was a time when parents would have to visit a centre or ask for a home visit by a specially trained representative of the nearest deafblind organization in hopes they could find the support they required. If a problem arose that had to be dealt with quickly, they could, of course, telephone the centre and, if possible, speak to their consultant or someone else who knew their child and in whom they had confidence to give them the information they needed. This is the way it has been done for many years. But a telephone call does not take the place of a visit and face-to-face discussion, demonstration of techniques to be used, and suggestions to the parents as they interact with their deafblind infant or child.

How can parents, intervenors, and others receive the service they so desperately need if distance, scheduling, and even agency financial constraints prevent

284 John M. McInnes

immediate and direct support by their consultant? Even a return telephone call often will not suffice. Today, if the parents have a computer, an inexpensive digital camera, and a modem, much better support is available. They now have greatly increased resources at their fingertips. By purchasing a small golfball-size camera and the appropriate software to run the camera, they can get in touch with the centre using a program such as Microsoft Netmeeting (free at the time of writing) and describe or demonstrate the problem and/or show the child's reactions. (This solution may be used even if a parent also has a hearing problem. Using the interactive setup, parents can communicate by 'BSL or ASL' Sign Language with the centre and reduce some pressure or stress they may feel when trying to describe the problem they are having.)

With the use of video and sound, parents can explain or demonstrate the problem and the adviser can see the problem and suggest a specific solution designed to meet the infant's or child's needs. Perhaps parents and the consultant could arrange a specific time every second week to have a discussion on ways forward for themselves and their child by using this interactive communication. It should also be noted, as long as the consultant has access to a laptop or desktop computer and a digital camera, he or she does not have to be at the deafblind centre to communicate with the parents over the internet. [This approach also can be used to reduce the number of consultant visits from once every two weeks to not less than ten per year. It will work, however, only when the consultant has first gained sufficient experience working with the child and the confidence of the family. JMM]

The computer can also provide additional ways for parents and professionals to find out information. There are many resources on the internet for information about deafblindness including a number of mailing lists. [A mailing list is a posting of questions and answers generated by members of the list usually using email. There is usually no charge for membership on a list or for using email other than internet connect charges. Email allows interaction with individuals all over the world without payment for long-distance telephone charges. See chapter 18, 'Resources,' for additional information.] It is very advisable for parents to join such a mailing list. Lists provide an excellent resource for parents of a deafblind child because there will be members who have come across the same problem and who would be more than happy to explain solutions they have found. Also, many members of such lists themselves work within deafblind organizations and are very knowledgeable about the field.

Parents may believe that to set up this equipment will be both costly and difficult. Prices of home computers are dropping, and, in addition, many large organizations are willing to donate older, but still very usable, equipment for such a good cause. It is said that in the computer field equipment becomes obsolete within two years but obsolete for big business does not make it worthless for home use. In some jurisdictions the cost of such equipment may be covered by government agencies or community service organizations such as Rotary or Kiwanis. In addition, this equipment becomes easier to install every day. The software practically installs itself.

The future will bring greater advances on this technology and for parents this will bring them the comfort of thinking that help is just a few seconds away no matter where they live within their country or in the world (e.g. John McInnes is interacting with parents in South America, Australia, the United States, and Germany at the time of writing as well as being a member of several lists).

Technology will play a large part in the life of all families in the future and because of this it will be important to introduce the deafblind child to computers and other technology as soon as possible. This is an excellent opportunity to teach him or her that one day this equipment will open doors and make communicating a bit easier. The child will begin to learn that the world is a huge place and that many people like him or her are out there too, and when he or she is older, the computer will perhaps bring them greater independence in later life.

So parents have nothing to fear about technology because they will find out that it can provide unbelievable resources and help to them and their child.

Summary

1. There are nine steps in developing preschool services.
2. Identification or referral is often delayed because the disability caused by vision and hearing loss is not recognized, or does not occur, at the same time.
3. Members of the medical profession and preschool visitors from centres for visually or auditorily challenged infants and children are prepared to refer clients if they are aware that a program to support infants, children, youth, and adults with deafblindness exists.
4. The initial evaluation should take place in the child's home.
5. The initial evaluation should be made by a team with highly specialized training in the area of deafblindness.
6. The team is composed of an interactor and a recorder.
7. During the six months following the initial evaluation a Personal Plan should be developed by the consultant.
8. The Personal Plan should be based upon formative evaluation.
9. Consultants should demonstrate, not tell parents, what to do and how to do it.

10. No Intervenor who is not a family member should be introduced until the family indicates that they are ready.
11. The parents should choose the preschool services in consultation with the consultant.
12. Preparation for entry into school should begin at least two years before the admittance date.

NOTES

1 Detailed suggestions are found in *Deaf-Blind Infants and Children: A Developmental Guide* (1982). The text is a comprehensive reference guide for teachers, parents, professionals, and paraprofessionals working or living with children who are deaf-blind. It provides day-to-day guidance and suggestions about techniques and methods for programming for and working with such children.
2 An in-depth discussion of all areas that will be addressed during the initial visit is provided in *Deaf-Blind Infants and Children* (1982).

REFERENCES

McInnes, J.M., ed. (1996) *The Developmental Profile for Use with Individuals with Congenital Deafblindness.* Brantford, ON: Canadian Deafblind and Rubella Association (Ontario Chapter)
McInnes, J.M., and J.A. Treffry (1982, 1993, 1997) *Deaf-Blind Infants and Children: A Developmental Guide.* Toronto: University of Toronto Press

10

The Community-Based School Option

CAROLYN MONACO and LINDA MAMER

The Community School: A Viable Option?

The community-based school can be and is a viable educational option for many students who are deafblind. There are a number of components or factors that must be in place to ensure the success of this option. Within this chapter we shall discuss the educational needs of a student who is deafblind and the supports that are required to ensure that the school personnel, the Intervenor, and the family are able to design, implement, and evaluate a program that will effectively meet the needs of the student who is included in their community school. This educational option and any school-based program comprise one component of a Personal Plan that is designed to support a student who is deafblind and encompasses home, school, and community.[*]

Making the Decision

There are a number of possible options for the educational placement of students who are deafblind. Each possible option available to a student should be explored by both the parents and the professionals prior to any final decision. Possible options in your locale may be the following:

---

*Editor's note. In this chapter it is assumed that the reader has read chapter 2 and thus understands that the authors are focusing upon one aspect of a Personal Plan developed for the deafblind student who is living at home and attending a community school. *They should not be seen as advocating that adequate support for the deafblind student will be found within a traditional IEP or similar document.* The program described in such documents is but one aspect of a Personal Plan. Other aspects of the Personal Plan have received comprehensive treatment throughout the text and thus only brief mention is made of them in this chapter. A Personal Plan addressing all aspects of the student's overall participation in the family, community, and school is essential.

1. Community school – regular classroom with classmates of the same age
2. Community school – regular classroom with classmates of ages other than that of the student with deafblindness
3. Community school – regular classroom with special education classroom opportunities
4. Community school – special education classroom with regular classroom opportunities
5. Community school – personal program utilizing any meaningful school-wide opportunities
6. Community school – personal program utilizing any combination of meaningful school or community opportunities
7. Congregated school – students all of whom have some level of disability, who travel to the same location
8. Congregated class within a community school – students all of whom have some level of disability, who travel to the same location
9. Residential school with residential placement
10. Residential school with day placement only
11. Home-based placement.

The exploration of all possible placements will enable persons to put the options into three categories:

1. Definite prospects
2. Potential prospects
3. Unsuitable prospects.

It is as important to explore those options, which on the surface seem to be unsuitable prospects, as it is to explore the definite prospects, in order for every-one to feel an informed decision has been made. Initially, some persons may have preconceived ideas or definite views on placements and into which of the three categories of prospects they may fall. Yet those placements that may ini-tially appear to be unsuitable could, in fact, be potential prospects once all of the information has been gathered and the site visited. There is a danger that people might base their final decision on inaccurate or outdated information, or on information received from a third party. The process of gathering this infor-mation and visiting all of the sites can take much time and effort. It is such an important decision in the life of a student with deafblindness, however, that it cannot be stressed enough that parents should take an active role in the process. The educational placement provides the foundation upon which the program will be designed and implemented and therefore warrants the time and effort required. The strength of the foundation will affect the success of the program and ultimately the success of the student.

Elements to Consider in Potential Placements

The following elements should be considered in the choice of a placement.

1. Amount of intervention provided
2. Availability of trained personnel in deafblindness
3. Welcoming attitude of the school principal and school personnel
4. General knowledge of deafblindness or willingness to learn about deaf-blindness
5. Previous success of the school with students with disabilities
6. Access to meaningful programming within the school
7. Types of programming that the school provides or is willing to offer
8. Amount of time spent on transportation to and from the placement
9. Physical accessibility of the school environment
10. Availability of support personnel if required, for example, therapists
11. Willingness to accommodate medical needs, if applicable.

It is important to remember that each placement will have individual issues or factors; thus no one element listed above should be weighted so high that a decision is made solely because of it. For example: Physical accessibility: do not discount a particular school if it is not accessible at the time of the visit but the administration is willing to develop strategies to compensate, such as building a ramp or providing personnel or equipment to lift a wheelchair.

The decision should be made by an informed team (defined in the following section) consisting of the parents, school personnel, and student, if appropriate. Parental preferences should be given serious consideration. The decision should never be considered final. The placement should be re-evaluated on a regular yearly basis to ensure that it continues to meet the needs of the student. This yearly re-evaluation allows the team to feel confident that they made the best decision they could, based on the information available at the time. The more informed the team members are at the time of the decision, the more secure they can be in the knowledge that they have made the best possible decision. Decisions made without current and accurate information can be a deterrent to providing the best Personal Plan to meet the needs of the student. As new information becomes available, the decision can be reviewed.

An Effective Team Approach

The Members of the Team
The parents/guardians, a consultant who is a specialist in deafblindness (here-after called the consultant), Intervenors, classroom teacher, and student (where appropriate) all should be a part of every student's educational team. Where the needs of the student warrant, the principal, vice-principal, special educa-tion teacher, resource teacher, special education coordinator, substitute Inter-venors, classmates of the student, in-home Intervenor, educational assistants, medical services coordinator, physiotherapist, occupational therapist, speech and language therapist, technology specialist, health care provider, optome-trist, audiologist, and orientation and mobility instructor should be members of the team.

The Benefits of Developing an Effective Team Approach

Creating an effective team approach provides the best possible opportunity for the following:

1. All personnel involved to meet each other on a regular basis
2. All personnel involved to develop an understanding of each other's roles and level of involvement with the student
3. All personnel involved to learn about deafblindness and intervention
4. Sharing in the challenges and the successes that occur within the educational program of a student with deafblindness
5. The Intervenor to receive consistent and coordinated input and direction
6. Reducing the potential for conflicting and or contradictory information that may arise from any of the professionals who see the student on an individual basis
7. Personnel and family members to feel part of a supportive, committed group of people focused on the specific needs of the individual with deafblindness.

The Roles of the Members of the Team

The team around the student ensures that the many facets of the student's edu-cational program are considered when the Personal Plan is written.

Parents/Guardians
The parents will be the constant in their child's life, unlike the vast number of professionals, whose involvement will be periodic or temporary. For this reason

they should be considered permanent members of the educational team. Their role on the team should encompass the following:

1. Advocating for their child's needs as they understand them
2. Providing a historical perspective about their child's development, when it assists the team to understand more clearly the student's strengths, needs, and areas of growth
3. Sharing pertinent information about the ongoing medical status of their child
4. Sharing information to assist with goal setting and to maintain consistency between home and school with regard to methods of communication, expectations of student, and strategies for skill and conceptual development
5. Providing feedback on those concepts and skills that are transferable between home and school
6. Giving information about training in the following areas:
   a) training that may be currently occurring within the home
   b) additional training that they feel may need to occur within the school
7. Providing a parental perspective on strengths, needs, and progress.

Consultant in Deafblindness
Individuals who design educational programs for those who are deafblind must have specific training and experience in deafblindness and intervention. In order to facilitate adequately the delivery of a program to both home and school they must also have considerable training in family dynamics, the grieving process, consulting skills, effective team membership, and training personnel. Programs for individuals who are deafblind cannot be adequately designed by persons having training and experience only in blindness / low vision or deafness / hard of hearing. The consultant's role on the team should encompass the following:

1. Assisting the team to develop an understanding of the needs of students who are deafblind
2. Assisting the team to understand the philosophy of intervention
3. Gathering input to develop the Personal Plan
4. Gathering input from the team to assist with the evaluation of the program
5. Assisting the team members to develop an understanding of the specific methods and techniques relating to deafblindness which are pertinent to their particular area of expertise
6. Providing current and relevant information from the field of deafblindness, in the areas of research, upcoming events, conferences, related agencies and services.

Intervenor

The Intervenor plays a vital role on the team, since the Intervenor implements the Personal Plan on a day-to-day basis. The Intervenor's role on the team should encompass the following:

1. Providing verbal and written feedback on the day-to-day implementation of the program
2. Assisting the team members to understand the needs of the student as they pertain to the student's educational program
3. Assisting in the coordination of the visits of the support personnel to the educational program
4. Informing the team of any concerns or issues regarding the educational program.

Classroom Teacher

The classroom teacher's primary roles are to provide and implement the curriculum for the students in the classroom and to provide the Intervenor with sufficient information regarding the day-to-day classroom activities or subject areas to allow him/her adequate time to make any adaptation or modifications that would be required. The classroom teacher's role on the team should encompass the following:

1. Providing feedback about the student's involvement in the classroom curriculum
2. Providing input based on their observations of the student
3. Informing the team of any concerns or issues they may have regarding the educational program.

Student (Where Appropriate)

Whenever possible the student should be encouraged to become an active member of his/her educational team. The student's role on the team should encompass the following:

1. Identifying his/her needs and wishes to the members of the team
2. Advocating for his/her needs and wishes
3. Developing an understanding of the roles of the various team members.

Additional School Personnel

There is a variety of school-based personnel who would be valuable members of the educational team. The titles and the job descriptions may vary from one geographical area to another. It is important that there be school personnel, in addition to the classroom teacher and the Intervenor, on the educational team in order to provide consistency of information from year to year. For example, the special education teacher from the school could be the case manager for the student as he/she is more likely to continue on in that role from one year to the next, whereas usually the classroom teacher will be different in the following school year. The case manager's role on the team should encompass the following:

1. Chairing the educational team
2. Ensuring that minutes from each meeting are taken and distributed
3. Ensuring that the team's recommendations are implemented
4. Ensuring that educational team meetings are held regularly and that members are informed
5. Providing feedback to the team from other personnel within the school or school system
6. Ensuring that access to the deafblind consultant is available to any member of the team who may have specific questions or concerns about deafblindness, intervention, or the Personal Program.

The Educational Program

The student's Personal Plan should be 'designed according to his/her needs, interests, abilities, past performance and present level of functioning. It should be delivered at the rate, in the depth, and by the methods best suited to his/her learning style and evaluated in terms of his/her improved level of functioning' (McInnes and Treffry 1982, 18).

Educational Program Development

An individual who has been assessed as deafblind requires a complex, comprehensive educational program. Implementation of a program necessitates the consistent application of those specialized methods and techniques that have been designed to address the individual's combined loss of vision and hearing.

A student who is deafblind, by definition, is 'one who has a combined loss of both vision and hearing such that neither can be used as a primary source of learning.' Over the years, the individual's inability to gather all of the necessary visual and auditory information results in many partial or distorted concepts. We should assume that the individual has the ability to process information as long as he/she receives it in a consistent and meaningful manner that is formulated to compensate for visual, auditory, and conceptual deficits. The role of intervention is one of providing the visual and auditory information that an individual is unable to gather independently. Thus, there is a need for a trained Intervenor, whose primary role is to provide the individual who is deafblind with the visual, auditory, and conceptual information that his or her classmates are able to gather on their own. This will provide the individual with the best possible opportunity to formulate concepts, complete tasks, make choices, and make decisions as is deemed appropriate. This Intervenor will require ongoing training from the deafblind consultant so as to ensure that the methods and techniques utilized, program modifications, and day-to-day program are as pertinent as possible. It should be stressed that Intervenors may be hired who have a range of experience:

- no previous experience
- experience with a few individuals
- a broad base of experience with extensive philosophical, technical, and practical training.

Each individual who is deafblind is unique and may be unlike other individuals with whom the Intervenor has worked. The deafblind consultant will have had experience with a number of individuals who are deafblind and thus the ongoing training and input from the consultant allows for a truly individualized educational program for the student.

The level of participation in each activity or subject area possible for the individual who is deafblind must be evaluated by taking into consideration the following factors.

Course Content
The number of new concepts and/or skills that will be taught within the regular school curriculum far outweighs the amount of time required to teach all of the components that would enable him/her to develop complete concepts. Therefore, within each activity or subject area, it is necessary to choose those concepts or skills that will be most meaningful and relevant to the individual. All of the concepts and skills that are addressed should be documented in *experiential, visual, tactile,* or *conceptual books* that are developed in conjunction with the student. These books will form an ongoing library designed for his or her future reference. All of the concepts and skills that the team identifies as primary goals should be documented within the *binder system* (to be explained later).

Prior Conceptual Knowledge
Within all of the student's courses at grade level, there will be learning situations that arise that will be dependent on prior knowledge and skills that the stu-

dent who is deafblind may have had limited or no exposure to in the past. Consideration should be given to the amount of prior knowledge required for the student to maintain a reasonable level of understanding and success in any given subject area or activity. The concepts and/or skills should be introduced by the Intervenor on a one-to-one basis prior to the classroom teacher's presentation to ensure that the student benefits as much as possible from the class instruction. The student will also benefit greatly from time spent one-on-one with his/her Intervenor in reviewing the class material. This will provide an opportunity to confirm that the initial concepts and all related concepts are understood. It will also provide time to ensure that the student is able to apply those concepts in a way that is meaningful to him/her. Thus, the Intervenor will require a weekly or monthly schedule in advance, in order to be as prepared as possible for the upcoming activities and related concepts.

Physical Demands of the Task
Consideration must to be given to the visual, auditory, and motor demands required for each individual subject area or activity. The amount of effort required by the student to use residual vision and hearing is extensive and fatigue will often result, particularly in the late afternoon. In many cases, alternative strategies will be required, to compensate for difficulties. In conjunction with the deafblind consultant, the Intervenor will need to develop observational skills in the areas of functional vision, functional hearing, and tactile ability and be able to provide learning situations that take into consideration the student's sensory abilities. At other times, the conceptual demands may be great and take much energy. The Intervenor may need to provide the physical supports that will allow the necessary time and energy required for the student to develop a complete understanding of the concept. The Intervenor may need to discuss the primary purpose of a specific lesson that is being presented to the class in terms of learning ability of the student who is deafblind. For example, a typical classifying activity in a grade one classroom might consist of colouring a page of pictures of fruits and vegetables, cutting each of the pictures out, deciding which are fruits and which are vegetables, and gluing them onto the appropriately titled page. A student who is deafblind with some residual vision may indeed be quite capable of completing all of the steps within this task. It is unlikely, however, that he/she will be able to complete them within the allotted time frame. The Intervenor and classroom teacher must then decide whether the time required to complete the task should be taken, thus missing something else that the class may be involved in, or whether the primary lesson is one of classifying rather than colouring, cutting, and pasting, which may be done at another time. If the latter is the case, then they could have available pictures already coloured and cut out, use pictures from magazines, or use actual fruit and vegetables and

work strictly on the classifying component of this task. At another time, colouring, cutting, or pasting may be the logical primary task for the student.

Experiential Learning
Initially, most students who are deafblind learn best by 'doing,' provided adequate, accurate feedback is available immediately. Subject areas or activities that provide 'hands on' learning will be of the greatest interest to the student. Students can gain an extensive number of concepts and skills through this type of teaching and learning. They are then able to be assisted to relate that knowledge to similar learning experiences. As new situations arise that are dependent on a knowledge base that the student has not acquired, some type of experiential learning will be required. For example, if the class is studying plant growth from seeds, the student who is deafblind would benefit from the hands-on experience of planting the seeds and regularly monitoring their growth in order to develop a complete concept.

Incidental Learning
Incidental learning, which is the ability to gather information from the environment and develop concepts based on that information without being formally taught, occur quite easily and readily in the sighted/hearing student. Often social skills are acquired in this manner. For example, students learn how to enter a play situation by watching what others do as they approach the play area and then imitate what they see. They do not have to be formally taught (have their attention directed to the acquisition of specific knowledge) how to enter the established group or activity. Because of a deafblind student's combined loss of vision and hearing, however, incidental learning is much less likely to occur. To compensate for this deficit, much of the knowledge that is acquired by other students on an incidental basis must be specifically taught to the individual with deafblindness. Once this formal teaching is complete, the student will require exposure to actual situations in order to apply that specifically taught knowledge. For example, a student who is deafblind first needs to know that the others are playing and what activity they are playing; then he/she can make a choice or be assisted to make a choice about participation. If the choice is to participate, appropriate questions and behaviours must be learned before he/she approaches the group.

Designing the Educational Program

Designing the educational component of a Personal Plan for a student with deafblindness who attends a community based school must be a collaborative effort by the deafblind consultant, the Intervenor, the classroom teacher, and the parents. There may be additional personnel, such as therapists or an orientation and mobility instructor, who may also provide input to the design of the program. This educational component is only one part of the student's Personal Plan. It will identify the objectives that can be worked upon during school-based activities and will complement home- and community-based activities. This school-based component should not be seen as the total program but rather as an important part of the whole.

Within the community-school based program, the daily or weekly educational curriculum is focused on academic areas such as language arts, math, science, and so on. This can create problems if the writing of the program's five-year goals and yearly objectives is based on developmental areas and its delivery is based on activities or subject areas. It is the responsibility of the consultant both to ensure the development of a comprehensive Personal Program and to ensure that the school personnel (teacher, department head, administrative staff) understand how their school-based program forms part of and contributes towards the achievement of the five-year goals and yearly objectives of the total program. When properly supported, the teacher will be able to enunciate both five-year goals and academic objectives as they pertain to his/her specific student and to identify how various subjects will contribute to that child's achievement. A student's Personal Plan may have as a five-year goal, a statement as broad as 'John will enter the High School in September 200–' or as specific as 'John will be able to add and subtract whole numbers by June 200–'. Each goal will result in curriculum-based objectives and again may be as broad as 'Mary will obtain a pass mark in Science,' or as specific as 'Jean will be able to count to 100 by 1s, 2s, and 5s.'

When the place of the school program is misunderstood and the school program is seen as being the total, or even a major part of the student's program, pressure is put on an Intervenor and a classroom teacher to assume the responsibility for the student's overall development rather than primarily for his/her academic progress.

When the educational aspect of the students overall program is being developed, the following points should be addressed.

1. Define and/or review the goals (using the process outlined in chapter 2) that have been identified in the areas of vision, hearing, communication, and socialization for that student. Then, the specific objectives related to the developmental areas of fine motor, gross motor, life skills, cognitive devel-

opment, and orientation and mobility will be defined as they relate to each of the school activities or subject areas in which the student is involved. In this way the Intervenor and the teacher understand both the five-year goals and the specific objectives identified in the areas of vision, hearing, communication, and socialization and how they 'fit' into the student's program throughout the day. These objectives should be addressed in every area of the program. The developmental skill areas of fine motor, gross motor, life skills, and orientation and mobility can be incorporated within certain activity or subject areas. Goals and objectives identified in the area of cognitive and conceptual development will now be defined primarily within the 'academic' content of the class and supplemented by additional goals and objectives that pertain to the home and the community.

2. Using the classroom teacher's weekly class schedule, the classroom teacher, Intervenor, and consultant will determine the student's level of participation in each of the activity or subject areas.

3. Once it has been determined that the student will participate in the activity or subject area, the student's specific learning objectives in the areas of vision, hearing, communication, and socialization, as they relate to each specific activity or subject area, will be reviewed.

4. The specific objectives related to the areas of fine motor, gross motor, life skills, cognitive development, and orientation and mobility will be identified as they relate to each activity or subject area.

5. Occasionally there may be an activity or subject area that is deemed to be inappropriate for the student, that is, foreign language class or an activity that for medical reasons is not viable. In such a case the team will suggest an alternate activity. This may be an appropriate time to incorporate aspects of the student's program that are not available within the regular class curriculum, for example, orientation and mobility, daily-living skills, therapies, community trips, swimming or horseback riding, if these activities are to take place during the school day.

6. Once steps 1–5 have been addressed, each aspect of the classroom curriculum will have been modified for the student in order to ensure that his/her specific learning needs have been met.

7. Members of the support team should keep in mind that the school program is one part of the student's Personal Plan. It is often wise to stress that the student attends school for approximately thirty hours a week of his/her more than 100 waking hours and that in most jurisdictions he/she will attend school usually less than forty of the fifty-two weeks in the year.

8. Team members should also be reminded that home- and community-based

activities that take place in the out-of-school hours should not be a duplication of school- and classroom-based activities. The level and intensity of activity in these environments must reflect both the interests and needs of the student and the resources available to the family.

Personal Plan Binder for Students with Deafblindness

A binder system outlined as follows will provide a means for documenting the program, the activities and the progress of the student throughout the school year. It is also a system that is easily duplicated for use at home. Some sample sheets and blank sheets for the binder appear as an appendix to this chapter.

Contents

The documentation binder is divided into sections. The following sections should be included each binder.

1. A copy of a *yearly calendar* with the visit dates of the deafblind consultant and therapists highlighted
2. A copy of a completed *information sheet* providing names and addresses of pertinent persons or services involved, as well as visual and auditory information regarding the student's abilities at a glance
3. Deafblindness and intervention
   a) the definition of 'deafblindness'
   b) the definition of 'intervention'
   c) the principles of 'intervention'
   d) the role of the 'Intervenor'
   e) additional articles as deemed appropriate
4. Summary of medical and educational history to date
5. Deafblind consultant's visit sheets with suggestions or comments arising from the visit
6. Student's weekly schedule or calendar of activities
7. Personal Plan goals
8. Personal Plan outlining
   a) *present level of functioning sheets* for each activity or subject as well as the developmental areas of vision, hearing, communication, and socialization

b) *concept and skill sheets* for each activity or subject as well as for the developmental areas of vision, hearing, communication, and socialization
c) *progress sheets* for each activity or subject as well as for the developmental areas of vision, hearing and communication
9. Articles of interest relevant to deafblindness

Students whose program is of a more academic nature would have identified subject areas and a section in the binder for each subject of current study, such as environmental studies, science, math, etc.

Parents, Intervenors, and classroom teachers are invited to have input into this process of developing the most appropriate program for the student. Owing to the ongoing nature of the process, we hope they will feel more comfortable providing input. This system provides the following benefits:

1. Classroom teachers, Intervenors, and families are able to provide more input and feel more a part of the student's program because the program is written on an ongoing basis.
2. Intervenors have a better idea of what is expected of them during each activity or subject and know exactly what they are to be working on and why, since each activity is delineated with specific objectives for the student.
3. It is helpful for substitute Intervenors, who may arrive on short notice, since they will have specific direction of what to do during each activity or subject.
4. The time line for goals and objectives runs within the same time lines that the regular school year runs, that is, September to June.
5. The teachers, who must complete report cards at the end of each term, can refer to the progress sheets for input.
6. Similar sheets can be produced for the families and home Intervenors for specific areas if desired by the families.
7. The families have a clear understanding of what is being worked on at school and the strategies that are being utilized.
8. Once the system is set up, the information on the progress sheets from the year before becomes the present level of functioning for the following year, provided there have been no major changes over the summer.
9. School personnel are better able to document the progress of a student from one year to the next as a result of the very specific objectives and regular efforts to document progress and to measure success.

The Five Key Factors for Effective Inclusion

The effective inclusion of a student with deafblindness into a community-based school system requires the following five key factors:

1. A knowledgeable and supportive family or primary caregiver
2. Supportive school personnel at all levels
3. An appropriate educational placement and program
4. Supportive community personnel
5. Appropriate Intervention.

A Knowledgeable and Supportive Family or Primary Caregiver

It is not by accident that this factor is listed first, since a supportive and knowledgeable family or primary caregiver is the *key factor*. Parents must have an awareness of the specific learning needs of their child as well as an awareness of the needs of individuals with deafblindness in general. Parents will frequently be asked to explain their child's needs to school, medical, social service, and funding personnel as well as to friends and relatives. Parents must also be knowledgeable of the methods and techniques involved in interacting with students with deafblindness and the philosophy behind intervention.

Teachers, Intervenors, and other professionals will come and go throughout the student's life, but the parents will remain the constant. There are often a number of hurdles to overcome when a student with deafblindness is included in the community–school–based system, and it helps the deafblind consultant, Intervenors, and school personnel to know that they have the support of informed and knowledgeable parents.

How We Can Encourage Knowledgeable and Supportive Families
1. From the beginning, the parents/families should be involved in developing an awareness and an understanding of the impact of a combined loss of vision and hearing on the development of their child.
2. Regular opportunities should be provided for parents/families to acquire an understanding of and the skills to compensate for this combined loss of vision and hearing.
3. Full explanations should be provided – not only the *how* but the *why* of what is being done.

4. The parents/family should be involved in setting five-year goals for their child.
5. Parents should be encouraged to attend medical appointments and their understanding of all information and reports should be ensured.
6. The deafblind consultant should make regularly scheduled visits to the home.
7. Parents/families should always be treated with respect and be empowered to be the integral component in their student's life that they truly are.

Supportive School Personnel at All Levels

Attitudes around inclusion and disabilities usually filter down more readily than they filter up. For this reason, the school board/district administrative personnel as well as the school principal need to be openly supportive and committed to the effective inclusion of the student. School personnel refers to everyone who attends or works at the school, including the students, volunteers, teachers, paraeducators, custodians, secretaries, bus drivers, and librarians. The attitudes of the school personnel can often 'make or break' the entire inclusion experience. It is essential that there be a coordinator or case manager to orchestrate the process. Ideally, this person would have experience in the areas of both inclusion and deafblindness. Socialization, interaction, and peer friendships are very important aspects of inclusion and should be included in the objectives designed for the student. The classroom teacher needs to take the same ownership of the student with deafblindness as he or she does with the other students in the class.

How We Can Encourage Supportive School Personnel at All Levels
1. School personnel should be given plenty of lead time, so that everyone can be prepared and start to become comfortable with the idea of having a student with deafblindness attend the school.
2. The student, Intervenor, and parents should make a few visits to the school prior to entering school. This often assists everyone with the transition process.
3. The classroom teacher can be helped to adjust to the idea of having another adult (the Intervenor) in the class as well as a student with deafblindness.
4. When the student with deafblindness is placed in a regular or special class in the community school, the family, classroom teacher, and administrative

personnel all should understand that the teacher is not expected to become an expert in deafblindness and will continue to present the same program to, and give the same amount of attention to, each student in the class as they would receive if the student with deafblindness were not present.

5. Workshops can be offered for all school personnel. They may include simulation experiences of deafblindness and intervention.

6. Simulations and information can be provided for the classmates at a level they can understand. This will promote awareness and interest.

7. Interaction between the students, school personnel and the student with deafblindness can be promoted by instruction in sign language and communication techniques. Often a sign-language club is a positive experience for students who demonstrate an interest.

8. Adequate time should be spent on an ongoing basis discussing the roles of everyone involved.

9. The classroom teacher should not be expected to be the case manager or coordinator, but should be involved in every aspect of the student's educational process.

An Appropriate Educational Placement and Program

An array of educational placement options should always be considered and explored by both the family and the school personnel. It is only through exploring these placement options that all concerned will know what is most appropriate and what is not. Any placement without intervention is not a viable option for a student who is deafblind. It is important for the team first to decide what the needs of the student are and then to decide where a program should be delivered to meet those needs. The program should be designed by a specialist in the field of deafblindness in consultation with the Intervenor, the family, and the school personnel. The program must be evaluated regularly and on an ongoing basis. This evaluation should once again be the task of the person with expertise in deafblindness in consultation with the Intervenor, the family, and school personnel.

How We Can Ensure that the Student Receives an Appropriate Educational Placement and Program

1. The parents and the deafblind consultant need to take time to explore all of the options. This will ensure that the most suitable placement is chosen.

2. It should be remembered that at different stages of the student's life, different options may be more appropriate.

3. The day-to-day program should be implemented by a well-trained and monitored Intervenor.
4. The overall program should be a well-developed collaborative effort by the family and school personnel.
5. The program should encompass objectives both within the developmental areas, as well as in all of the activity or subject areas.
6. The importance of the involvement of a specialist in deafblindness who looks at the total student cannot be overstated.

Supportive Community Personnel and Services

By community personnel we are referring to occupational therapists, physical therapists, speech and language therapists, orientation and mobility instructors, as well as those people who may come in contact with the student with deafblindness as a result of community-based programming, for example, swim instructors, scout and guide leaders, job placement supervisors, and persons working in restaurants and stores. In order to provide support for the student with deafblindness, community personnel need to have a basic understanding of the impact of deafblindness. Community personnel also need to understand that communication is the most critical element in interactions with the person who is deafblind.

How We Can Develop Supportive Community Personnel
1. The knowledge that therapists bring to the team as it relates to their specific field should be recognized. They will require assistance to understand the impact of deafblindness as well as the specific needs of the student. Awareness workshops and simulations are very informative and help to encourage a positive attitude.
2. Community personnel will need to learn the methods and techniques associated with the particular student they will be interacting with as it relates to their specific area of speciality. For example, a physiotherapist may find it very helpful to know about physically cueing a student and some of the basic signs the student uses prior to beginning a physiotherapy program.
3. Because communication is so important for the student who is deafblind, family and Intervenors may need to teach people in the community some basic communication strategies.
4. Frequent visits to the same restaurants and stores will help the staff to know the student with deafblindness and to become more comfortable interacting with him/her.

5. When appropriate, thank-you letters – made by the student if possible – can be sent to show appreciation.

Appropriate Intervention

It is essential that we keep in mind the definition of an Intervenor. Intervention provides the best possible opportunity to compensate for the vision and hearing loss. This loss results in the inability to gather non-distorted information. It is important to recognize and define appropriate intervention as it relates to each individual with deafblindness. It is also important to recognize, and to have the student recognize, whenever possible, that a skill or concept has not been mastered until he/she understands when he/she needs to ask for intervention in relation to the skill or concept and does so appropriately.

Designating a one-to-one worker to a student does not make the worker an Intervenor. It is essential that the Intervenors be trained. We need to appreciate that the training takes time. It is an ongoing process. The issue that intervention may result in the student's becoming dependent on the Intervenor is often a concern for persons not familiar with the philosophy of intervention. While the student and the Intervenor certainly develop a bond or a relationship, intervention does not result in a personal dependence but rather a healthy interdependence and a recognition of the importance of the information that is being relayed to him or her by the Intervenor.

How We Can Ensure Appropriate Intervention
1. Specific training should be provided for the Intervenor with each individual student.
2. The majority of the training should occur in the natural environment of the student.
3. Additional formalized training with regards to the philosophy of intervention and the specialized methods and techniques related to communication strategies must also occur on a more formal basis.
4. Personnel should be assisted to understand the needs of the student, so that they will have a greater understanding of the important role that intervention plays.

Commonly Asked Questions/Issues about School Intervenors

Is there a union of Intervenors?
Currently, in most countries, there is not a union specifically for Intervenors.

School-based Intervenors are typically grouped in a contract category with educational assistants or para-educators. In some jurisdictions, such as Ontario, Canada, the Intervenor Organization of Ontario (IOO) has developed an Intervenor Code of Ethics as a guideline for Intervenors.

How is seniority addressed among Intervenors?
Since there is not a specific union, the group or category that the Intervenor belongs to would have terms of reference or guidelines for employment, including sick pay, long-term illness, working hours, seniority, and so on. The Intervenor is bound by those terms. Some school districts recognize the specialized training that Intervenors receive either on the job or at college courses or workshops, and they may 'protect' the Intervenor's status when seniority issues arise.

Is the Intervenor allowed to transport the student in his/her personal car?
The school district may have guidelines for the transportation of students in personal cars. The school may agree to allow the Intervenor to transport the student as long as the parent signs a legal waiver permitting this action. However, the legal aspects should be thoroughly explored by the Intervenor, the school, and the parents. Intervenors may need additional automobile insurance if they transport students.

Is there a specific budget for materials that the Intervenor will need?
The educational team would need to identify sources of potential funding for items such as special materials or pieces of equipment. The school or school district might have such a fund. If there is no funding available, other sources of funding could be explored, such as government agencies, social services, or charitable organizations.

When there are entrance or attendance fees to programs or programs that the student will attend, who pays for the Intervenor?
Since the Intervenor is attending the program for the educational purposes of the student, he/she should not be responsible for the costs. The team should have access to funds if there will be costs incurred during the program. These would include bus, taxi, or train fares, entrance fees to athletic facilities (swimming, bowling, etc.), rental of athletic equipment (skis, skates, etc.). If a mealtime occurs during the time when the Intervenor and the student are out in the community, the Intervenor should not have to pay for his/her own meal if typically lunch is brought from home on work days.

When the Intervenor is in the community, who takes responsibility for
the activity, the Intervenor, and the student?
An Intervenor who goes with a student into the community for aspects of the student's program is still under the employ of the school. The school is responsible for the Intervenor. The team would have deemed the outing as necessary for the programming of the student. Thus, the Intervenor would go into the community only with the approval of the team.

Does the school Intervenor work in the home as the home Intervenor as well?
In our experience, the optimal situation is when there is a separation between the school Intervenor and the home Intervenor. The school Intervenor is employed by the school district, while the home Intervenor typically is employed by social services or privately by the family.

Does the Intervenor write in the communication book that regularly
goes back and forth between the school and the home?
The overall responsibility for the student is with the teacher; thus, the communication book is the teacher's responsibility. Some teachers do write in the book, but this task can take several minutes each day, and often the classroom teacher is not fully aware of the specifics of the day's events. Some teachers will ask the Intervenor to write in the book and then will read what the Intervenor has written and initial the entry each day.

Summary

1. With the proper supports in place, inclusion in the community school is a viable educational option for students who are deafblind.
2. Parents should be supported to make an informed decision as to their student's educational placement.
3. An educational team that works together effectively can be instrumental in the success of an individualized educational program for a student who is deafblind in an inclusive setting.
4. The ongoing involvement of a consultant who is specifically trained in deafblindness, intervention, and consulting skills, and who has extensive hands-on experience with a wide variety of students who are deafblind is essential.
5. The ongoing philosophical and hands-on training of Intervenors in deafblindness and intervention is critical.

6. The school program forms only part of the student's day, week, and year, and thus represents only part of a total Personal Plan.
7. There are five key factors for effective inclusion.
8. A number of commonly asked questions and issues arise concerning Intervenors working in a community-based educational setting.

REFERENCE

McInnes, John M., and Jacquelyn A. Treffry (1982, 1993, 1997) *Deaf-Blind Infants and Children: A Developmental Guide*. Toronto: University of Toronto Press

Appendix
Personal Plan Binder Sheets

PRESENT LEVEL OF FUNCTIONING

Student's Name: Hanna Stroud

Subject, Developmental Area, or Activity: Lunch

1. Using a palmar grasp, Hanna will independently eat finger foods that are bite size (i.e., pieces of cookie, cracker, cheezies, or grapes)

2. Hanna will tolerate hand-over-hand feeding.

3. Hanna will independently hold a spoon.

4. Once the spoon has been hand-over-hand loaded and brought half-way to her mouth, Hanna will bring it to her mouth, remove the food and return the spoon to the bowl.

5. Hanna will carry her lunch bag to and from her lunch table.

6. Hanna uses her left hand to bring finger foods to her mouth.

7. Hanna will independently drink from a straw that has been placed in a drink box.

PRESENT LEVEL OF FUNCTIONING

Student's Name: _____

Subject, Developmental Area, or Activity: _____

CONCEPTS AND SKILLS

Student's Name: Hanna Stroud

Subject, Developmental Area, or Activity: Lunch

Date	C or S	CONCEPTS AND SKILLS	METHODS
Sept. 1998	S	Hanna will develop the ability to load food onto the spoon independently.	Gradually reduce the amount of physical support
"	S	Hanna will develop the ability to bring the loaded spoon to her mouth independently.	Repetition Natural cause and affect Modelling
"	C	Hanna will associate the sign for 'eat' with the activity it represents.	Consistency
"	S	Hanna will locate her lunch bag on the shelf in her bucket in response to 'get lunch.'	Classmate demonstration
"	S	Hanna will visually attend to the food in her bowl while loading her spoon.	Cue her to look

CONCEPTS AND SKILLS

Student's Name: _____

Subject, Developmental Area, or Activity: _____

Date	C or S	CONCEPTS AND SKILLS	METHODS

PROGRESS REPORT

Student's Name:___Hanna Stroud_____

Subject, Developmental Area, or Activity:_____

Term One
1. Hanna has begun to bring the loaded spoon to her mouth, removing the food and returning the spoon to her table, with only minimal initial cuing.
2. Hanna has begun independently to reach into her open lunch bag and remove her cookies and juice box.
3. Hanna has begun briefly to look at her spoon when she brings it to her mouth and there is no food on it.

Term Two
4. Hanna will drink independently from her new plastic juice box.
5. Hanna has become much more aware of others sitting on either side of her during lunch time and will reach out to their food if it is something that she likes.

Term Three
6. Hanna will independently scoop and bring the spoon to her mouth in order to eat her favourite foods of applesauce and pudding.
7. Hanna is visually attending to the spoon in the bowl each time before she scoops.
8. On a number of occasions Hanna has begun to smile when told '*time to eat*' using sign language presently visually.
9. Hanna has occasionally gone to and stood in front of the shelf where her lunch bag is located.

PROGRESS REPORT

Student's Name: _____

Subject, Developmental Area, or Activity: _____

COMMUNICATION

Word or Concept	Concrete Cue Receptive	Concrete Cue Expressive	Picture Receptive	Picture Expressive	Sign or Gesture Receptive	Sign or Gesture Expressive	Verbal Receptive	Verbal Expressive	Print Receptive	Print Expressive

MEDICAL AND EDUCATIONAL HISTORY

Student's Name: _____

Date (of latest entry) _____

11

The Residential School Option

SUSAN CAMPBELL, MARK DEMERLING, JANIS McGLINCHEY, and ELIZABETH VAN KIMMENAEDE

Introduction

Throughout this chapter, when the term 'residential school' is used, it will be referring to either a setting dedicated specifically to the education of deafblind children or to a deafblind unit of one or more classes with separate accommodation within a residential setting that has been developed to meet the needs of students challenged by other handicaps. In no case is it suggesting that an infant, child, or youth with deafblindness should be placed in a class or program designed to ameliorate other handicapping conditions. In the past twenty years there has been a shift in the type of education a child who is congenitally or early adventitious deafblind, receives. This shift has been worldwide. In Canada there are very few residential educational programs for children of school age. Instead of attending a specialized school or program, these students are being educated as students with deafblindness in schools within their home community.

The movement to the local school has created several educational problems for this low-incidence population of deafblind students and their families. When the local-school option is chosen, some of the problems that arise are as follows:

a) A lack of staff in the local school with training as a specialist teacher of the deafblind
b) A lack of understanding by the staff of the local school as to why the child is identified as deafblind
c) Little or no understanding of the problems faced by the child with deafblindness

d) An insufficient number of teachers trained, or being trained, as specialist teachers of the deafblind

e) An insufficient number of consultants trained as specialists in the education and support of infants, children, and youth with deafblindness and their families

f) Bureaucracy, including school and board administration, with no, or faulty, perceptions of the needs of the student with deafblindness

g) A lack of specialized program development covering twenty-four hours per day, 365 days per year

h) A lack of funding for intervention outside school hours,

i) A lack of resources with knowledge of deafblindness within the child's home community.

Successful integration requires support for the family and student in the hours after school and on weekends. Intervenors, whether they are family members, volunteers, or paid professionals, are needed to continue to work on program objectives during personal maintenance routines, family activities, and community activities. Without this continued intervention the child lives in a non-reactive environment until school resumes the next day.

The Residential School

The option for a residential-school-based education needs to be available to all children who are deafblind. The ideal situation is to have a demonstration school combined with a resource and training centre. This demonstration school would provide students with a Personal Plan, implemented with intervention throughout the child's entire day while he or she is in residence. The resource centre would also

- house a resource library with publications concerning deafblindness, for the use of families, lay workers, and professionals
- provide a meeting place for national and regional parents' associations
- provide workshops for families and professionals
- be the training centre for Intervenors working both in the home and in the school
- provide ongoing training for teachers and other staff of the demonstration school.

In addition to the main resource centre, where geographical distances dictate the need, there should be regional, satellite, residential centres to support children who are deafblind, so they can be closer to their home area. Such schools should be funded adequately to suit the unique programming and staffing needs of the student who is deafblind. No additional charges should be made for parents and families who choose to have their child attend a residential school.

What to Consider in a Residential School

All parents and students should be provided with non-biased information concerning the choices available to them for the education of their child. It is a difficult decision for parents and students to make, and it is a decision that requires careful consideration of advantages and disadvantages of all educational approaches.

When parents are looking at a residential-based program as an option, they should ask specific questions to see if it will meet their deafblind child's needs. Seeking answers to the following questions will provide important information for the parents and help them to identify the appropriate educational setting for their child who is deafblind.

1. What is the level of family involvement?
2. Are goals and objectives written for each student in consultation with the parents?
3. How are goals and objectives implemented and evaluated?
4. What is the staff to student ratio?
5. How is consistency maintained between home, school, and residence?
6. Is there support to assist the student and the family in planning for the future and for transition from school to an adult living situation?
7. What support services are available within the residential setting?
8. What is the level of staff training and expertise within the setting?

Family Involvement

Learning continues to take place during all of a child's waking hours when he is at home, at school, or in the community. It is important to develop a team approach with a strong home-school partnership because parents and siblings of the deafblind have a unique insight relative to deafblindness. 'There is no substitute for the understanding that comes from living each day with a deafblind son or daughter. The interests and welfare of the deafblind will be enhanced when parents share information with one another and with professionals' (Petty 1983).

Parents must be encouraged to contribute information and insight about their child at all times through constant interactive communication with the teacher and residential staff. Such communication may be accomplished through

- phone calls
- letterbooks in which both the parents and the teacher share information on a weekly basis
- school visits by parents and relatives
- regular, planned home visits by teachers
- written or pictorial communication between the student (with assistance from the teacher where necessary) and his/her immediate and extended family
- in-depth anecdotal report cards
- picture report cards containing pictures of activities that the student is working on at school, along with a written explanation of the activities and intervention techniques used.

Education and training of parents, siblings and extended family members should be an ongoing process. Family members and friends should be encouraged to visit the residential school classroom and residence on a regular basis throughout the school year and to participate actively in activities with their child under the guidance of the teacher and other school staff. The most effective way to promote understanding and confidence is to involve family members as Intervenors for their child, working 'hands-on' during a variety of activities. The appropriate school staff should demonstrate the intervention techniques to be used, the language involved, and the communication techniques required. Parents and family members should have an opportunity to practise the techniques with their child in the appropriate setting when the professional is present. This ensures that they will understand not only the techniques involved, but also the reasoning behind their use as they apply to their child. Another means of disseminating information and training is workshops given by school staff either at the school or in the home community, and through home visits by teachers. 'Most parents accept responsibility for taking on their share of the special care and training needed during the early years; for being actively involved in educational planning and decisions; in obtaining provision for the adult years and in seeing that the rights of their children are met' (Freeman 1986).

The school should continually be working on improving communication skills between family members and their deafblind child. Keeping family members informed about the signs that their child is learning and demonstrating individualized adaptive signing techniques and other communication techniques that the child is learning and using at school, will help the family to communicate more effectively with their child. By participating in activities with their child and learning the communication and intervention techniques used in each activity, the family learn communication skills and intervention techniques that can be used at home. This provides a more consistent approach. Active participation develops in the family the ability to recognize the progress that their child is making and to delight in his/her accomplishments. Family members' interest and enthusiasm increase the child's feeling of belonging within the family unit as well as his/her self-esteem. In turn, his/her motivation to continue trying and learning is increased.

Parents and family members should make the teacher aware of what motivates the deafblind child to attend to objects and participate in activities, as well as which objects and activities the child seems to prefer while at home. This information is useful in establishing transition and consistency for the child between his/her home and school.

Parents, siblings, and extended family members should be welcome to visit the school at any time and to stay for several days. Not only does this approach provide an opportunity to share knowledge between members of the home-school team, but it allows the child to show his/her family what he is working on and what he has learned; introduce his/her family to his/her friends and Intervenors; show off 'his' school and residence; and feel the same sense of belonging to his school as his siblings feel for their school(s).

Regular visits to the residential child's school are also vital to building and implementing the child's Personal Plan. When parents and teachers agree on the long-term goals and yearly objectives for the child and participate in writing these goals as a team, the approach and intervention techniques are likely to be consistent. This consistency will ultimately lead to greater learning and skill development by the child. The more knowledgeable that parents are about their child's programming goals and objectives, communication techniques, and intervention techniques, the easier it is for them to hire and effectively train home-based Intervenors to support their child on weekends and holidays. The Intervenor working in the home and in the home community with the deafblind child is ultimately responsible to the parents for program implementation. These Intervenors will receive the majority of their training and/or guidance from the parents.

Teachers can also promote the development of parent networks in which small groups of parents come together to share information. These groups may initially be facilitated by a teacher and later by the parents themselves. Topics of discussion may include practise of communication skills; sharing useful intervention techniques; and sharing information about local community activities that their children could participate in while they are at home.

'During the lifetime of an individual with deafblindness, he/she will need and benefit from the help of many people with professional qualifications. None of these will be more important to the individual with deafblindness, nor be in a position to provide him/her with as much support, as his/her family' (Freeman 1986). The participation of family in the residential school program is an essential ingredient for success. It is a win-win situation when both family members and professionals are able to work as a team toward the education of individuals who are deafblind.

The Development, Implementation, and Evaluation of a Personal Plan

All parents and relatives of infants, children, youth, and young adults with deafblindness have hopes and aspirations for them. Thinking about and discussing these helps parents to project into the future, to dream dreams as they do for their other children. Not all dreams become reality and not all dreams will become long-term goals. Unless the professional knows of and aids the parents in identifying the boundaries of these dreams, however, he or she will not be in a position to identify long-term goals or to plan a course towards their achievement.

Development of a Personal Plan
Five-year goals should be established by the teacher and parents when the child first enters school, if they have not been previously established by the consultant who worked with the family in the preschool years. Once established, these goals should be reviewed yearly and added to or revised as necessary (see chapter 2, 'Programming'). Areas of importance that the family may wish to see addressed may include toilet training; interaction of the deafblind child with his siblings or relatives; using intervention to interact in community-based activities with peers, for example, clubs; eventual return of a child to a local school program with intervention; as well as the seven developmental areas. The knowledge, skills, and attitudes required successfully to achieve identified goals should be included in the yearly objectives of the school program. Each set of yearly objectives may be viewed as the first of five steps to reach an identified goal.

Teachers should meet with parents to prioritize goals in each program area. Once these goals have been identified and agreed upon by both parties, the teacher should write the five-year goals and present them to the parents for approval. These goals should be reviewed yearly and modified, confirmed, added to, or removed, as appropriate. New and existing goals should be melded to establish the direction of the child's program over the next five years. When reviewing the existing five-year goals and identifying future ones, the parents and teacher must take into consideration which goals have already been achieved; goals that will be achieved within the next one-year period and therefore should be written as one-year objectives; goals that would no longer be appropriate because of medical or other problems; the child's and family's priorities for the child's future; and the identification of any new goals that are necessary for a well-rounded program for the child.

Short-term or 'yearly' behavioural objectives are the steps towards achieving the five-year goals. The purpose of yearly behavioural objectives is to identify the specific means by which progress will be measured. These behavioural objectives will be achieved during the daily routines and activities that appear in the teacher's weekly plans when the child is at school and during the routines and activities carried out when the child is home on weekends and holidays.

Yearly objectives should be written by the teacher in cooperation with the parents, in terms that describe the success indicators that will be observed when the objective is attained. After discussion with the parents to determine which skills need to be emphasized at home, and after goals have been established and the teacher has assessed the child's present level of functioning, the teacher writes objectives based on all of this information. Teachers may write yearly or term objectives, as appropriate. Discussions should be held with the parents during their visits to the school and the teacher's visits to the home, about how the yearly objectives can be worked on in the home setting by family members as well as by home-based Intervenors.

Objectives should be evaluated at the end of each school year at a meeting attended by all members of the module team and the parents. Each objective should be reviewed to determine if it has been attained and whether the focus of the program should continue in the same direction or be adjusted to meet the changing needs of the child more effectively.

Implementation of the Personal Plan
No two children who are deafblind are identical in their needs or in their style of learning. Therefore, no one approach is applicable to all children. When planning the implementation of the individual student's Personal Plan, all staff must take into consideration the varying degrees of vision and hearing loss, differing experiences, the expectations of their family and community, as well as the differing community and family resources available during weekends and school breaks and after they have completed their education. 'The purpose of the Personal Plan is to help the child lay the groundwork for development and continued growth throughout his lifetime. Through intervention and a plan designed for the individual student, the student will experience, orga-

nize and react to external stimuli within his environment. The student will be taught to use his residual vision and hearing, to develop essential motor skills, concepts, and an effective means of communication as well as the living and mobility skills necessary to be a member of their community' (McInnes, 1993).

It is important to remember that it is the 'total approach' to the child's twenty-four-hour Personal Plan, not the setting in which it occurs, is what ensures continued development. One setting in which the child's program may take place is the residential setting. Since students remain at the school twenty-four hours per day, the residential school is able to provide an activity-based program throughout the student's entire day for at least five days per week. Individual areas focused on during an activity are designed for each student, based on individual objectives. Two students, while participating in the same activity, usually are working on different objectives. The student's success in each activity is evaluated on an individual basis. Focus areas during an activity will change as the student's level of functioning changes.

Students with deafblindness usually require concrete experiences to develop concepts, language, and skills. The residential program is able to provide these experiences within the appropriate setting. It provides a consistent level of intervention to support individual needs and facilitates active participation in a variety of daily activities from hand washing to bathing; from tricycle riding to rollerblading; from computer skills to school dances; from participation on the wrestling team to work experience in the community; from setting the table to eating in a restaurant; from use of a local pool to doing laundry; and from physiotherapy to long-distance running. The list goes on, and on, and on. There are few limits as long as a Personal Plan has been developed and appropriate intervention is available.

Activity-based programming is essential, since most students who are deaf-blind cannot be taught either life skills or academics in isolation. They must have concepts taught in functional terms through a variety of situations, owing to their reduced ability to generalize from one situation to another. Simple concepts are gradually expanded upon once language and meaning have become attached to the activity.

A Personal Plan must be implemented in a reactive environment for it to be successful. The degree to which an environment can be reactive for a child is dependent largely upon having intervention available for the entire school day. Many feel a residential program, with the appropriate staffing ratios, is able to provide a reactive environment that will facilitate learning.

Specific success indicators are identified in daily plans. All staff are responsible for evaluating the success of the student with whom he/she consistently works. The plans support the use of specific techniques to promote development. The teacher and residential staff strive to provide situations that will encourage the child to interact with the environment, to solve problems, and to attempt to communicate with others. A reactive environment is also necessary to provide social and emotional growth. It reduces frustration and provides the student with an environment he/she can understand and control.

A residential program provides a reactive environment and consistent levels of intervention during the child's entire day, as well as selected activities designed to provide an opportunity to work on the individual student's objectives. This environment also promotes the development of necessary social skills through planned interaction with an expanding group of adults and peers. This expanding group will include classmates, other school staff, and students. In addition, it will also come to include members of the community, such as cashiers, restaurant personnel, bus drivers, doctors, dentists, recreation centre personnel, and new friends. This planned interaction promotes social growth through experiences that are meaningful and positive. These positive experiences motivate the student to want to repeat the experience.

Often, owing to the slower development of concepts and language and the lack of an ability to anticipate what will happen, the student's behaviour is looked upon as autistic-like or neurotic. In the residential program it is the duty of staff to identify the specific behaviours exhibited by the student that require further development or replacement by more appropriate coping mechanisms. The deafblind student lives a very stressful life because of his limited access to direct information about his environment and his interaction with it. This is particularly true if he has limited communication skills or no established routine. Trained residential school staff are always on hand and can look at behaviours carefully to see which events preceded a child's response, what happened during the situation, and what occurred after the behaviour. This evaluation will include the language and concepts attached to both the incident and the follow-up so that consistency will be maintained while attempting to instil a more socially acceptable response. The residential school environment will facilitate communication among staff and with the home in order to establish a consistent approach to behaviour.

Life skills form an important part of the student's Personal Plan. It is important for life skills to be taught within regular routines. They will not be effective if taught in isolation. For example, shoe tying from 2:15–2:30 pm every Tuesday, is not a meaningful or functional way to teach children with deafblindness. Shoe tying is taught every time shoes are put on and tied up and an imaginative Intervenor can create many reasons that the child will want to put on his shoes and tie them up. Basic life skills will also include, for example, bathing, grooming, eating, toileting, dressing and cooking, choosing clothing appropriate to the activity or weather, care of clothing, and managing money.

Learning basic life skills is necessary before more advanced skills can be taught. Using the Presentation Sequence (awareness, acquisition, application, and generalization) will help to ensure that skills are learned (see chapter 3). The residential school provides an uninterrupted opportunity to teach these skills without having to worry about meeting other family responsibilities. To illustrate how the Presentation Sequence facilitates the learning of life skills, the routine of teeth brushing will be used.

In the initial awareness stage, the child needs to understand the purpose and function of brushing his teeth. It happens at regular times throughout the day and thus is built into the child's routines. Through appropriate communication and positive feedback, the child will learn to understand the outcome of the activity. Initially, the Intervenor will go through the process with the child. He will communicate what is going to happen (*It's time to brush your teeth.*); what is happening during the various steps (*First, get the toothpaste, now take off the cap, turn on ...*); and after the child has completed the routine, talking about what he/she did with the child, communicating that he/she did a fine job and that his/her teeth look good.

The use of the Total Communication Approach provides the positive feedback necessary for the child to feel successful. In the beginning, this activity is usually tolerated because of the Intervenor rather than an understanding of the outcome. Initially, it will be done hand over hand, with the Intervenor manipulating the child's hands throughout the process, accompanied by the appropriate language.

In the acquisition stage, where the child him/herself is doing more, the Intervenor provides the motivation, again through appropriate communication and positive feedback. The focus shifts from language acquisition to the child's learning of the steps in the process as he is doing them. He also continues learning language, and communication continues to be developed around the activity.

It is a whole/whole process. It is not broken down and taught in pieces with individual isolated actions. You brush your teeth as one activity. Acquiring the motoric skills is a process, not a series of isolated events. If necessary, the Intervenor manipulates the child's hands throughout the process:

- getting the toothbrush and toothpaste from the cupboard
- unscrewing/screwing the cap
- turning on/off the water
- putting the brush in his mouth and brushing
- returning the toothbrush and toothpaste to the cupboard.

Once the child is able to go through the steps of brushing his teeth and the activity is automatic within the routine, the application level has been reached. The Intervenor decreases any remaining manipulative support and introduces several 'problems' for the child to work through. These problems should be ones the child may naturally encounter during the activity. The toothpaste tube may be empty, the cap may fall on the floor, the toothbrush may not be in the cupboard. It is important always to make sure that attempts to solve the problems are met with success and that the child does not become frustrated. One of the things that the child is also learning during this stage, is when and how to ask the Intervenor appropriately for assistance.

Now that the skills of 'brushing teeth' are learned and the process is automatic, expansions and modifications need to be put in place to reinforce generalization. Such activities may include brushing teeth at home, at grandma's, and while on an overnight outing with schoolmates or family members. The skill of teeth brushing should also lead to other skills in activities such as shopping for toothbrushing supplies, packing for a trip, and so on.

The residential school is consistently able to incorporate these steps into the child's regular routine. The Personal Plan allows for time and opportunity to go through such activities at the child's pace and to teach such life and other skills at the appropriate time and in the appropriate circumstances/settings. Because staff are assigned to work with specific children throughout the school year, necessary consistency in expectations, approach, and support in all areas of development are assured.

A residential school program provides excellent opportunities to promote motor development during functional activities throughout the child's day. Without intervention, deafblind children often are not motivated to participate in motor activities because they are unable to use their vision or hearing to anticipate the movements that will be required and are unable to pattern their movements after those of their peers or to know if they have been successful or not.

The deafblind child develops through many or most of the same stages as any other child, but usually at a much slower pace. For example, when appropriate intervention is available, the child moves through the stages of random play, to parallel play, to interactive play, developing specific leisure activities that are enjoyable. Every child who is deafblind should be exposed to a variety of leisure activities and should be allowed continued opportunity to develop the same social and creative skills as their peers. Success, as defined by themselves, their peers, their teachers, and their family, will lead to expectations of future successful and confident participation in the activity. Constant frustration and failure will lead to withdrawal and learned helplessness.

In a residential setting, access to a variety of leisure activities should be available. Students should have easy daily access to swimming pools (both school and community), therapy pools, gymnasiums, parks and playgrounds, pottery classes, sewing equipment, fitness centres, bicycles for two, skis, skating areas, and so on. They also need opportunities to revisit some activities that may not have been their favourite ones. It is possible that with expanded language, improved motor skills, expanded or new concepts, and improved self-image, the activity would have more appeal.

Physical exercise is essential for good health for everyone. This is particularly true for the infants, children and youth with deafblindness and especially for those who have additional medical complications. A program without adequate emphasis on activity throughout the day can cause additional complications. A physiotherapist who has training in working with deafblind individuals is a definite asset to the residential program, and is an excellent resource in assisting in developing specific programs to meet the needs of individual students (see chapter 15).

The development of skills involved in orientation and mobility plays an important role in promoting awareness and independence of the deafblind child within his environment. Orientation refers to the ability to locate one's place in space. Mobility refers to the ability to move through space and arrive at a desired destination. Children who are deafblind often lack curiosity about the world around them (see chapter 5). This may stem from a fear of movement, lack of sound or visual stimuli, an inability to learn by visual example or modelling behaviour, and/or little or no satisfaction being derived from initial attempts at exploration. The result is a lack of motivation to interact with the environment.

Since sensory information may not be present or may be distorted in children who are deafblind, learning to move about the environment at will may not come naturally to them. Deafblind children need instruction in concepts related to themselves and their environment, in addition to instruction in specific travel skills and techniques. 'Orientation and mobility is commonly referred to as "O & M." O & M encompasses such things as sensory awareness (gaining information about the world through the senses); body awareness (understanding the parts of the body and how they move); spatial concepts (realizing that objects exist even if they are not heard or felt, and understanding the relationships which exist between objects, up/down, close/far); searching skills (locating items); independent movement (includes rolling, crawling, walking); sighted guide (using a person to aid in travel); and protective techniques (skills used in specific situations which may provide added protection to the traveller)' (Alsop 1993).

'The goal of purposeful movement is to be able to travel in whatever mode possible for a desired outcome. Students who do not develop purposeful movement skills may be unable to go anywhere or do anything without assistance, thus limiting their ability to develop and express their independence. Teaching students to travel independently or with guidance increases their awareness of their surroundings and their self-confidence, as well as their mobility skills. Simply leading students from place to place teaches them to be passive and to wait to be moved. It does not motivate children to satisfy their curiosity through independent exploration of their environment with intervention' (Huebner et al. 1995). Put more simply, the deafblind child who has been led, carried, or transported from place to place and denied appropriate intervention enabling him or her to acquire and practise appropriate orientation and mobility skills, is developing learned helplessness and probably will develop severe behaviour problems.

Concepts that need to be taught in order to achieve meaningful independence in movement include awareness of the child's surroundings (knowing that people, places, and things exist and understanding their nature and the child's physical relationship to them); initiating and sustaining movement (knowing that one needs to start moving to reach a desired location and to continue moving until the destination is reached); recognizing the destination (recognizing and identifying the destination and knowing when it has been reached by responding appropriately); protecting oneself from danger (recognizing obstacles in the path and dealing with them safely); and making decisions (choosing when and where to go and how to get there).

Communication systems need to be individualized for teaching O & M and for conveying information about movement. Language needs to be taught while exploring environments, to help the child label what he sees, feels, hears, and explores. The meanings of touch cues and object cues should be connected with activities and locations. Tactile communication systems should be portable, so that object cues can be carried with the student when necessary.

The most important thing to remember is that O & M instruction for children who are deafblind should occur during routine daily living activities in natural environments. Skills and techniques taught in natural environments and real-life situations are more meaningful to the child and are easier for him to understand and remember than those taught in contrived instructional settings.

Initial orientation and mobility skills should be taught in familiar environments by familiar adults, using appropriate intervention techniques, in order to foster a sense of security and safety in the child. As the child becomes more secure in his/her own abilities and begins to explore his/her immediate environment, the area that he/she is exploring should be expanded. If the area is gradually enlarged, the child will begin to form ever expanding cognitive maps of his surroundings and community. For example, to build on O & M skills learned in the preschool years, the child may begin by exploring his bedroom in the residence and his classroom. Exploration of other areas in the residence and school helps to expand the child's cognitive maps. As the child becomes more familiar with his/her surroundings inside the school buildings, he should be encouraged to explore outdoor areas and routes to routine familiar areas in the buildings. Exploration of the school's grounds and other buildings, as well as the neighbourhood and local stores, playgrounds, and recreational facilities, will encourage the child to form more complex cognitive maps of the community surrounding the school as well as improving his/her skill to build cognitive maps in general.

The child should also learn the necessary skills to use public transit, including communicating with the public; route planning; use of schedules and timetables; money management; map reading (tactile or visual maps); boarding and disembarking; judgment of time and distance; and problem solving.

In addition to gaining the necessary skills to travel with an Intervenor successfully, O & M instruction should involve teaching children to use special travel tools, such as long mobility canes. Mobility devices will enable the child to gather information regarding his/her immediate surroundings. However, the child must have the necessary motor skills to use the tool and must understand both the purpose of the tool and the limitations that the disability of deafblindness places on its use.

Residential school staff are able to focus on the area of perceptual development in a child's Personal Plan. The child who is deafblind often is sensory defensive, or sensory selective, and is unable to tolerate the use of more than one sense at a time. The child often must be taught how to use his/her residual vision and/or hearing through planned activities. The child can be taught how to integrate and process the sensory information that he/she receives. This is often a slow process. If the wearing of hearing aids or glasses is introduced but does not 'pay off' for the child, he/she will soon refuse to wear them. The staff in a residential school setting should always be aware of the importance of having the student integrate the use of his/her senses. They have the opportunity carefully to develop and implement a program promoting the student's use of vision and/or hearing during all daily activities in the classroom and residence. Once the use of this vision or hearing is rewarding for the student, it is often a puzzle to professionals about how the student uses what he has in order to function as well as he does. Quite often there is a great disparity between the student's functional vision and/or hearing and the medical assessment of his disability. In a residential school setting, the Personal Plan also focuses on activities throughout the day that promote the development of language, communication, and concepts outlined in the objectives identified for each student. Children without any disability are like sponges. Every moment throughout the day they absorb sights, sounds, and other information from the environment incidentally. This visual and auditory interaction reinforces, expands, or introduces new language and concepts. Incidental learning is almost non-existent for the deafblind child. It takes much longer to introduce or develop a concept for a child who is deaf-blind than for his peers who are not challenged by the disability of deafblind-ness. The information that peers acquire incidentally must be identified and taught in a systematic manner.

The extended length of time required to educate a child who is deafblind implies that the need for the Personal Plan approach should continue beyond the educational time frame established for the general population. The residential program should support transition from the educational setting to living within an adult-supported, independent living situation in the student's home community.

Communication is one of the most important aspects of our lives. By utiliz-ing a Total Communication Approach, the residential school can provide a consistent environment that will promote the development of the child's com-munication skills throughout the day while the child is at school as well as sup-port the parents in their development of the child's communication skills while he is at home. This approach is an effective way of teaching the child to com-municate. It provides the child with the maximum opportunity to obtain infor-mation and then to understand it. The child often has difficulty transferring language between activities, situations or persons. For this reason, experiential-based learning is important for language development. In the early stages, lan-guage and communication should evolve from the interaction between the Intervenor and the child during the child's daily routines (see chapter 4).

Creating a reactive environment using a Total Communication Approach is essential. This approach helps to create a reactive environment that responds to the child, allows time to comprehend the information, provides security, and promotes the child's ability to make choices and exercise control over his world.

An approach that has been found very successful is initially to develop lan-guage through Total Communication, with the use of Signing Exact English (SEE) as the base, supported by other forms of Total Communication. At the most advanced level, SEE means that at all times you sign and speak everything you want to say. This includes suffixes, prefixes, and tenses. The use of endings gives a much better understanding of past, present, and future. The Total Com-munication Approach, which includes SEE, is adapted to meet the child's indi-vidual needs, according to his/her visual loss and motor skills. This form of communication could be called Adapted Signing Exact English (ASEE). The development of language is crucial for the deafblind. He/she will not read or otherwise be exposed to syntax sufficiently to enable the structure of the language to be taught as a second language at a later date. ASEE provides an important base that offers an opportunity for advancement academically. It reinforces syntax, which, in turn helps to develop the ability to read and write print, script, and Braille. As a result, many forms of modern technology become accessible, such as computers, TDDs, and Closed Caption machines for the television.

It is important to repeat at this time that the use of signs and gestures with spoken English while using the ASEE and the Total Communication Approach, does not mean that the child will automatically understand. Implementation of the student's Personal Plan includes the development of special techniques to use with the student to help to develop an understanding of language and thus the ability to communicate.

The residential school staff have the expertise to develop the child's vocabulary and individual communication techniques after careful analysis of the child's visual and auditory functioning, physical problems, and general level of functioning. Home, school and residence are able, through consultation, to provide a consistent and comprehensive communication environment by always having staff available who know what to look for when the child tries to initiate communication and can respond to such attempts immediately and appropriately. Every effort is made to ensure that teachers, Intervenors, and parents use this type of environment.

Evaluation of Student Progress
A progress report should be written at least three times a year. The first report should outline the child's progress in his new program and should give detailed information about activities that the child participates in and his/her level of functioning in each developmental area, as well as specialized intervention techniques being used. This information will provide a written resource for parents and home Intervenors to follow in the home setting.

The second progress report may be more informal and may consist of a written and pictorial update on the child's progress in each area of his Personal Plan. The pictures serve as an excellent means of showing the child actively involved in a variety of activities and of visually recording the child's school program for family members and friends in the home community to see and to read about.

The final report should be written after the meeting of the module staff and parents. The report should document the child's progress in each objective identified. The use of behavioural objectives ensures that evaluation is in terms of an improved level of functioning. All reports should include suggestions on appropriate activities during extended school breaks, reflecting the objectives identified in the child's Personal Plan and suggesting how such activities may be used to work on specific objectives.

The most important thing to remember when writing the child's Personal Plan is that if the child could fit into the normal school curriculum and did not require special techniques, methods and an expanded curriculum, he/she would not require the support that a deafblind program offers and could use a standard reporting format. Because the Personal Plan approach is different from that experienced by the child's parents, and because the parents have no other source to turn to for an explanation, it is the responsibility of the staff to develop and explain in detail the items contained in the specific Personal Plan designed for their child and his or her overall development during the school year.

The Staff to Student Ratio

Program implementation begins when the child wakes up in the morning. He/she requires one-to-one intervention to allow for optimal learning, communication, and interaction to take place. The activity-based program, with a large portion of the programming taking place in the community as well as in various parts of the school other than the classroom (pool, residence, sewing room, woodworking room, kitchen, gym, school grounds), requires a one-to-one ratio to provide adequate intervention necessary to carry out the activities. Without this ratio, it is impossible to support the child's making choices and decisions and then of turning these choices and decisions into actions.

Intervention is necessary to provide the constant feedback that permits the child to determine his/her level of success in activities, to motivate him/her to continue trying; to initiate communication, interact with others and with his/her environment; to utilize any residual vision or hearing that he/she may have, and to ask for assistance appropriately.

The reactive environment is not created for only a few minutes or hours each day. For optimal learning to take place, intervention must always be available from an Intervenor who has an comprehensive knowledge and motivating relationship with the child, so that the child's attempts at communication may be responded to appropriately. Without appropriate intervention, the deafblind child will cease to interact with his environment at an appropriate level. Since the same objectives are used while planning and carrying out activities in the residence after school and when the child is at home, adequate intervention ratios are essential.

Intervention is the process between the person with deafblindness and the person who is providing him or her with support. A ratio of two staff acting as Intervenors to three children provides opportunities for the minimum level of intervention required for a child's programming needs to be met. Such ratios, if maintained, will begin to place limits on the child's development. Any lower ratios (e.g., one to three or greater) reduces the amount of support available to the child to a level that may result in the development of severe frustration, inappropriate behaviours, and limited progress.

In addition to appropriate staff:student ratios, Intervenor consistency is an important factor for maximum learning and interaction to take place. The emotional bond formed between the Intervenor and the child will be one of the decisive factors in determining the child's rate of progress and success. Settings in which staff are switched between residences or even between modules are inappropriate.

In the residential school setting, consistency in staffing can be achieved by formulating a module team that works cooperatively as a unit. In the authors' experience, the best organizational pattern for a module is a teacher, three students, and three or more Intervenors. This does not mean a teacher plus three adults. The teacher is also an Intervenor and demonstrates techniques and methods as she works with each student. Volunteers and long-term placement college students may be used to boost the Intervenor:student ratio where necessary. It is important to keep the volunteer or placement student with the same module throughout the year, and to provide appropriate training in educational theory and intervention techniques as applicable to the specific child or children with whom they will be working.

Intervenor shifts should rotate through a cycle. In this way each Intervenor could spend one period of their cycle in the classroom with the teacher. This enables the Intervenor to keep up-to-date with changing objectives, intervention techniques, and progress made by each student in the module. During this period, the teacher is also able to work on improving the Intervenor's knowledge base and intervention techniques with the students. During the second period of the cycle, the Intervenor works in the residential setting outside of school hours. He or she works on the objectives found in the Personal Plan using activities different from those used in the classroom. The third stage in the cycle finds the Intervenor working nights and, if necessary, on weekends.

Communication between the teacher and the Intervenors is easier when all members of the team are working together, and it ultimately leads to a more cohesive team. Regular module meetings in which all staff members of the module meet to discuss the student's program and progress are essential for maintaining a consistent approach to programming. Module meetings provide an excellent forum for sharing ideas and gives the teacher an opportunity of providing professional development for the Intervenors.

Depending on the setting of the residential school program, a variety of difficulties may arise for the individual who is providing one-to-one intervention for a child who is deafblind.

1. If the deafblind program is housed in a residential school for the deaf or for the blind, the higher staff:student ratio in the deafblind program may lead to resentment from the staff in other parts of the school. Having staff from other parts of the school become familiar with the deafblind program, the uniqueness of the handicap, and the difference in the role of the Intervenor vs that of a classroom assistant should assist them in recognizing the need of a higher staff:student ratio within the deafblind program.
2. Stress caused by shift rotation is another major problem faced by Intervenors who are rotating shifts on a weekly basis. Frequent rotation between shifts may lead to problems with sleeping patterns, inability to concentrate, greater susceptibility to illness, and possibly family problems. Information should be made available to employees on ways of coping with shift work.
3. High staff turnover may result when Intervenors face too much stress. Regular staff training sessions should include workshops on stress management, and staff should be encouraged to discuss problems with their supervisors.
4. Physical problems may arise because of lifting students, repetitive strain injuries from continual hand-on-hand signing with the students, and dealing with inappropriate student behaviour. Regular staff training sessions should include information on appropriate lifting techniques, work breaks, and techniques for managing aggressive behaviours.
5. Communication styles become quite individualized when two people work together consistently for long periods of time. The child becomes used to the Intervenor's signing speed and style and acquires most of his receptive and expressive vocabulary from his Intervenor. It is important for the child to communicate with a variety of Intervenors, so that he will be able to understand and communicate with a wider number of people.
6. Most students use adaptive signing techniques, designed to meet their motoric abilities. Since modified signs can be highly individualized, it is important to keep accurate lists of signs and how they are formed, so that others may communicate with the child as well.
7. Intervention is a social interaction of support. Intervenors not only provide contact with the outside world; they may inadvertently become the deafblind child's main 'friend.' Most of the child's contact with the outside world is through his Intervenor, and the child's perception of activities and people

may be influenced by the Intervenor's attitudes and preferences. Overdependence on one Intervenor may restrict the child's overall social growth. The module approach, the training of family members, and the use of home Intervenors helps to ensure that a number of Intervenors interact with each child.

8. Unionization of Intervenors has its benefits as well as its drawbacks. All employees feel more protected when they are members of a union, but strict union guidelines may interfere with or limit student programming.

Staff Training in the Residential School Setting

Intervenors and teachers working in the residential school setting for students who are deafblind will require an extensive, ongoing, in-service training program. In chapter 16, 'Intervenor, Teacher, and Consultant Training,' approaches to Intervenor and teacher training are outlined. The following are a few additional essential components necessary for people acting as Intervenors in the residential school program.

As the school's instructional leader, the principal or program director should be provided with administrative training focusing on the role of the principal as staff developer. The specialist teachers of the deafblind who will be involved in the site-based in-service training of Intervenors should also receive further training in staff development skills relating to workshop preparation and presentation, collaborative team building, adult learning styles, and so forth.

The in-service training program for Intervenors should include the following components.

1. A two-week training session should be delivered on site during holiday breaks or during the first two weeks of the new school year, including:
   • the entire education team
   • large group and small class settings
   • a variety of instructors and presenters
   • a curriculum geared towards developing and expanding a basic understanding of deafblindness, programming for students with deafblindness, specialized methods and techniques utilized with students who are deafblind, intervention, and communication skills and techniques.
2. One-day training sessions throughout the school year should include additional topics such as CPR, First Aid, Lifting Techniques, Use of Assistive Devices, and Behaviour Management.
3. Ongoing in-module training should be scheduled throughout the school year. Each specialist teacher should coordinate regular short sessions to present information specific to the student in his/her module to the Intervenors

working with those students. These sessions could be scheduled during shift changes, on professional development days, or at other appropriate times (e.g., Friday afternoons if students travel early). Sign language classes need to be held weekly, or bi-weekly, according to staff needs and scheduling arrangements.

4. Training should be reviewed annually in relation to the experience and needs of the present Intervenors on staff, the numbers of new Intervenors, the changing needs of the program, and the needs of the student population.

For site-based training of Intervenors to be successful, it is necessary that central office staff provide support, expertise, and options. An essential component of any residential school program is staff who are specifically trained to develop and implement individual programs designed to meet the needs of the students who are deafblind and their families.

Consistency of Approach

Consistency in programming must be maintained between home, school, and residence. Teamwork is the cornerstone of a successful program, especially for a student who is deafblind. Consistency can only be achieved if school staff, families, and home Intervenors work as a team, with common objectives and techniques to achieve the desired outcomes. In many residential school programs, the child will spend five school days and nights in the residential school, travelling home on weekends and school holidays. The child is usually at school from 180 to 200 days a year. Therefore, the program must cover the child's needs twenty-four-hours per day while the child is at school and also during the time when he/she is not. The teacher and residence staff must work together to plan complementary activities that provide consistency in programming objectives. The activities in the residence must incorporate the objectives and skills worked on in the school program, so that the child will learn how to transfer skills he has learned in school to other situations in the residence as well as in the community.

The teacher is the team leader who coordinates programs at school, in the residence, and in the student's home. It is the team leader's responsibility to communicate with the family and Intervenors, design goals and objectives in consultation with the family, establish techniques to achieve these goals and objectives with the school staff and family, and plan an organized school day for the student that will help to promote the accomplishment of these objectives and goals. The teacher also is responsibile for helping to train Intervenors to work with the students in their module. The teacher encourages both Intervenors and families when progress slows down and reviews the program to see what adaptations may need to be made. Another responsibility is to communicate with the parents and to assist in designing an in-service training program for the home Intervenors. The teacher, as team leader, is responsible for daily plans for each individual student, report cards three times per year, as well as weekly journals to parents. He/she is responsible for making home visits during the school year. The teacher is a resource for the families and will attend medical and other appointments with the student and the family if this is requested.

Teachers should make a minimum of two visits to the child's home each year in addition to the visits that family members make to the school. This will give them the opportunity to see how the child interacts within the home setting and to discuss the child in greater detail with his parents in a more relaxed atmosphere. They will also gain insight into the family's resources and thus make activity suggestions that are suitable to the home setting. Parents are often more willing to share information and concerns with teachers when they are in the secure environment of their own homes than they are while visiting the school. Home visits also provide an opportunity for teachers to demonstrate intervention techniques to family members and home Intervenors, both in the home setting as well as out in the home community. Teachers can initiate or enhance training of home Intervenors during home visits while participating in activities that the child enjoys while at home.

Home visits also allow the parents to demonstrate activities the deafblind child does independently at home. Many children are able to complete activities independently at home that they will not complete at school without assistance or cueing, and vice versa. The teacher will be able to gain new insight about the student simply by observing the child in his/her home environment and watching how the child interacts with his/her family members.

Home visits also provide an opportunity for parents and teachers cooperatively to identify and investigate activities within the home community that the deafblind child can participate in with intervention. Activities within the community should stress communication, recreational and leisure skills, and peer interaction. Activities in which other family members can also participate are ideal for promoting interaction within the family group. Locations to investigate in the community may include public swimming pools, bowling alleys, summer day-camps, horseback riding stables, roller skating arenas, fitness clubs, and so on. Many offer, or can be persuaded to offer, special rates for individuals with handicaps and/or their Intervenors.

The teacher is the contact with resources within the school, for example, nurses, physiotherapists, principals, residence coordinators, and counsellors. The teacher is responsible for the student's program twenty-four hours a day,

365 days a year. Last, but not least, he/she works hands on with each of the students in his/her module to educate other staff by example, on a daily basis throughout the school year. It is recommended that a student stay with the same teacher for at least two years. This promotes a stronger bond between the student and the teacher and helps the family to become better acquainted with the staff. Staff assignments of longer than two years often benefit the child and family.

The teacher should ensure that module meetings are held at least every six weeks with the entire module team in order to review techniques and approaches and to discuss any needed program modifications. These meetings serve as an opportunity to

- share detailed information and to coordinate the approach used by all members of the module
- identify areas in the child's program that may need to be modified because the child has already attained an objective, or because he/she has developed health problems that may temporarily prevent him from working on an objective
- identify areas of the child's program that require more attention; this information can be very useful to the teacher when future yearly objectives are written
- remind staff of the goals and objectives for the child's program and to suggest ways to incorporate work towards these objectives into daily activities for the child. Ideas on how the objectives can be incorporated into residential activities and other daily routine activities will help to plan effective activities that teach the child to use his/her skills in a variety of situations

Residence Workers

Who May Be Designated Aides, Residence Counsellors, or House Parents? Residence counsellors or residence supervisors, house parents, and school or residence aides, who work as Intervenors and should take turns rotating through the classroom setting. The basic concept is that everyone working with the child spends a week in the classroom with the teacher on a regularly scheduled basis. The residence counsellors' primary function is to support other staff during the afternoon, night, and weekend shifts when the children are not in school, and counsellors must be able to demonstrate correct methods of intervention. They are also available to interact with teachers if there are concerns about staff working on their shift. Counsellors are also responsible for the handling of medications and communicating directly with medical personnel about medications and other medical treatments. They are responsible for evaluations of school aides on their shifts and for making suggestions and demonstrating techniques to improve the aides' professional skills. The residence counsellor reports to the teacher about module matters and reports directly to the program director or residence coordinator concerning broader residence issues.

The program director, sometimes called the principal, is responsible for the residence as well as the school program. He/she is responsible to all staff, all students, and all families and for all the business administration of the program in the residential setting. Depending upon the size of the program, the director will need a support person to assist him/her in the school area and one to assist in the residence area.

All of these people work as a team with the family and the student. Each student has, on his team, at least three Intervenors, one teacher, one counsellor, the program director, and the family. The family has a very important role with this team. Family members must commit to communicating with the school on a regular basis, following through on the goals and objectives that they have established in consultation with the teacher. They are responsible for hiring, training and supervising Intervenors that work out of their homes during the weekends and holidays. It is the responsibility of the program director and school staff to make the parents feel welcome and comfortable with contacting the school whenever they have problems or concerns, whether it is about school programming, their child's behaviour on weekends, or with resources in their home community, that is, doctors, health issues, funding. This keeps a two-way communication line open and gives the school a complete overview of the student and the concerns of the family. It is essential for all team members to communicate through the proper channels and to keep these lines of communication open so that the student's program is successful. It is also important that the privacy of the student and the family be maintained and that only pertinent matters that have a direct impact on the student's program be discussed at module meetings or with other staff in the school.

Transition from the Residential School to an Adult Community

According to the dictionary, transition can be defined as 'A change or passage from one place to another or a development that forms part of a progression.' These meanings are fundamental to the overall program for young persons who are deafblind in a residential school. In the following description of an approach to transition developed by the staff of the W. Ross Macdonald School, Deafblind Unit, however, transition will pertain to students approximately sixteen years of age or older, who are involved in a specialized three-stage Deafblind

Transition Program. This program focuses on preparing students for entry into adult life and must address problems that will be caused by changes in routines and structure, the environment, personal contacts, and the student's expectations. The thrust is to continue development in the following areas: communication, self-maintenance skills, recreation and leisure, socialization, experiential placement, and the concept of intervention. The provision for appropriate intervention services and a Personal Plan prepared by education professionals are integral factors in the success of the transition process.

As alluded to in the introduction, the transitional format is organized, planned, and structured to meet the needs of each individual student. At the age of sixteen, students can enter the following stages.

Stage 1: The Pseudo Apartment Setting

At this point, students participate in a residential apartment based project. To appreciate this initial stage fully, one must be rather imaginative and flexible in the perception of apartment living. A supervisor once called this project, in its earliest conception, 'The Emperor's New Clothes Apartment.' Anyone familiar with this tale will remember that although the emperor rode about the streets virtually naked, it was the perception of all those around him that he was attired brilliantly. Thus, it is imperative that the staff accept the premise of the Pseudo Apartment Setting and augment it with an experiential hands-on program for the students. In reality, the apartment project is housed within the residential setting at the school. The students have individual or shared bedrooms, a community room for leisure pursuits and meals (their own combined living room and dining room) and access at pre-scheduled times to a nearby kitchen. The program evolves around the apartment setting, from which students, with the support of their Intervenors, have the option of utilizing on-site school activities or venturing out into the community. This preparatory stage provides the necessary building blocks to be successful in adult programs.

Stage 2: The Transition Housing Project

The second stage of the transition format is the Transition Housing Project. This program is available to those students eighteen years of age and older. In this intermediate stage, students have the opportunity to live in a house located in the community and to continue to develop the skills that will allow them to be successful in attaining appropriate adult placement. The essence of the program is that the home and the surrounding community are being utilized as an educational setting to prepare the students for future living. Three students live in a home and twenty-four-hour staffing is provided to meet the individual needs of each occupant.

It is interesting to note, however, that the format for this program is structured around extraneous factors, which seem arbitrary to the program itself, such as age (sixteen–eighteen–twenty-one), funding (disability support), and the legislation (Education Act). Juxtapose this format against the concept that for this unique population learning must be a supported lifelong process, then one can say that the education system itself is only a transitional phase in a lifetime of experiential learning for persons who are congenitally and early adventitious deafblind.

When students are ready to participate in the off-campus Transition Housing Project, the program does not move away from the seven developmental areas, but is presented in an adult developmental format. The adult format attempts to reflect growth in the following areas:

- Communication
- Intervention
- Maintenance
- Experiential Placement/Education
- Leisure and Recreation
- Socialization

These same areas are the focus of the five-year goals for young adults. Students are provided with a program that mirrors the daily lives of adults. This is done through an activity-based program providing functional, concrete learning scenarios. For example, the local community is used for activities such as grocery shopping, fitness, continuing education, banking, medical appointments, and work placements. In addition, the home provides a natural setting to work on other facets of adult developmental areas. Life skills, as well as skills of daily living, are accomplished through a multitude of maintenance activities, such as personal hygiene, cleaning, and meal preparation. Hands-on activity-based programming allows the individual numerous opportunities for experience-based learning, the development of problem-solving skills, and a foundation for the decision-making process.

During stage 2, the Personal Plan is prepared by a specialist teacher of the deafblind. During the implementation of the program, the Intervenor acts as the facilitator, allowing the individual who is deafblind an opportunity for growing independence within his/her environment by providing the necessary information and support. It is of the utmost importance that intervention not be intrusive, threatening, or directive in any way. This intervention is pivotal in providing young persons who are deafblind with the necessary support to pilot their own existence by making informed and responsible decisions.

Communication is also fundamental. The ability of the individual to receive, comprehend and act upon information by expressing ideas, perspectives, and decisions is of paramount importance. The threads of intervention, communication, and self-expression are intertwined throughout all aspects of the program in the off-campus Transition Housing Project.

Stage 3: Transition to Adult Services

This final phase should take place in the last year of the student's attendance at the residential school. During this time, the school works in cooperation with the individual, the family, the adult service provider, and other government agencies to assist in the slow process of transferring the person who is deafblind into specialized adult services in the home community. Staff members, along with parents and the adult service provider, coordinate what is termed a 'transition timetable.' This stage can include training, support, and on-site consultation from school personnel. In addition, a temporary exchange of staff and a video package are provided. The concept is that a gradual change, allowing for consistency and continuity for both the individual who is deafblind and staff persons, will be of the greatest benefit to everyone. In addition, this final stage is of the utmost significance to the parents and/or alternative caregivers. The process allows vital time for the parental figures to deal with the changes in their son's or daughter's life as their child makes the transition from education to adult services. It should be understood that the parents' feelings during this stage will be similar to the first day that their child entered the residential school; they held out hope, had feelings of guilt, and were suspicious of any person who claimed to know what was best for their child. Professionals must not forget that parents will continue to be the greatest resource available, next to the deafblind individuals themselves. Throughout the years, within the educational system and on into adult life, parents remain a vital part of the lives of their children.

Once stage 3 is completed, the school must provide follow-up consultative visits. These resource visits can provide an additional source of extensive knowledge and expertise for graduates receiving adult services.

Prior to graduation, the school will assist individuals, parents, and/or agencies entrusted with the care of the students, to prepare an Adult Individualized Proposal (AIP). The concept behind the AIP is that government sources are provided with information specific to a person who is deafblind with regard to possible future placement options. This proposal gives the government the necessary documentation for the school leaver to qualify for needed funding.

When the government recognizes the need and agrees in principle to the proposal, the next step is to negotiate an annualized budget with the potential service agency. This may sound like a rather simplistic perspective, but basically, the AIP acts as a bridging mechanism between the government and service providers, promoting dialogue and ultimately negotiations to enter into a long-term service agreement.

Like many situations in daily life, there is, on the one hand, the theory or philosophy and, on the other hand, the reality or concrete application. In this instance, the reality is the long and arduous process of proposal preparation and presentation. The building and preparation of the proposal requires a team approach between the individual who is deafblind, parents, and professionals. The initial stage in the process begins approximately three years prior to the student's leaving the residential school program. The first step is a meeting to discuss proposal planning and responsibility for sections of the proposal. The preparation of the proposal requires that all parties work closely together and share information in the early stages. As has always been customary, within the very underpinnings of this philosophy, the individual, parents, or significant others have the final responsibility to make all decisions. With empowerment, however, is the weight of responsibility for preparation of the proposal. The role of the residential school is to expedite matters, such that the Adult Individualized Proposal may come to fruition. Unless all parties are prepared to participate, the process of proposal preparation cannot go forward.

Following the initial meeting, the individual or parents must do the following.

1. Contact the service providers who they hope will administer the contract should they receive funding from the government. (In many jurisdictions a branch of government will not provide funds directly to the congenitally deafblind adult or to his/her family.)
2. Attempt to secure special individualized funding for the adult who is deafblind from government or other sources.
3. Acquaint themselves with an individual or an agency that will assist in advocating on behalf of the special adult needs of their son or daughter. Advocacy and support can be of great assistance to both the individual who is deafblind and their parents. Ultimately, individuals and their parents are their own best advocates, and professionals can only direct them to the door, which they will have to open for themselves. In some jurisdictions, the school itself cannot be involved in direct advocacy, since doing so would be deemed a conflict of interest, and it is essential to establish the integrity and objectivity of the AIP.

To say that the proposal format ensures adult services would be ludicrous. Nevertheless, it provides a useful platform for discussion and negotiation in procuring optimum services to meet the specific needs of the individual who is deafblind, coupled with a budget that is both feasible and economically responsible, which thus meets the criteria of the government. The Adult Individualized Proposal attempts to close the gap between the ideal and the real.

The proposal format involves several parts and, from the initial meeting to completion, may take up to three years to prepare. It follows closely the format of the Personal Plan as outlined in chapter 2.

Prior to the student's final year in the residential school, a final set of five-year goals is created along with twelve-month objectives. These are included in the student's Personal Plan in order to provide the student with direction. The five-year goals will be of assistance to both the individual and the adult service provider in that their use will maintain continuity and, in essence, acts as the conduit between educational services and adult programs. Setting long-term goals is relevant for the young adult in that such goals provide a sense of direction and continuity within the support program. This format takes into consideration, whenever possible, ideas from the individual who is deafblind, as well as parents, caregivers, and professionals in the field of deafblind education.

If we think of our lives as a long and adventurous journey, then goals are our destination and objectives are the signposts on the route map we follow towards this destination. In our travels we can follow a variety of routes to reach a final destination, which will affect the time required to get there. When we arrive is not the key factor: what is important is that we continue on the road and in the direction of our destination.

Success is found not in the destination chosen, but in the quality of the journey taken to get there!

Is the Deafblind Transition Program successful? Yes! The positive response is based on several very concrete indicators. First, there are individuals who are deafblind, who through their actions or formal communication impress upon us that this transition format is both positive and productive. Students who are deafblind thrive in an environment that, through contemporary adult-oriented programming, fosters growing independence. Having one's own room, paying rent, being responsible for household duties, and buying groceries provide a sense of ownership and of self-worth. Documentation of sources and written evaluations, such as report cards and day books, also indicate the success level of the program. Regular contact and follow-up, both written and verbal, with parents or other caregivers help to ensure that we are maintaining a positive direction. Post-graduation consultative follow-up with adult service agencies is yet another good indicator of success. By doing student follow-up, not only can we be of assistance to the individual and adult placement, but we can evaluate the viability of the transition format with these adult service provision agencies.

Finally, our placement rate indicates success. This very high rate is indicative of two factors: (a) these young adults are well prepared for adult services, and (b) there has been a high level of commitment by the government to adult program provision for graduates of this school.

As the program continues to grow and evolve, there is no doubt that changes or modifications will be necessary, given a variety of extrinsic pressures. The concept is fundamentally sound, however, and the Deafblind Transition Program will persist in laying the foundation for young adults to develop and continue on the path of lifelong learning.

Support Services

It is recommended that a community liaison worker and a communication coordinator be appointed. Their functions are key supports to the residential-based deafblind program. The community liaison person has the following responsibilities:

- Assisting teachers to locate jobs and work experience placements within the school and the community
- Working on transition goals and objectives with the family, student, and the teacher
- Updating staff on changes in areas that affect students, such as government funding resources, advocacy, new policies related to adults with disabilities, and the status of present transition plans
- Organizing the input from families, students, and school staff to prepare a proposal to fund a supported independent living program from government or other agencies
- Directly assisting with the transition plan for the deafblind student by providing support to the module during transition.

The communication coordinator has the following responsibilities:

- Assisting staff and families to keep their communication skills at an optimum levels; the coordinator provides classes to maintain the proficiency level of staff at an established level of manual communication, for both signing and two-handed finger spelling, adapted to meet the needs of the individual students
- Teaching Braille to staff and families
- Teaching the use of other assistive devices that are used to communicate with others

- Holding communication classes or workshops for parents and siblings of students who are in the residential setting
- Holding communication classes or workshops for home Intervenors in their home communities, or holding weekend workshops at the school for families and their Intervenors.

The residential school should have good support services that address other student needs beyond those of direct programming. There should be a registered nurse on duty at all times to look after daily medical needs and to be the first contact during additional medical concerns. The nurse is a support for staff who are responsible for giving medications. The nurse is also a resource for the teacher regarding medical information about eyes, ears, and congenital syndromes and their characteristics. A medical doctor should be available to make visits to see a student who is ill to and to decide whether the student should be admitted to the local hospital, be prescribed medication, or be sent home to recover. There also should be easy access to a clinic that specializes in low-vision testing and is willing to work with hard-to-test children. This is necessary so that progress in the use of residual vision can be tracked, the appropriate assistive devices can be prescribed, and their use can be followed closely by professionals in this field.

An audiologist and assistive devices technician should be connected with the deafblind program. From their varied experience with children who are deaf-blind, these individuals are able to provide practical suggestions and recommendations on audiological assessments and amplification. The formal test situation may need to be repeated many times before results are obtained that accurately reflect the student's functional level of hearing with and without amplification.

The residential school should have a physiotherapist attached to its program. The physiotherapist should work hands- on with the students at least once a week and supervise module staff as they learn exercises and techniques to use both on land and in the therapy pool. The physiotherapy objectives and activities should be incorporated into the child's Personal Plan and therefore the activities that the child participates in throughout the week. The physiotherapist should meet with the teacher to discuss progress on a regular basis, as well as be involved in team meetings with the module team and with the family.

Conclusion

The residential school offers many advantages to parents of children who are deafblind for the education of their child. Trained staff, adequate levels of intervention, a carefully developed Personal Plan designed to meet the specific needs of their child, and ongoing family consultation and support are but a few of the advantages available when this option is chosen. The residential school is not the only option, but it is one that should be carefully considered. In fact, the ideal approach for many children is a combination of the residential-school option and the community-school–based option in order to obtain an educational experience that will best meet their needs.

Summary

1. The term 'residential school' refers to either a residential plan for deafblind children or a unit for deafblind children with separate classes and residential accommodation within a residential facility serving the needs of a different population.
2. Other facilities of a residential school should include a resource centre, a resource library, meeting facilities for parent groups and support and advocacy groups, workshops for families and professionals, and staff training.
3. There are at least eight areas that should be considered when looking for a program to meet the needs of a deafblind child.
4. Family involvement is essential for program development and the education and training of family members and community support workers.
5. Teachers should support networking of parents and family members.
6. Families must be involved in setting long-term goals and yearly objectives.
7. Objectives must be written in behavioural terms.
8. Teachers should provide comprehensive anecdotal reports at least three times a year.
9. The residential school can provide
   a) an activity-based program with identified success indicators
   b) a reactive environment
   c) communication training throughout the child's day
   d) life-skills development
   e) motor development
   f) comprehensive, ongoing orientation and mobility training
   g) appropriate intervention by trained staff with an in-depth knowledge of the child and his needs
   h) a cohesive team approach facilitated by the module staff
   i) a consistent approach throughout the child's day.
10. The teacher has overall responsibility for the development, implementation and evaluation of the child's program. He/she must train staff, assist par-

ents through regularly scheduled home visits, conduct module and program meetings, and consult regularly with parents.

11. The principal or plan director has overall responsibility for all programs and assists with support for the children and their families.

12. Transition from school to adult life involves three stages: the Pseudo Apartment Setting; the Transition Housing Project; and Transition to Adult Services.

13. Specialized training is necessary in order to work with children who are deafblind.

RESOURCES

Meshcheryakov, A. (1979) *Awakening to Life*. Trans. K. Judelson. Moscow: Progress Publishers.

Chess, Kom, Fernandez (1971) *Psychiatric Disorders of Children with Congenital Rubella*

Collins, Michael T. (1993) 'Educational Services.' In *Proceedings of National Symposium on Children and Youth Who Are Deafblind*, ed. J.W. Reiman and P.A. Johnson. Monmouth, OR: Teaching Research Publications

– (1994) 'Assessment of Today's 301.77 Program' *Deafblind Perspectives* 2:2, 1994–5

Intervention Task Force Report, Queen's University, April 1992

Fredericks, Bud (1994) 'The 307.11 Program in the New Millennium' *Deafblind Perspectives* 2:2, 1994–5.

REFERENCES

Alsop, Linda, ed. (1993) *A Resource Manual for Understanding and Interacting with Infants, Toddlers, and Preschool Age Children with Deaf-Blindness*. SHI*HI Institute. Logan, UT: H.O.P.E.

Freeman, Peggy (1986) 'The Family and the Professionals.' *Proceedings of the Second Canadian Conference on Deaf-Blind Education and Development*. W. Ross Macdonald School, Brantford, ON, 16–18 March

Haebner, Kathleen Mary, Jeanne Glidden Prickett, Elga Joffee, and Theresa Rafalowski Welch (1996) 'A Self Study and In-Service Training Program for Individuals Who Work with People Who Are Deafblind.' In *Rehabilitation and Educational for Blindness and Neural Impairment* (Winter). Washington, DC: Heldref Publications

Heubner, Kathleen Mary, Jeanne Glidden Prickett, Theresa Rafalowski Welch, and Elga Joffee (1995) *Hand in Hand*. New York: AFB Press

McInnes, John M. (1993) 'Educational Services: Reaction.' In *Proceedings of the*

National Symposium on Children and Youth Who Are Deafblind, ed. John W. Reiman and Pattie A. Johnson. Monmouth, OR: Teaching Research Publications

McInnes, John M., and Jacquelyn A. Treffry (1982, 1993, 1997). *Deafblind Infants and Children: A Development Guide*. Toronto: University of Toronto Press

Petty, Robert H. (1983) 'Parents As Partners.' In *Proceedings of The First Canadian Conference on the Education and Development of Deaf-Blind Infants and Children*. Brantford, ON, 28–30 March

12

Community-Based Adult Programs

CONNIE TAYLOR-SOUTHALL and LAUREN SMITH

Introduction

It is expected that all adults who are deafblind will be provided with the opportunity to develop to their full potential while participating as a part of the community through personal planning. That they will be allowed to live their lives in the way they choose, with intervention and with as much independence as possible through intervention. That they are given the opportunity to make, and are given all the necessary information to follow through with, their own choices and decisions. That they have an awareness of what is available, constantly working towards more choices and control of their world. Communication is essential to deafblind persons and carries on throughout their lifetime. Even those who have not developed communication skills earlier on can develop them throughout their adult lives.

The basis for Community-Based Adult Programs was described in previous chapters. In a Community-Based Adult Program we need to consider the following topics:

- Background
- Transition
- Personal planning, including life skills, recreation, and vocational
- Implementation of the personal program
- Calendars
- Challenging behaviours
- Late Manifestations of Rubella
- Sexuality
- Intervention

Background

There are two main groups of adults challenged by deafblindness, Those with acquired (adventitious) deafblindness and those with congenital or early adventitious deafblindness. Both main groups contain subgroups. Our focus in this chapter will be upon adults with congenital or early adventitious deafblindness. Individuals with acquired deafblindness have some of the same but also many different challenges than those faced by adults who are congenitally or early adventitiously deafblind, and they should be the subject of a text that focuses on them and their specific needs.

For the purposes of this chapter, the authors will talk about those adults who have been challenged with deafblindness since birth or early childhood. Those who have been diagnosed with this disability fall into several identifiable groups, although many have a history that bridges at least two groups.

These groups are as follows:

a) Adults who were identified as deafblind and who received support to some extent during preschool years and as a residential pupil in a deafblind program during most of their school years
b) Adults who were identified as being deafblind and have received support to some extent during their preschool years and who received appropriate support as they lived at home and attended their local school during all or most of their school years
c) Adults who lived at home, attended a local school, were placed in a program designed to support children with other disabilities, and received little or no adequate support during preschool and school years
d) Adults who were placed in institutions or other care facilities as infants or children and who received little or no support designed to meet their needs as a person with deafblindness
e) Other.

Each group presents specific challenges as well as many common ones. Most important, regardless of background, we have found that most, if not all, are capable of continued learning and overall development. As adulthood approaches, it is necessary to look at the future and what it might encompass for each of these groups.

Adults Who Have Received Appropriate Programming and Support

Youths who are deafblind and were diagnosed at an early age may have been fortunate enough to receive services designed to meet their unique needs. Some may have attended a residential setting for individuals with deafblindness. Others, who lived at home, may have attended school in their local community while receiving support from consultants or teachers with expertise in deafblindness.

These individuals will face both different and similar challenges. Those who have lived away from home in a residential setting will likely have the challenge of learning about a new community, as will the other group. Both will have to adapt to changes in routine. They will now receive seven-day programming, twelve months of the year. Those individuals who attended a residential setting will no longer be at home for the long summer break. Those who have lived at home will have to adjust to a move away from home and to a completely new environment without the daily support of the family network.

Adults Who Have Been Home Based without Appropriate Support

There are also those adults who have remained at home with inappropriate support. They face many of the same challenges, particularly those of leaving the family home and moving to a new community in an environment that has very different expectations of them.

Communication will also be a great challenge for these individuals since they will likely have very minimal communication skills or may have developed their own method of making their needs and wants known. They will also face the challenge of accepting a program that involves being an active participant in the community.

Adults Who Have Come from an Institutional Setting

The individuals who have been moved from an institutional setting to a community-based setting face some of the greatest challenges of all. Not only are they going to have to adapt to a new living environment, which includes intervention, communication, and programming, but they are most likely to be extremely resistant to this new way of life.

As is the case with the previous group, it is unlikely that many expectations have been placed on them. For survival purposes, they may have developed routines and a way of coping with day-to-day life that involves very little interaction with the rest of their world. They will quite likely have withdrawn into themselves or have developed such severe behavioural problems that medication may have been used to alleviate the problems. It then becomes a challenge for those involved to encourage them to adjust to life in an adult community-based setting.

Transition

Advanced Planning

As individuals who are deafblind approach adulthood, plans should be put in place that will provide a lifestyle which will meet their specific needs. When planning for the future, the person who is deafblind should have the same opportunities as their peers who are not challenged by disabilities. A team must be assembled, consisting of the deafblind person, his/her advocate, and professionals with expertise in the area of deafblindness. Options need to be explored, as they are with any young person, before any decision is reached as to what is optimum for this individual.

Some questions should be asked: Does the young adult with deafblindness want

- to live alone, with other individuals who are deafblind, or with other young people?
- to live in the city, the suburbs, or the country?
- to live in an apartment, a townhouse, or in a home?
- to live close to their families and/or advocates?

All these questions must be given due consideration in developing a plan for the future. It is important to begin planning several years before the young person leaves school, since it may take time and active lobbying to achieve the funding sources and find the personnel with the required expertise to develop and implement an appropriate Personal Plan.

Parental Concerns

This is often a very difficult time for families. Their child who is deafblind is growing up and ready to graduate from school. Parents have been heard to comment: 'My child has spent all those years at school and he is still deafblind!' They are angry! This may be a time when they once again realize that their dreams for this child's achieving their hopes and aspirations for the future will never occur. They will go through the same feelings of anger, fear, denial, and so on as they did when the child was born and again when he started school. No, the educational program could not cure the child of his deafblindness, but it did prepare them for an adult lifestyle which will allow them to become contributing members of our society.

The Medical Aspects of Transition

Another aspect of the transition phase must include medical services. It is quite likely that young people who are graduating from school have received medical services from children's hospitals, pediatricians, and family doctors. Because of their age and other considerations, the young adults now will no longer be able to access these services. New medical practitioners and other community service personnel will have to be identified and educated. This aspect becomes particularly important, since most of the young people, such as those with Congenital Rubella Syndrome, have ongoing medical problems and continue to develop new medical problems. This issue will be discussed in further detail later in the chapter.

Transitions for Young Adults Who Received Appropriate Services

Throughout the school years, regardless of whether the young adult attended an appropriate program in the local school or a residential-based program, he/she has been home on weekends, on school holidays, and during summer and has been very much a part of the family. Now, plans are being made for the young adult to live in his/her own home and have a life apart from the family. We must remember to include the family in the transition plans and make them part of his/her adult lifestyle. There are several factors that must be considered, such as location, medical support, introduction of new staff, as well as the kind of lifestyle that the young person wishes to have.

Once the transition team has decided on a course of action and the funding has been obtained, it is time to put the transition plan in place. Transition must be planned with a gradual move from the present setting to the new setting and new staff of Intervenors. Optimally, the transition phase should consist of visits back and forth between the two locations, involving former Intervenors and new Intervenors. It is beneficial to utilize known Intervenors while the new community is being learned about. Training of the new staff should occur during this time and should be conducted by people who have expertise in deafblindness. It should also involve the individual who is deafblind and the family and/or advocates.

Transition for Young Adults Who Did Not Receive Appropriate Services

Transition for young adults who did not receive appropriate programming and support is often more difficult. This may be a whole new way of life for them.

Again, involvement of the families/advocates is imperative in determining how smooth the transition will be. A gradual introduction to the new environment and staff, allowing the individual to familiarize him/herself slowly will be of benefit. Each will have to develop a bond and learn to trust the new staff of Intervenors. Programming will have to be adapted to meet individual needs, allowing the young adult to get to know the new home before moving out into the community.

Adults Moving from an Institutional or Other Care Facility

Those individuals who are deafblind and have lived in institutions, some for many years, may have great difficulty in accepting a transition to a new environment. The individual may not wish to participate, since it may be a very frightening experience for them. The transition must be gradual and involve both known staff and new staff. New Intervenors may have to spend a great deal of time with the individual in the institution, getting to know him/her and trying to develop a bond. As this trust grows, the person who is deafblind and the Intervenors should start spending more time in the new home environment until the individual begins to accept the new home and surroundings.

The level of functioning for these young adults may be learned helplessness. It is likely that few expectations relating to their progress have been placed on them, and they will have gradually learned to ignore their environment and all in it. They may exhibit severe behavioural problems when requested to become re-involved. This behaviour, then, becomes a challenge for those working with them in an adult community-based setting.

Other

Adults with congenital or early adventitious deafblindness that fall into this nebulous category often present the biggest problems. They may have been placed and failed to progress in a residential school or local school classes designed for pupils with other challenging conditions. By the time they reach adulthood, they may be coping by exhibiting challenging behaviours, completely withdrawing from the world, or simply by functioning far below their abilities in many areas.

Usually there will be major deficits in communication, self-care skills, and life skills. Like all congenitally deafblind adults, when programmed for appropriately and when skilled Intervenors are available for support, progress will be made towards a personal feeling of self-worth, an ability to make decisions, recognize consequences, participate in the community, and form new relationships. Progress will be slow at first, but progress will be made.

Programming

The same steps to create a Personal Plan as outlined in chapter 2 are used when dealing with adults. The emphasis should be on decision making, calendars, and learning to take part in developing a Personal Plan within the home and community.

Basis for Personal Plan Development

When developing and writing a Personal Plan, the deafblind adult should be the starting point and his/her goals are the primary concern. As well, the involvement of all people who interact with the client is essential to ensure all areas are included. The implementation of the plan includes the requirement that each of these individuals have an understanding of the Personal Plan's goals and objectives, which will reflect the varying abilities of each individual. The previous background of the adult will have influence on the content of the program but not on how the program is developed. (Refer to the 'Developing a Personal Plan' chart located in chapter 2.)

The main change of emphasis in working with the adult who is congenitally or early adventitiously deafblind is a conscious and continuous effort to include him/her in, and eventually to turn over to him/her the responsibility for, writing his/her Personal Plan. As the adult's ability to contribute to the plan's development increases, care must be taken to ensure that he/she understands the reason for the plan and how it will enable others to provide appropriate support. The level of functioning of the adult when he/she enters a support program will determine his/her involvement.

Sources of Information

The previous Personal Plan, if one is available, is an extremely valuable source of information. Like any adequate program, it should contain a statement of the important points of medical, developmental, and educational history; a description of his/her level of functioning as it was a year ago; a statement of five-year goals; and sets of objectives for each of the goals. A review of the previous plan's goals and objectives and the preparation of a new description of his/her level of functioning as it is now will lay the groundwork for identifying where future progress may be made.

The deafblind adult, his/her parents, nuclear and extended family members, Intervenors, community workers, and medical professionals all can provide information that will be helpful in program development. The person developing the program must obtain permission from the deafblind adult or, where this is not appropriate, from the individual who acts as their advocate to gather such information. Many community and medical professionals will refuse to discuss information concerning a specific adult unless permission has been obtained in writing.

Once the initial Personal Plan has been written for the adult in his/her new setting and the time covered by the first set of objects has passed, usually a year, Intervenors who are working with the deafblind individual should be looked upon as a valuable source of information. When providing support for the deafblind adult, Intervenors working hands on with the individual will gain valuable insights into the needs, abilities, and aspirations of the individual. Such practical information is essential in identifying goals and setting objectives.

Identifying Key Result Areas

Once all the information is assembled, the areas that are to be focused upon should be identified. Each key result area (KRA) will be reflected in a five-year goal and a number of objectives that will represent progress towards the goal. The process involved in writing a Personal Plan is described in chapter 2.

Plan Content for the Congenitally Deafblind Adult

Variations in the Personal Plans that will depend on the abilities of the individual, as is demonstrated in the following examples.

Life Skills
There are a number of guides available that list life skills and break them down into steps. The authors have found *The Developmental Profile for Use with Persons Who Are Deafblind* (McInnes 1996) a useful tool for this purpose. Life Skills is a broader classification than the traditional 'Living Skills' designation. Because of the available material, only banking, designing menus, home maintenance, and shopping, will be addressed.

Banking
Banking, like budgeting, is an abstract concept that can be successfully taught at various levels. The concept of where to obtain money can appear simplistic to the deafblind adult. The bank gives you money when you ask. The concept that it is not an unending supply, however, must be taught. The concept will be developed when the deafblind adult and his/her Intervenor go to the bank, where they will:

- open an account
- deposit money that has been received or earned and that he/she has person-ally carried to the bank
- fill out and sign deposit and/or withdrawal slips, cheques, and other forms.

The development of this type of concept will require many repetitions and will be accomplished only if time is taken to explain and discuss each step in the process every time the bank is visited. During the initial stages, obtaining money should be restricted to one method and one bank branch to avoid confu-sion. Banking machines, cheques, and cards should be introduced one at a time, when the basic concept of the bank as a place where you can save money and get it back as needed has been established. Also, it is wise to explain to the bank staff what is happening, to avoid using the bank during busy times, and to use the same teller if possible. The process should begin well before the individual is functioning at a level where he/she can be expected to grasp the concept and initiate and carry out the process independently.

Budgeting
The motivation to learn budgeting may be introduced through the experience of not having enough money available to make desired and/or necessary pur-chases. It will take many repetitions and a variety of experiences before such concepts are formed and acted upon. The first step in budgeting may be putting aside a small amount of money, preferably earned, each week towards the pur-chase of a specific desired item. A second step may be the establishing of a 'Needs List' and a 'Wants List.' The concept of budgeting also involves learn-ing to wait for a purchase of a desired item and to anticipate the pleasure that will be derived from its final acquisition. Dialogue is essential at all phases of the development of this concept if it is to be grasped.

Menus
Designing weekly menus is another opportunity for the adult to exercise control and choice even where he/she is functioning at a low level. Initially the adult may not make more than one or two choices for the week. Hamburgers for lunch tomorrow may be a place to start. Menu planning can help to develop communication, anticipation, and provide motivation to carry out the activity: 'I will make mom a hamburger for lunch tomorrow when she visits me.'

   The use of menus is not confined to those created by the individual and his/her Intervenor. Going to restaurants and using their menus is also important in developing the concept. Where the deafblind adult cannot read the menu him/herself, the Intervenor should read the menu and communicate its contents.

Unfortunately, sometimes adults supporting the deafblind person feel that by limiting the choices available through not giving access to all the information is an appropriate approach. Only a few items on the menu are communicated, or only one or two choices of meals are provided. This approach destroys the trust in, and the usefulness of, an Intervenor should the deafblind adult find there were other choices available. The Intervenor would never put up with such treatment when out with a husband, wife, or friends; therefore such an approach cannot be justified in supporting a deafblind adult.

Home Maintenance
The deafblind adult should be involved, with the support of his/her Intervenor, in the daily maintenance of personal and shared space at the same level as a peer who is not challenged by the disability of deafblindness. This activity can also be viewed as a volunteer, or paid, position for a specific deafblind adult with all the decisions and responsibilities normally attached thereto. Common sense must be used when selecting activities for which the deafblind adult will be responsible.

Shopping
Shopping involves many levels and varieties of activity. Shopping may be for an item that is required or desired immediately or it may grow out of an activity such as daily or weekly meal planning. Activities such as the acquisition of items required for personal care, household maintenance, purchase of clothing for personal use, or choosing gifts provide many opportunities to develop this concept.

Shopping first for specific items, then from a personal list, and finally from a list designed to meet the needs of all those living with him/her can be a realistic activity. For individuals who cannot read print or Braille, a list can be developed using concrete or semi-concrete cues. Concrete cues could be a selection of used containers or representative items that are taken to a store. These items would then be exchanged for things they represent. Semi-concrete representations might be a front panel or part of an item, a picture of an item taken from a magazine or photograph, a model of an item, or a drawing made by the adult. In all cases the relationship of the semi-concrete item to the item itself will have to be developed.

Recreation

Recreational activities are as varied as the individuals. One of the best ways to obtain information concerning what an individual likes to do is to introduce numerous activities with enthusiasm. As the adult progresses from awareness, and even dislike of the activities, through the Reaction Sequence to a level where he/she can initiate the activity, sufficient information about the activity will be obtained to allow him/her to choose or ignore it.

Recreational activities must be related to the abilities and interests of the deafblind adult. It is very important to allow each adult to indicate where his/her interests and preferences lie. For example, once the deafblind adult has had sufficient exposure to an activity such as bowling to decide whether or not he/she likes it, the Intervenor should not take one, two, or ten individuals bowling merely because it is in the plans or because the Intervenor is sure it will be enjoyable for them. In fact, when a group of individuals are going out together for any activity, the one question that should be asked is when did the deafblind adults (not their Intervenors) get together and make the decision. Until congenitally or early adventitiously deafblind youth or adults reach a high level of social functioning, it is likely that the staff, not the deafblind individuals, have made the decision leading to a group outing. Occasional group outings are both desirable and fun for all concerned. Frequent groups of deafblind youth or adults, all being herded to the same destination, point to either staffing level problems or a lack of understanding of the needs of the deafblind individual and/or the purposes of intervention.

The deafblind adult, with ever widening interests and improving social skills, demonstrates over and over again that limitations should not be placed on recreational opportunities. Activities like those in Table 12.1 provide many opportunities to work on a variety of objectives.

The only limits are those that apply to the adult's non-challenged peers when an appropriate level of intervention is available and provided that the deafblind adult knows when to ask for intervention once the activity has been established as part of the available alternatives from which he/she can make choices.

'Age appropriate' is a phrase sometimes used when looking at judging the suitability of activities for deafblind adults. This term can be misleading or applicable. It should not mean that deafblind adults are deprived of activities they enjoy because they are too old, too young, or too challenged. Activities can be adjusted to being age appropriate for any individual.

Reading and writing are not always a relaxing, enjoyable means of passing the time, owing to eye fatigue and/or limited background experience. Both stories and movies can provide a basis for a safe discussion of a fictional character's actions and the development of a recognition of individual and societal expectations concerning behaviour. These activities also can be useful in developing the skills needed for writing letters, a journal, notes to Intervenors and others, and for some, things such as poetry or stories both for their own enjoyment and for others to read.

TABLE 12.1
Varieties of Recreational Activities

Outdoor activities	
snowshoeing	skiing
snowmobiling	nature walks / hiking
horseback riding	fishing
camping	swimming
canoeing	picnics
roller/ice skating	cards
Indoor activities (home)	
video games	cards
badminton	ping pong
TV/VCR	
Crafts	
woodworking	copper tooling
rug hooking	model building
flower arranging	candle making
jewellery assembly	knitting
crocheting	sewing
Community	
fitness classes	yoga classes
Tai Chi classes	judo classes
music therapy	massage therapy
churches	outdoor concerts
dances	bar scene
movies	theatre
fairs	garden shows
theme parks	craft shows
public gardens	exhibitions

Individual craft items can be used as models. Initially, an item may be completed by the adult and the Intervenor working together. The finished item can provide motivation for the deafblind adult to want to make other items and will provide a model with which the adult can compare the next attempt. The Intervenor's enthusiasm for the project and people whom the deafblind adult cares about admiring the finished craft are important components of the activity.

An interest in various crafts created in the home can lead to involvement in community craft classes. By participating in such classes the deafblind adult is not only enjoying an activity, but also having an opportunity to socialize. Many community facilities and gathering places for young adults provide an enjoyable atmosphere and an opportunity for social interaction. They start with the

Intervenor acting as a companion (social intervention). After a few sessions the deafblind adult will suggest that the Intervenor be separate, but available. The authors have found congenitally deafblind adults are able socially to interact successfully and find acceptance with a variety of non-disabled peers provided they are supported with appropriate intervention.

Vocation

For adults with deafblindness attempting to obtain employment can be frustrating. The difficulty should not prevent identification of either volunteer or paid employment as a goal. Once employment is identified as a goal, objectives can be written around obtaining and maintaining employment experiences.

Knut Johansen (1997) notes: 'For congenitally deafblind people in particular, I suggest that the term 'employment' also relates to the work carried out in sheltered workshops, adapted workplaces, and individual arrangements for developing meaningful activities that will not necessarily lead to income of some sort.' The July–December (1997) issue of *Deafblind Education* (Eileen Boothroyd editor), in which this article appears, is devoted to employment for the deafblind adult and is well worth reading.

The first step in obtaining employment is to identify things the adult enjoys doing. This list could start at home and then expand. For example: An adult who is deafblind loves to organize, socialize, and imitate peers. This individual volunteered at the Parks and Recreation office in his neighbourhood. This position led to a nomination for 'Volunteer of the Year' award by his peers, and he received it. This is a position where his abilities have been recognized and could possibly lead to a paid position.

Visits to a variety of work sites should be planned and carried out. Where there is a high degree of interest, and where the opportunity is suitable for the deafblind adult, further visits should be made, which eventually will include an opportunity to meet the potential employer. To introduce options, it is best to expose deafblind adults to numerous opportunities, therefore enabling them to make informed decisions. When they have experienced different job settings and employers, they can indicate which they would prefer. This makes it more probable that they will enjoy their employment and be successful. Now is the time to introduce the résumé. The second step is to compile a résumé. The résumé can include pictures instead of, or in addition to, the typed, written, or Braille wording. Braille résumés should be interlined and pictures suitably arranged and titled to make a coherent presentation. Pictures are often very persuasive.

Now that the résumé has been produced, volunteering should not be overlooked and can be used as a training process. Many employers are more likely to experiment if the introduction is not going to cost them money. As they become more aware of the capabilities of the deafblind adult, paid positions may develop. Even where a paid position does not develop, if the attitudes of the Intervenors and advocates are supportive, the deafblind adult will gain satisfaction and community recognition through the experience.

Another alternative might be to develop a supported small-business operation within the support agency. These operations may be staffed by deafblind adults and their Intervenors or a combination of deafblind adults and personnel with and/or without other disabilities. Such operations may produce and sell products manufactured by deafblind adults; may be re-sellers; or may contract to perform services such as garden preparation, grass cutting, small appliance repairs, or any other service that the individuals staffing the operation are capable of performing either independently or in partnership with others.

Other deafblind adults may operate independently. They can produce crafts in their own home and sell them at craft shows or on contract. Some deafblind adults can contribute successfully to a family business provided he or she has appropriate support and that the family sees him or her as someone who can, rather than someone who cannot because of the disability of deafblindness. The possibilities are only limited by the imaginations of the support staff and, as the adult with deafblindness develops a wider exposure to the work-a-day world, by his/her own wishes.

The measurement of success is different when one is looking at employment of the deafblind adult. The motivation for working is often enjoyment, raised self-esteem, and other intangibles such as opportunities to have increased levels of socialization and meaningful communication. When the money earned is attached to buying something, the money itself can become more of an incentive. The concept of, and the pay-offs from, having a job is extremely complex. The adult who works is usually viewed by the society in which he/she lives in a positive way.

Implementing the Personal Plan

Plan Ownership

Once written, the Personal Plan should be presented for approval to the deafblind adult or, where more appropriate, to his/her advocate. This approval should include permission to share the program contents with Intervenors, support persons, and others. From the beginning, the Personal Plan must be seen as the property of the deafblind adult, his/her parent, or advocate, as appropriate.

Professionals have a duty to provide the best information and advice, organize it, and add information based on professional training and experience. There is also an obligation to support the decisions of the deafblind adult and/or parent or advocate concerning the goals and objectives that are identified. The decisions of the deafblind adult who has attained an appropriate level of functioning, however, must be respected. It should be stressed that the information supplied by parents, advocates, and Intervenors should in no way limit the input from the individual with deafblindness.

Two Underlying Goals

There are two goals implicit in all such programs. They are to have the adult with deafblindness reach the stage where he/she

- will be able to write all or part of his/her own program
- will be able to participate in the hiring and training the individuals who will provide him or her with intervention.

Utilizing Activities

Activities that will be utilized to achieve the objectives identified in the Personal Plan include everything from home and personal maintenance to understanding and interacting with the world. By the time the young person becomes an adult, many basic life skills have already been established. As he/she moves from a home- and educational-based lifestyle to a supported independent lifestyle, he/she will apply previously learned knowledge, skills, and attitudes in new ways and will experiment to find out what still works, what doesn't work and needs adjustment, and what is no longer applicable. For the adult who is congenitally or early adventitiously deafblind, this is a major task, which will present many difficulties before it is accomplished.

Each activity will provide the young adult and his/her Intervenor with the opportunity to work on many objectives. The following example will illustrate that a number of objectives can be worked upon during one activity. Objectives in the areas of communication, anticipation, problem solving, cause and affect relationships, planning, and social and emotional behaviour all will be addressed.

As a teenager, JG had learned to make coffee but had relied on others to solve problems such as not having any coffee in the cupboard when he decided to make a cup for himself or to serve to others. A problem like this presents an opportunity for a variety of responses and numerous decisions.

a) Will he make something else instead?
b) Will he go out immediately and buy more coffee?
c) Will he become angry and attempt to focus his anger on others?
d) Will he devise a system so that he does not run out of coffee next time, such as putting coffee on a grocery list.

Problem Solving, Decision Making, and Understanding Consequences
Life is full of problem solving, decision making, and assuming responsibility. Understanding consequences begins to play an important part in the life of the deafblind adult. Learning to solve such problems will permit the adult to have more control over his/her life and surroundings. It would seem that common sense would dictate such an approach.

Problems that arise in caring for personal and shared space help the young adult to achieve a sense of accomplishment and pride. Such activities also provide opportunities for the Intervenor to promote the making of choices.

There is a point when it is necessary to learn what happens when a task is not carried out. Such learning may take place through personal experience or through the Intervenor's explaining the consequences. Everything cannot be learned by the deafblind adult through experience alone, and thus the close relationship to an Intervenor becomes very important. Deadly microbes are difficult to identify on a kitchen counter, in a cupboard, or in refrigerator. It is important, however, that these areas be given a good cleaning frequently. Most deafblind adults will not have sufficient vision even to see common dirt or mould in these areas and none of us will see microbes. This is one area where the deafblind adult can, and should, ask for assistance without in any way limiting his/her independence.

Some would say that individuals with deafblindness are not capable of making choices beyond a level of 'juice or milk.' It is felt that it is easier for the Intervenor, parent, or advocate to make the important decisions, thus protecting the deafblind adult from making mistakes or becoming frustrated. Adults with deafblindness experience the same issues and are required to make and must be supported in making the same type of decisions as the general population. It is important that they feel they have control over their lives at a level at which they can understand and function. Choices are able to be made successfully only when all necessary information has been communicated.

The development of an appropriate level of control by the adult over his/her life can start with something as basic as choosing what to wear in the morning. Choice does not have to be limited by the degree of disability or the lack of formal language. For example, if an individual with no vision or hearing is to make choices concerning what to wear, one might introduce the idea by putting a pair of jeans on one knee and a pair of corduroys on the other. Provide the language necessary for communication if it has not already been established. If the adult who has not yet developed formal language indicates, through gesture or body language, that the corduroys are preferred, support him/her by communicating that you understand. Use this as an opportunity to 'talk' about the fact he/she liked the feel of the corduroys.

If time is taken for the development of communication around this choice consistently, the adult will begin to understand the concept behind making this choice. Of course, this interchange is only a beginning, and eventually it will lead to the following kinds of activity. The adult

- organizes his/her clothing in a way that will enable him/her to make such choices independently
- identifies particular clothing with specific activities and seasons
- identifies clothing that needs care or repair
- knows when to ask for assistance, for instance, in choosing coordinating outfits if this is beyond his/her personal level of visual functioning and clothing organization

The idea of being able to make a choice, even if it is not always the most appropriate, is a difficult concept to grasp. Understanding and accepting the consequences of decisions must be learned through experience.

After such an experience, it will be easier for the deafblind adult to understand that decisions have consequences and he/she will begin to anticipate the them. This result is less likely if he or she is prevented from making important choices or does not receive support for a decision.

In some cases deafblind adults may make choices or decisions that would put them in an unsafe or an extremely inappropriate position. In such situations Intervenors have an obligation to indicate the reason and to ensure that actions arising from the decision are not carried out. Such actions are no different from those the law of most countries expects of any of us, for instance, when a guest in our home has consumed too much alcohol and announces the intention of driving home. We are expected to prevent that person from putting his/her life, or that of others, in danger.

Motivation
Motivation is a very important aspect of routine activities. Many deafblind adults are not motivated to do mundane tasks around the home. The only way some will be motivated to complete such tasks is if there will be recognition from, or positive comments by significant others. Socially acceptable values

must be explained to the deafblind adult by an Intervenor with whom the adult has built a relationship such that he or she will care what the Intervenor thinks.

Social Relationships
Another area of concern when a Personal Plan is implemented is helping the young adult to gain an understanding of the responsibilities and consequences of social relationships. Concepts must be addressed and questions answered concerning appropriate behaviours with a friend, a stranger, an acquaintance, or a significant other by those supporting young men and women who are deafblind. Some Intervenors and advocates avoid discussing this area, feeling that *what deafblind adults don't know, can't hurt them*. It has been noted that adults with deafblindness experience the same feelings and have the same questions as adults not challenged by the disability of deafblindness. When they are experiencing these natural feelings, it can be very frustrating if they are unable to understand what is happening, particularly if no one seems to care.

Relaxation
Adults who are congenitally deafblind often have difficulty understanding the concept of relaxation. Relaxation must be identified at the goal, objective, and activity levels. Activities designed to incorporate relaxation should be identified and utilized. Sitting and having a cup of tea is a legitimate activity upon which can be built the concepts of relaxation, doing things for others, and many objectives identified in the areas of social, emotional, and conceptual development.

Physical Exercise
Without appropriate, enthusiastic intervention, it is very difficult to design and implement an adequate exercise program for congenitally deafblind adults. Without such intervention, they may lead a semi-sedentary lifestyle, which will have serious consequences for their overall health and physical well-being. Motivation through participation in the company of someone who enjoys the activity is an important component of exercise with deafblind adults.

Calendars

A factor in reducing the amount of stress in anyone's life is knowing and anticipating upcoming activities. Calendars are a rich source of information for individuals with deafblindness. They can range from concrete to Braille and from visual pictures to the written word.

The Calendar Process

Use of calendars is an ongoing process: evolution of the calendar format and of the items used to represent the activities will take place, but progress in one area is not necessarily dependent on progress in the other.

Step One

Place a representation of each activity on or in a suitable medium such as a shelf or in a box as each activity is completed. Most important, at the end of a specific time period (a shift or a day) take time to talk about what the individual with deafblindness and you and others have done, using the 'calendar' for reference. Time must be set aside to communicate. If necessary, shorten or drop other activities.

Initially the representations will probably, but not necessarily, be concrete in nature, for example, a washcloth to represent morning pre-breakfast activities, a plastic plate for meals, a soap scoop for measuring soap for clothes washing. Such activities may be broken down into finer representations (tooth brush, wash cloth, etc.) according to the level of functioning of the particular individual. Over an extended period, the concept will evolve from identifying each specific part to becoming an all-inclusive symbol indicating all routine activities that take place prior to breakfast.

The next step is to begin to place the representations of the activities in a 'day' format before they are carried out. It is at this point, when a day is being preplanned, that choices as to specific special activities and their sequencing will begin. A day may be any twenty-four hour period, not necessarily from 12 midnight to 11:59 pm. It could be from 2 pm one day to 1:59 pm the next. The choice will be more dependent upon who will conduct the discussion than on clock time.

Step Two

When step one is firmly established as an *enjoyable activity*, leave the daily record up, and as a conclusion to talking time, plan what you (the Intervenor and the deafblind adult) will do tomorrow. As each activity is discussed by the partners, have the deafblind partner place its symbolic representation in the appropriate time slot beside those for the 'day' just completed. The amount of time needed will increase to allow the partners to discuss both what was done today and what will be done tomorrow. It cannot be stressed too strongly that this must continue to be an enjoyable, relaxed activity. If it appears onerous to the deafblind adult, all or most of the usefulness of the 'calendar approach' is lost. The concepts that will be introduced at this stage include 'tomorrow, then yesterday, today, and tomorrow'; the predictable reoccurrence of some events, such as morning activities, meals, and daily chores; the occurrence of special activities scheduled by others and over which little choice is available, such as a trip to the doctor, going to a parade or party, or the time that a specific Intervenor will be available; and the making of choices in advance, not only immediately prior to or during an activity.

When concepts are being introduced, representations of some activities may become more refined. This change should take place slowly and be based upon the level of function of the individual. The stress is upon understandable communication based upon a mutually shared understanding of the representations. The evolution of the complexity of the 'calendar' does not necessarily parallel the evolution of representational material. The final part of step two is to expand the calendar so it represents yesterday, today, and tomorrow.

Step Three
Gradually, the process of leaving up completed 'days' evolves into a full week's representation and accompanying discussion about important things that happened during the week. These discussions will begin to focus on two topics. The first will be about what we did today and what we shall do tomorrow. The second will be the combination of what shall we do tomorrow and what were the important things that happened during the week. In step three, time for these discussions should be shown on the calendar part of the overall weekly plan and most, or even all, afternoon (or morning or evening if more appropriate) will be set aside for the discussion.

The next development will be to leave the week in place and begin to record plans for the next week below or beside it. Remember, it is the direct and total involvement of the deafblind adult, through discussion and physically placing the representations on the calendar, that is important. At this second stage, weekly planning sessions will begin at a routinely specified time. Activities will be identified according to type.

It is suggested that fixed activities of daily living be placed first. Next, place special activities for the week, ensuring that sufficient 'discussion' takes place to have the activity understood and anticipated. Finally, symbolic representations of 'choice' activities should be placed. The stress during the communication must be on understanding the choices to be made. Eventually, it is often useful to have more options than time to fill them. Discussion should now focus not only on *what* the activity will be but also upon *who* will provide the intervention.

Evolution in the representative media should continue. It must be stressed repeatedly, however, that the ability to understand the concepts of calendar, planning, and recording is not tied to the level of the representative media being used. The ability to use sophisticated representations, such as the printed or written word, may be well in advance or significantly behind the ability to understand the complexities of the 'calendar approach.'

A week does not necessarily have to run from Monday to Sunday or from Friday to Thursday. Where staff work with more than one adult, it is probably better for each deafblind adult to have an individual weekly cycle so that sufficient time can be given to the discussions arising around his/her calendar.

The weekly calendar is not the final step.

Step Four
Monthly calendars are introduced and special events are noted on them. The relationship of the weekly calendar to the monthly calendar must be taught. Discussions should now include a review of the special activities that took place in the week just passed, and of the activities in the week to come, as well as a look ahead to special events in 'so many days' and eventually 'so many weeks.' Finally, down the road, the goal is also to have the deafblind adult placing family birthdays, identifying special holidays, and so on, on a yearly calendar.

Step Five
The calendar should evolve into a 'book' form with a version of the 'daily planner approach' suitable to the individual's level of symbolic communication. The onus and responsibility for developing weekly and monthly calendars should begin to shift to the adult. It should be seen as his/her record and as a way to control his/her world.

A diary (a written, drawn, picture book with photographs and drawings, including titles when appropriate) should be introduced. Initially, this will be a record that can be used to explain to other Intervenors what is going to happen today, or when you will be here on Thursday of this week, and so on. He/she should be encouraged to discuss this record at first, but the ultimate objective is that he/she will decide if the diary is to be shared, and with whom. In some cases the diary may be partly or wholly computer generated.

The focus of this approach is complex, but one of its most important aspects is to be able to look back over several weeks or even months and recall enjoyable activities.

Points to Remember

1. *Without discussion stressing both receptive and expressive communication, The 'calendar approach' is probably a waste of time.*

2. If too many choices are offered initially, it can be frustrating for the deaf-blind adult. Possibly cut back to providing two choices for each area on the calendar. Certain daily routines and weekly events occur regularly.
3. Keep events such as morning routines, meals, and jobs in place, thereby reducing the overall number of choices to be made.
4. Make sure that new events are introduced using the Presentation Sequence and Total Communication.
5. From time to time introduce new options and gradually increase the number and variety of choices, eventually moving to the point where the individual needs your input only about special events happening within the time frame for which they are planning. This recommendation also applies to increasing the number of days in the calendar.
6. Variations of calendar format will occur because of the individuality of the person utilizing it. A totally deafblind individual will use concrete cues, such as a bathing suit symbolizing swimming. This can eventually be changed to a piece of an old bathing suit that the individual can feel. Braille can be introduced, provided the adult can make the fine distinctions necessary, using concrete cues to identify the word.
7. An individual with some usable vision may use photos or drawings of activities. As his/her vocabulary increases, printed words can be added beneath the pictures. From this step he/she can then proceed to using simply the printed word. Involving the adult, by having him/her take the photo that will represent the activity or the adult with whom it will be done, often adds meaning and aids recall and identification.
8. The deafblind adult can, and will, change his/her mind occasionally. This can happen when it is time to carry out an activity that was put in the plans as they were being developed. The deafblind adult should be supported when making the changes required by his/her new decision. If it is important that the activity be carried out, then the Intervenor, not the deafblind adult, has a problem, one of providing motivation that will ensure the activity is carried out, either at that moment or at a new time arrived at through dialogue between partners.
9. One important final thought: the important part of any activity is the deaf-blind adult, not the plan, the process, or the calendar.

Challenging Behaviours

It has been our experience that if you do have an individual who is experiencing challenging behaviours, you should re-evaluate closely each of the three areas of communication, health, and programming and then develop a strategic plan with which everyone is in agreement. If inappropriate behaviours are occurring, staff should investigate as follows:

1. Reassess the communication that is taking place to ensure that a Reactive Environment exists and that both receptive and expressive, not merely directive, communication is being used by the Intervenors.
2. Check medical records for probable causes or possible trends.
3. Check to see if there has been a change of routine or program imposed without explanation.
4. Check to see if an expected Intervenor failed to show up, or worse, if an Intervenor was scheduled to work with another person, and the deafblind adult is unaware of the fact.
5. Review the Personal Plan and its implementation to see if
   • the person is being underchallenged
   • too much is being expected at this particular time
   • the program is meeting the person's needs
   • the person has an appropriate degree of control during its implementation.
6. Review special shift or daily reports for possible causes, such as staff-client conflicts, location, sleeping patterns, time of day, and specific activities.
7. Assemble the above information and then consult with the individual's medical practitioners and family and/or advocate.

The routine examination of the above points will help staff to arrive at some answers that will lead to changes in administrative practices or intervention techniques.

Communication and Challenging Behaviours

Challenging behaviours often pose difficulties for the individual with deafblindness, Intervenors who are working with him/her, and family members and/or advocates. When problems occur, we should look at why they are happening. Usually, through good documentation, observation, and discussions with staff and families and/or advocates, the problem can be traced to one of communication, health, or programming, or sometimes a combination of these factors.

The development of both language and communication skills does not stop when the individual who is deafblind becomes an adult. It is often assumed the person with deafblindness understands our communication, or we may incorrectly think we know what he/she is trying to tell us, when in fact we have completely misunderstood. When poor communication takes place, frustration sets in and inappropriate behaviours may occur. *It must be emphasized that when problems with communication exist they are our problems, not those of the deafblind adult.*

Many of our young people who are deafblind lack sophisticated communication skills and may require objects of reference and concrete cues throughout their adult life. Daily, weekly, and monthly calendars, or, where appropriate, Personal Plan books, and utilizing objects of reference, will frequently help to eliminate many of the uncertainties the deafblind adult faces and thus enable him/her to anticipate what is going to happen. This approach is an essential part of a Reactive Environment. It will promote a feeling of control over his/her life.

Congenital Rubella Syndrome and Challenging Behaviours

When challenging behaviours do occur, it can be an indication of a health-related problem. Many deafblind adults currently being supported have a medical history of Congenital Rubella Syndrome (CRS). Studies have been done in an attempt to look at the 'Late Manifestations of Rubella.' Such problems are very difficult to diagnose, since few medical practitioners have much experience with CRS. Again, through observation, good documentation, discussion with families and/or advocates, and the involvement of an understanding medical practitioner we go through a process of elimination to attempt to arrive at a diagnosis. There are times, too, when the medical diagnosis is more problematic than the situation itself. In such cases it is essential that all involved work together to arrive at a compromise that is suitable to everyone. At the same time, it is important to keep in mind that the person who is deafblind and his/her advocate have the final say concerning any remediation. There are other times when there is no medical solution and the lifestyle of the deafblind person may have to be altered dramatically to meet the ongoing challenges of a community-based program.

Challenging Behaviours in the Community

A question that has often been posed 'Is how do you deal with challenging behaviours in the community.' There are no easy answers to this problem, but keeping the individual at home is not a solution. The person who is deafblind will not learn from such an approach. The authors have a practical approach whereby we examine all possible reasons for the behaviour to identify the best ways to eliminate any further occurrences. By sitting down with those involved, discussing the situation, and looking at all the possible approaches we can arrive at a practical solution that is supported and will be used by all. Until the problem has been solved, we try to offer back-up support to the Intervenors who are going out into the community with the individual in question.

Late Manifestations of Rubella

The authors and others work with and observe Rubella children growing into their adult lives. As these deafblind adults continue through the aging process, it is evident to all who support them that there are new and unexpected manifestations of the Rubella Syndrome occurring. Most of what has been learned has been taught to us by our young people who are deafblind.

A study was done by Nancy O'Donnell of the Helen Keller National Centre in 1991. In her survey she identified seven categories according to problems that were reported to her. They were as follows:

1. Auditory Disorders
2. Ocular Damage
3. Cardiac Problems
4. Endocrine System (Diabetes and Thyroid)
5. Degenerative Conditions
6. Esophageal/Gastrointestinal Symptoms
7. Miscellaneous.

O'Donnell's findings, combined with the observations of others and records of these young people, some of whom we were directly involved with, seems to indicate the following.

a) Some members of the Rubella population appear to escape further damage and also show areas of continued growth and development when they receive appropriate programming and support.
b) Some show signs of physical and physiological deterioration.
c) Some, identified as NOT having had Rubella also show signs of the same type of such deterioration.
d) In some cases this deterioration may be a result of premature aging.

In attempting to diagnose some of the medical problems that occur as these young people age, it is usually through behaviour, that one begins to suspect there may be something wrong. For example, in one or more cases these findings were noted.

a) Constant pounding of the head led to a discovery of glaucoma.

b) Several pairs of eyeglasses, broken for no apparent reason, led to testing for and diagnosis of a detached retina.

c) Onset of seizure activity led to a prescription for anticonvulsants,. This seemed to result in an inability to maintain the previously established level of mobility and alertness .When the individual was taken off all anticonvulsants, the previous established level returned. This result presented the parents/advocates and the doctor with the choice of seizure activity or alertness and mobility.

d) Constant thirst and ongoing inappropriate behaviours finally resulted in the individual going into a coma, and, as a result, diabetes was diagnosed.

e) Aggressiveness, unusual behaviours, and weight gain led to a diagnosis of thyroid problems.

Overall, degenerative conditions appear to be the most predominant. The situation is not the same for all individuals, but in the authors' experience, difficulties in walking and balance problems usually have been the first symptoms noted, and further degeneration has occurred subsequently. In only one case with which the authors are familiar has an individual developed Progressive Rubella *panencephalitis*, a slow neurological deterioration that is described as being extremely rare.

The authors continue to observe and document many problems in deafblind adults that appear to be medically related. Finding the answers to these problems is truly a challenge. This can be accomplished only through the support of understanding medical practitioners, families and/or advocates, and the Intervenors who are involved. It is essential to continue to observe, document, and consult in an attempt to arrive at viable conclusions.

Sexuality

In recent years, attitudes towards sexuality and individuals who are deafblind have changed. Human sexuality has become more accepted, as society recognizes that sexuality is part of being human, not something we do. To some adults who are deafblind, sexuality may be confined to dealing with self-care skills and to one-to-one relationships. To others, it may mean becoming aware of much more complex areas.

One approach to sexuality is suggested by Paul Andreoli of the Kalorama Centre for Deafblind Adults (1996).

Sexuality belongs to a person's private life and should, in most cases, not be a target of professional intervention, unless the person himself seeks help for sexual problems or information. Yet we have formulated some criteria for rules concerning sexual activity in our residential setting. The reason for this is that for some residents their level of 'sexual development' does not match their calendar age. Sexual education for these residents implies more than just information; on the one hand they need to have a safe space to discover this own sexuality, on the other hand they need to learn boundaries and values concerning this exploration. In sexual education it is important to avoid confrontation with undesirable situations, such as abuse, or confrontations with sexual activities of others which are not appropriate to the level of sexual development of the resident.

Concerning 'boundaries and values' we make use of the concept of 'most accepted values in our general culture.' This means that we try not to favor our own values concerning sexuality, be they liberal or conservative, but try to use those values which are most frequent in the general culture the client will experience outside the institute.

What Does This Imply for the Residents at Kalorama?

We have different group-homes for residents with different levels of development. In those group-homes with adults who have an age-appropriate level of development, residents are, in their private rooms, free in their sexual activities under the condition that these activities are not harmful to others.

In group-homes with adults who are still in a stage of 'sexual education,' sexual activities between residents are not allowed. How strict we maintain these rules depends on the estimated 'age-of-sexual-development' of the residents concerned. A deafblind person with an estimated age-of-sexual-development of about sixteen years will be allowed more room for experimentation than a person with an estimated age-of-sexual-development of eight years.

In groups with residents with different levels of sexual development we always ensure that the living environment offers protection for the resident with the lowest level of sexual development.

This well-articulated approach combines a recognition of the importance of community standards and the rights of the individual. It can serve as one model to be considered by those charged with the task of developing a policy for the education and support of the adult who is congenitally or early adventitiously deafblind in understanding his/her sexuality.

Regardless of the approach taken, a great deal of responsibility is placed on those who are involved with the development of deafblind adults, whether it be the Intervenors, the families, advocates, or any other person involved in their support. These people need to think about their own beliefs, values, attitudes, and what impact they might have on a program to be developed for a specific deafblind adult. It cannot be assumed that deafblind adults will learn about sexuality incidentally or during peer discussions. Therefore, we must ensure that a program is in place that will enrich their lives by giving them more understanding of themselves, their families, their peers, and society. Such a program and its presentation must not be a reflection of our own opinions and biases. If an appropriate program is not developed to enable deafblind people to learn about their sexuality, we can be assured that challenging behaviours will develop.

For the deafblind individual of any age, sexuality is something that must be taught. It will not develop through incidental learning, discussion with peers, and modelling the actions of others. We must be careful not to relegate individuals who are deafblind to a future of non-human denial of their sexuality through the imposition of standards that are totally different than those that the rest of society follows. (For further discussion see chapter 7.)

Intervention

The Need for Intervention

We shall confine our comments to that aspect of the process that is directly related to the deafblind adult. The principal purpose of the process of intervention is to provide the deafblind adult with sufficient non-distorted information to enable him/her to make appropriate decisions, with the motivation to act upon the decisions, and with the support necessary successfully to carry out the actions arising from the decisions within a reasonable amount of time.

Intervention will be provided by any person interacting with the deafblind adult. The question is not if intervention will be provided but rather will it be appropriate and useful. The goal of intervention for deafblind adults is to assist them to exercise their independence. This means allowing the deafblind adult to have as much control over all aspects of his/her life as a non-deafblind adult, functioning at the same level, has.

As deafblind individuals mature, more intervention will be needed to provide the information they need to have control over their lives and actively participate in the community. The more choices available, information received, and decisions made, the more the deafblind adult will avoid frustration.

Hiring an Intervenor

Although we do not always have the option of choosing who we want to work with, we do have an ability to decide with whom we will live and with whom we wish to engage in different activities. We rarely choose the same companion for every activity; therefore, this option should not be taken away from a deafblind adult. Routine activities, such as as work, can have the same Intervenor. Activities such as a special shopping trip, vacation, or going out on Saturday night, should provide an opportunity to choose the Intervenor.

The concept of control will eventually evolve into control over who will provide intervention for both special activities and routine daily living. After the deafblind individual has experienced choosing the person who will provide intervention from available staff, the next step will be to begin to involve him/her in the hiring process.

The Hiring Process

Step One: Introducing Strangers into One's World

The hiring process can be a complicated concept for a deafblind adult to grasp. It has been found that every deafblind adult has the ability to participate to some degree in making a decision in the hiring process, particularly if the process of information, observation, hands-on experience, and interview, as outlined in chapter 15, is followed. In the beginning , the deafblind adult will be unaware of the implications of interviewing, hiring, and firing and may even resist contact with these strangers who are introduced into his/her world. When deafblind adults are comfortable with these invasions, they have reached the stage where they may begin to participate in the interviewing process.

Step Two: Attending the Interviews

The deafblind adult should have his/her advocate attend the interviews with him/her to provide security. The deafblind adult may stay for only one or two interviews in the beginning and be visited by other interviewees while participating in activities at another location. The advocate, at this stage, should participate in the interview and be asked to form questions for the interview that target his/her areas of concern. This also eases the mind of the advocate when he/she is a parent, who is essentially leaving a 'child' in the hands of this person.

Step Three: Forming the First Questions

If the deafblind adult has reached a level of understanding that will permit him/her to participate in this way, then he/she either instead of, or in addition to, the advocate should provide one or two questions. The Intervenor will have spent considerable time discussing why they are meeting these strangers and will have shared his/her questions during the previous stage. The Intervenor should place stress on why he/she is asking the question.

When the deafblind adult reaches the stage where he/she can prepare a question or two that is felt to be important, he/she should be assisted to do so. Often such questions will concern likes or dislikes of the individual being interviewed.

Step Four: Beginning Participation in Discussion during Interviews
The next step would be participation in a discussion of the interview process that will be followed by the advocate and administrators. This stage gradually involves the deafblind adult in activities such as providing a variety of questions and actually asking the questions he/she provided, with an emphasis placed upon communicating all that is being said during each interview and ending the interview with a question to the deafblind adult enquiring if he/she has any further questions.

Step Five: Complete Participation
The highest level of involvement includes participation in posting the vacancy, going over each résumé, and along with others who will participate in the interview shortlisting the applicants. The deafblind adult would be consulted and involved in some or all of the other activities required before the interviews take place. These might include setting up tables and chairs, establishing interview times, and then gathering information for target questions. Such questions are easily formed when what the deafblind adult says he/she wants from a person working hands on with him/her is listened to. They can include topics such as employment background, hobbies, and availability. It is important that the interests of the deafblind adult are reflected in the questions asked at the interview. During the discussion of which questions to include and who will ask them, discussion and recording (and if necessary explaining) of expected answers should also take place. Next, there should be discussion of who will ask each question.

The day of the interviews can be a stressful time for deafblind adults experiencing the process of interviewing for the first time. Reassurances for the individual and breaks should be included in order to ensure success.

Following the interviews and when the finalists for the position have been identified and their references checked, a meeting(s) should be held with the interview team, including the deafblind adult, to discuss the final candidates. This process can require considerable discussion and numerous meetings may be necessary before the deafblind adult is able to make an informed decision, and it should be his/her decision to make. If required, once a decision is made, management can inform the successful applicant on behalf of the deafblind adult.

The involvement of the deafblind adult at the highest functional level he/she is capable of handling successfully is very important to ensure the best possible match. Having all the pertinent information to make a successful decision plays an important role in the hiring process. Once stage five is reached, no meeting should be held or decisions made without the informed involvement of the deaf-blind adult.

Experience has shown that many years may pass before level five is reached, but it can be reached by a surprising number of deafblind adults if they are supported through the process and if their input is taken seriously. In fact, one or two deafblind adults have reached a level that might be identified as stage six. They planned the interviews, wrote all the questions except those that were the responsibility of administration, chaired the interviews, and, after accepting recommendations from the interview team, made the final decision.

Training the Intervenor

Once an Intervenor is hired, an ongoing training process is initiated. Training of the Intervenor is a responsibility shared among the administration, team members who are supporting the specific deafblind adult, and the deafblind adult.

'Hands on' is an expression often used to describe working with a deafblind individual. This should not be confused with constant physical manipulation. 'Hands on' is the best form of training. 'Hands on' means working with and listening to the deafblind adult as well as to those Intervenors who have experience in working with him/her. Initially asking the deafblind adult using a form of communication compatible with his/her level of functioning and the observation of the adult interacting with a competent Intervenor is one of the best ways of beginning training.

Reading the individual's Personal Plan is essential for the newly hired Intervenor. The properly written Personal Plan will provide an insight into all aspects of the individual's program, particularly the objectives that the Intervenor will be working on during daily and special activities.

Communication skills are essential. Communication classes, in adaptive sign language, should be available to the new Intervenor. Simulations are another effective training tool. The authors have found they provide the best way to have new Intervenors gain some understanding of the world of deafblind. Simulations should include activities that occur in the everyday life of the deafblind adult, such as shopping, cooking, and recreation activities.

Simulations, lectures, and workshops are valuable for all Intervenors. Such activities permit them to upgrade their skills. Regularly scheduled communication classes and examinations as to competence should be routinely held for all staff. As the needs of each deafblind adult change, the required competences will have to be upgraded or acquired by each Intervenor. The deafblind adult's needs, not the skills of the Intervenor, will define the areas in which training will be required. The deafblind adult should be seen both as the person who can best indicate these areas and also as a source of expertise in gaining such training.

Conclusion

When appropriate information and control is available, the deafblind adult will be motivated to participate in 'life.' There is no place for learned helplessness in the world of the deafblind adult!

When an Intervenor has been hired, the deafblind person has the right to expect that he/she will be provided them with all the information and support necessary to participate meaningfully in the community. Receiving the information in no way obligates the deafblind adult to act upon the information, and no Intervenor should feel slighted if such information appears to be ignored. Advice should be given only when asked for by the deafblind adult. Information and advice are two different things. Again, even when advice is asked for and received by the deafblind adult, he/she still is not obligated to follow it.

We all learn from our mistakes, and the same is true of a deafblind adult provided he/she is allowed to make the mistake and then receives appropriate feedback, so that the consequences of the mistake can be understood. It is not the Intervenor's job or right to attach blame. Although it is our nature to protect the deafblind adults with whom we work, in doing so we prevent them from making informed decisions and experiencing the consequences of their actions. The role of the Intervenor is to support not direct, assist not do for, and to provide all information not decide which information is appropriate.

When looking at intervention, keep in mind the following points.

1. Successful Intervenors are more than professionals. They become friends, providing support and following direction.
2. As deafblind adults mature and grow, more intervention is needed to provide the information necessary for them to have control over the decisions needed in their lives.
3. Deafblind adults deserve to receive the amount of intervention when and how they decide they require it. Each adult's needs and aspirations are unique.
4. Intervention is the process of interaction between one person who is deafblind and one Intervenor. Intervention does not necessarily take place when one adult takes a number of deafblind persons on a group outing or simply because one adult and one or more persons with deafblindness are in the same room.

5. The ultimate goal when teaching any skill, routine, or process is for the deaf-blind individual to recognize when he/she needs assistance because of the disability and to ask appropriately for it.

Summary

1. Congenitally and early adventitiously deafblind persons enter adult programs from a variety of sources: residential schools, local schools with adequate support, local schools with inadequate support, and institutional or other care facilities.
2. Transition requires a change of residence, lifestyle, Intervenors, friends, routines, community services, and medical support.
3. A Personal Plan is required for the adult who is congenitally and early adventitiously deafblind.
4. The process of developing a Personal Plan involves assembling background information, identifying the key areas, and writing goals and objectives.
5. The Personal Plan is the property of the adult who is deafblind, not the support staff.
6. Each activity provides opportunities to work on a variety of objectives.
7. Activities will focus on life skills, recreation, and vocation
8. Activities should be at the level of, and be appropriate to, an adult lifestyle.
9. The deafblind adult should be supported, encouraged, and required to take part in the hiring and training of his/her Intervenor.

REFERENCES

Andreoli, Paul (1996) 'Deafblindness, Self-Determination and Mental Competence.' *Deafblind Education* (July–December) 18
Johansen, Knut (1997) 'A different Aspect of the Term "Employment."' *Deafblind Education* (July–December) 7
McInnes, J.M., et al. (1996) *The Developmental Profile for Use with Persons Who Are Deafblind (1996 Edition).* Brantford, ON: Canadian Deafblind and Rubella Association (Ontario Chapter)
O'Donnell, Nancy (1991) 'Late Manifestations of Rubella.' Paper produced by the Helen Keller National Center

13

Creating and Maintaining a Support System: An Analysis Based on Experiences at Sense

RODNEY CLARK and MALCOLM MATTHEWS

Introduction

It would seem to be a universal truth that when two or more people sharing specific and intensive needs meet, it is almost inevitable that a new organization will be born. Such was the case in 1954 when Peggy Freeman and Margaret Brock, both parents of children who were deafblind through Rubella, were introduced to each other and to other families by Wendy Galbraith at the Nuffield Centre, the Children's Hearing Clinic at the Royal National Throat, Nose and Ear Hospital in London. The combination of the drive, knowledge, and creativity of parents and the expertise and sustaining power of committed professionals is the key to the successful establishment and healthy growth of our family organization. It is hoped that this will be evident throughout this chapter, in which the essential steps needed to create a support system for congenitally deafblind children and adults from the family perspective will be considered.

First, a few provisos. As a family-based organization, Sense must be aware that all its actions must be practical and directly related to improving services, and hence the quality of life, for our beneficiaries and their families. The writers of this chapter have therefore attempted to convey their thoughts in a simple and universal fashion, accessible to readers anywhere, although it must be stated from the outset that Sense's work is very much grounded within the U.K. experience, of which the cultures, history and philosophies, policies and practices of service provision will be markedly different from those of other countries. Even where two countries have common or similar cultures and service practices, there is, of course, no single right way of providing support, so the following paragraphs should be read as indications of what we have found significant and valuable, rather than as a blueprint or model for organizational development elsewhere.

Finally, the brief for this chapter was 'Essential steps in creating a support system for individuals who are deafblind from a parent and family point of view,' with an implication that these steps are the critical elements in the establishment of a parent-based organization such as Sense. While this is largely true, at times the support needs of the individual families who come within the orbit of the organization will be in alignment with, differ from, or, as can happen on occasion, be in direct conflict with the organization's needs. It must be accepted that no organization will be able to encompass all of the support needs of all the families within its orbit, even though it is a commendable objective to try to do so. Inevitably, all that follows is written from the perspective of the writers' experience through the organization. But families will know that their support needs in different situations can be met in many varied ways from the whole range of human experience.

Contents

This chapter will begin with a description of the nature of service provision for people with disabilities in the United Kingdom, followed by a brief history of Sense, the National Deafblind Association, from those small beginnings to its 40th Anniversary in 1995, during which time it has grown to be a major service-providing agency with a multi-million pound turnover. Following this outline, consideration will be given to these points:

- the needs of young people and their families as they have been made manifest over the years and how these needs were addressed
- the pluses and minuses of being both an advocacy organization and a service provider
- attitudes towards Sense's young people and services, both of families and within society, and how they have changed over the years
- the essential elements necessary for the achievement of one's goals
- finally, conclusions and statements arising from the preceding text; Malcolm Matthews has contributed this final section of the chapter, not only with conclusions, but with some additional thoughts on the topic.

Since the chapter was conceived, it has become clear that some thoughts on fund raising for a support group and on staff development might be of value. Two sections have therefore been added before 'Last Words.' The writers are indebted to Jim Swindells for his contribution to the first and to Eileen Boothroyd, Lindy Wyman, and Virginia von Malachowski for their contribution to the second.

The U.K. Environment

In considering services for people with disability in the United Kingdom, we tend to consider four main areas: health, education, welfare, and housing. Employment services should also be included. Being a much smaller government activity, however, these services tend to be included within one of the above categories, education being the currently fashionable home, since the emphasis is on vocational training. The U.K. system of service provision, if a haphazard patchwork of historical arrangements can be called thus, is unique in the world, largely because of the size of its voluntary sector. This is the third of the three main sectors, the other two being, of course, the state and private sectors, which now exist in nearly every country, albeit in different states of development. The voluntary sector is distinguished from the private sector inasmuch as it is 'not for profit.' Its huge contribution to disability services, now reckoned in many billions of pounds per annum, dates from its early recognition in law. Charities, which make up much but not all of the voluntary sector, were first granted legal status at the start of the seventeenth century and ever since have been identified as key elements in that part of U.K. society concerned with welfare, education, religion, and the relief of poverty. While the state is undoubtedly the largest provider in all four areas above, the private and voluntary sectors are substantial, and their loss would undoubtedly be critical in terms of the country's ability to respond to the needs of its citizenry.

Historically, many services were pioneered by what we now call the voluntary sector, that is, by charities or similar institutions, such as the Church, and subsequently were taken over by the state when their importance was recognized by Government and when they saw that it would be beyond the financial power of the sector to provide generally. It is interesting that we are living at a time of immense change in this respect when services, still substantially financed by government, are considered to be more effectively provided by the other two sectors. This is demonstrated by the emergence of purchasers (or commissioners) and providers, and a welter of legislation, regulation, and procedures to keep them separate.

Health for people with disabilities was, and overwhelmingly remains, the responsibility of the National Health Service (NHS), which is organized into local purchasers (Health Authorities) and providers (Health Trusts). Income benefits are mostly a direct government service through a 'Quango,' a quasi-non-governmental organization. These 'quangos' represent government's attempts to privatize as many of its tasks as are not directly related to governing itself. This privatization is not a complete separation, but the creation of agencies, with their own boards, but wholly financed by government. Social work

HEALTH provided by National Health Service through local Health Authorities and Health Trusts *clinical* *medical* *long-stay hospitals* *nursing homes*	**EDUCATION** Local Education Authority *schools and preschool* or Central funds *further education*
	EMPLOYMENT
WELFARE National agency for benefits Local Authority Social Services Department *income support (benefits)* *social services* *community care* *residential homes*	**HOUSING** Local Authority Housing Department National and local Housing Associations

Figure 13.1   Organization of Services in the United Kingdom

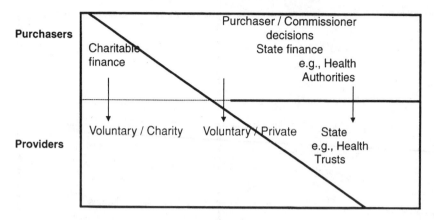

Figure 13.2   The Purchaser/Provider Split and the Voluntary Sector

and community care are financed and in large measure provided or funded by local government through social services departments, and the same is true for education through Local Education Authorities (LEAs). An increasing number of schools have an independent or semi-independent status, however, and further education is now financed directly by central government through a quango, the Further Education Funding Council. Housing is also provided by Local Authorities, although a substantial subsector is represented by Housing Associations, which are overseen by another quango, the Housing Corporation, but are generally held to be within the voluntary sector because of the freedom of action they enjoy. In the field of congenital deafblindness, residential services are largely the responsibility of the NHS, since Sense's beneficiaries were classed as mentally retarded and placed in the large hospitals that existed from Victorian times until recently in all parts of the country.

Within this strategic picture, charities play a very substantial role at local, regional, and national levels in the provision of services. Many provide money for the relief of poverty or for specific purposes such as obtaining special equipment. Others run their own schools and other educational services, while others act as agents for their social services departments, who have recognized the specific skills that they have in their fields. Deafness is an immediately obvious and relevant example, although one of the most sizeable is child protection services from organizations such as Barnardo's, the National Association for the Prevention of Cruelty to Children, the Children's Society, the National Children's Homes, and many others. Residential and housing services also are substantially provided for by charities who have specific expertise in the various disability fields or in other areas involving people with special needs, for instance, mental illness and the elderly. Sense similarly contracts with the NHS and Local Authorities to provide such services for deafblind children and adults, which are taken up because the purchasers recognize where the expertise lies and that charities are well able to respond quickly and flexibly to changes in need. Not all voluntary organizations are charities, but most try to achieve this status because of the tax advantages and fund-raising opportunities that it brings. The contribution of charitable funding, that is, donations from individuals or corporate bodies, remains significant – at present approximately £1 billion per year. It has long been a tradition for charitable monies to be used to pioneer new services or to provide services that either are not considered to be the responsibility of the state or are unlikely to be provided by the state. This is still the case, and, with the growth in contracts, the voluntary sector has become very careful to ensure that this 'privatization' of services does not inevitably lead to the transfer of responsibility from the state to itself.

Organization

The year is 1955, and Sense counts it as its starting date, since this is when the first twelve families met and when the first newsletters emerged from Peggy Freeman's rather battered typewriter. All the children were deafblind as a result of Rubella, and so the name 'Rubella Group' emerged. Useful information was shared during these early days, for instance, on the causes and ramifications of Congenital Rubella Syndrome (CRS), on practical matters such as toileting, feeding, suitable toys, and communication aids and on a wide range of issues relating to growth and development, sibling needs, available services, and so on. The parents and their professional contacts soon became aware of the need to advertise their children's existence and to campaign for the provision of appropriate services, principally educational at this time. Many of the families sought opportunities to speak at meetings and conferences, and the Association held its own first conference in 1962 at Condover Hall School. Books and leaflets were written; films were made; as a result of campaigning, deafblind school units were established and were financed through fund raising; and a substantial contribution was made to the research that led to the implementation of the government's Rubella immunization program in 1970.

The families of children whose deafblindness was from causes other than Rubella joined, and in 1961 Sense was first registered as a charity as the Rubella Group for Deaf/Blind Children. During the 1960s severely disabled children were still being classified as ineducable. They were denied schooling but were given 'Training' in centres run by untrained personnel within the

Local Authorities' mental health services. In addition to campaigning for specific deafblind school units to be opened, Sense, along with other parents' organizations, sought to change the law to require the provision of education to all children, no matter how disabled, and this goal was achieved in the Education Act of 1970. Long before, members had turned their attention to the two matters that were most exercising them. They were as follows.

1. There were no services at all for their children when they reached school-leaving age, when the option was to live at home (the family home, not their own) or to enter the grim wards of the large mental retardation hospitals.
2. What would happen to their children when they became old and after their death?

In the late 1970s, after years of seemingly fruitless campaigning, the members of what had become the National Association for Deafblind and Rubella Handicapped decided that the only course was to become a service provider, and so the die was cast and a residential service for twelve deafblind school-leavers was established in Lincolnshire in the east of England, the first of many in what was to become the largest of the services Sense was to offer.

At that time, the Association was the lucky recipient of funds from a children's TV program, and another long-sought dream became a reality: the opening of a Family Centre in West London. In the early 1980s, following a first review and strategic planning exercise, the work of this centre was refined into a service for families with young deafblind children. This plan determined that formal schooling should remain the responsibility of government, while Sense, as it then came to be known, would concentrate on the two areas where little or nothing was happening: preschool and post-school services, together with other family support services that could be identified and financed. Enormous expansion of the professional side of the organization took place during the 1980s and continues today. Further residential and day services were opened around the United Kingdom, in Birmingham, Glasgow, Exeter, London, Berkshire, Northern Ireland, and so forth, and today there are over 300 adult service users in Group Homes or attending Day Centres. The Family and Education Advisory Service has been extended through a growing network of Family Centres, and a Regional Advisory Service, offering welfare advice and support, has been established. Sense has continued to seek the creation of strategic deafblind school services by LEAs, which culminated in 1989 in the recognition, by the Department for Education and Employment (DfEE), of deafblindness as a distinct educational category and the awarding of grants totalling more than £6 million to LEAs to establish specific services. A wide range of holiday schemes is available to the families of deafblind children and adults of all ages, and Sense continues to develop advocacy programs for both beneficiaries and their families. Since the early 1980s Sense has been offering specific support programs for children and adults with Usher Syndrome, now the largest known cause of deafblindness other than aging, and more recently consideration has been given to services for adults with acquired deafblindness, including the elderly, for whom services are either non-existent or patchy in the extreme.

Need

No apology is made for quoting extensively from Peggy Freeman's marvellous history, *Good Sense*, which was published in March 1996 at a Buckingham Palace reception to mark the end of a year of celebrations for our 40th Anniversary: 'The more the child is disabled, the more he needs his parents. On the other hand, the more the parents have difficulty, the more help they need (Dr Salvatore Lagati) [Director, Lega del Filo d'Oro]. There were several reasons for the strong bond which held together the early members of the Rubella Group. Firstly, the common cause for the handicap, maternal rubella. Secondly, the dual handicap of deafblindness was very rare so that most of the professional people with whom we came into contact had little to offer us in terms of daily care and management, so we turned to each other' (107).

For a most perceptive description of the needs of families at the time of diagnosis, Margaret Brock's book, *Christopher: A Silent Life* (1976) is recommended. It is a telling account of the overwhelming effect of the birth of a disabled child on a family. Through her chronological depiction of the events following the birth of Christopher, Margaret shows how their lives were turned upside down and the awful accompanying shattering of confidence. Confidence, as ever, is the key to how well newly disabled families deal with life. Margaret demonstrates how, in the early days before the return of personal strength and equilibrium, the worst assaults on her confidence came from people who pitied or who over-sympathized. The best support came from those who treated her son no differently from any able-bodied child and who commented on all those things that make us feel pride in our offspring: their beauty, their cleverness. Throughout its forty-year life, Sense has found in almost every contact with disabled people and their families that their need is for practical information, practical advice, practical help, and then, above all, services.

Most of those families in the early days thought that they were the only ones in the world to have a child so affected, and the relief, indeed delight, of coming into contact with others so placed is greatly in evidence from their contributions to the early editions of the newsletter that Peggy Freeman produced on an occasional basis. Here, we will not try to duplicate what the parent contributors have written in chapter 8, but it will not be entirely possible to consider the creation of support systems without reference to the stated and perceived needs of the users and their families. Not only were those first parents trying to come to terms with their roles of rearers and educators in the face of extreme disability, but the multiplicity of their children's impairments brought them into confusing touch with a plethora of professionals. Their approach was usually not to treat the children as a whole person but to concentrate on their particular specialism, as a result of which much information and advice, often conflicting, had to be absorbed and sorted. The emergence of Sense as a self-help group meant that families then had a trusted source of information, a sympathetic shoulder to cry on, and new social opportunities, very important in those days when the birth of a severely disabled child often led to social ostracism. In most cases, families know exactly what it is that they need and whether or not an association like Sense can meet it. Involvement with the organization will grow or lessen according to the degree that changing needs are recognized and provided for.

It is not unrealistic to state that there are as many needs as there are families; these needs have to be met in a variety of ways, only some of which an organization might be able to respond to. It is a rare family that is not greatly affected by the birth of a disabled child, and in most cases family dynamics will be markedly changed. The relationship between husband and wife will often take a battering. It is commonly remarked that the birth of a disabled child will make or break a marriage. There are families who have joined Sense whom it has been unable to help because the unstated, usually unrecognized, need has been for help with their anger, guilt, or inability to come to terms with what has happened to them. Often in such cases, what is on offer is not viewed as helpful, and so the organization is viewed as letting them down, just like everyone else. Undoubtedly, many will in time find a positive way forward, while others will be permanently damaged by the experience.

Because deafblindness was, is, and ideally always will be, a low-incidence disability, family members were always few in number and widely scattered. As a result, it was rarely possible for the growing Association to organize on a local basis. From its early days, therefore, families were encouraged to join the local branches of other disability groups, which might help with financial support or in providing or campaigning for local services or which could otherwise provide a more intensive support service. Sense has always been indebted to the network of groups within the National Deaf Children's Society (NDCS), the Royal Society for Mentally Handicapped Children and Adults (MENCAP), and Scope, formerly the Spastics Society, which have added substantially to what

Sense, as a tiny organization during its first twenty-five years, was in a very limited position to offer.

As Peggy Freeman writes in *Good Sense*, 'the parent to parent contact was vital to the development of the Association; moreover, it was the freely shared information that kindled the interest of the professionals and ultimately their involvement. The contact between parents was to ebb and flow over the years but the need for it remains. The fact that professional expertise is available does not mean that there is no place for the comfort and understanding one parent can give another. Inevitably there are feelings and domestic problems which it is not always possible to discuss with anyone but a parent in similar circumstances' (1996, 108). Some families came and went during those years, since Sense did not have the means to support them in a practical way, although happily many have become known again as Sense was able to extend its ability to offer services. Margaret Brock expressed this so well in *Christopher: A Silent Life*. She writes:

In May [1955] we had a first meeting of rubella parents at our house. We were by then in touch with twenty families, and Mrs Freeman was duplicating a three-monthly newsletter of the children's progress, which kept us in contact with each other ... Later in the year Mr and Mrs Hutchinson held a northern meeting at their house in Huddersfield, with twelve parents from the area and three experts. These two small meetings really convinced us of the need for greater efforts, and also that the strength of our group must be in parent-to-parent communication – for in the early days of devastation, only someone who has themselves been through a similar experience can be of help. The time for expert help really comes a little later, and the greatest comfort to parents can easily be the confidence which, when asked about some bizarre aspect of your child's behaviour, you can say, 'Oh, all rubella children do that' – and realise that you have joined one of the world's most exclusive clubs, that of rubella children's parents. It is impossible to convey the sense of relief that one feels when coming into a room full of such parents, knowing that there is no necessity for the endless explanations usually needed before any rapport is established, no need to contradict all the categorical mis-statements or to correct the misapprehensions that so wear one down over the years. So the few of us who were becoming conscious of the upholding effect of such an association felt we must search out and share our feelings with the many more we knew existed. (1976, 64–5)

Since 1982 Sense has undertaken strategic planning on a regular and increasingly sophisticated basis. This is an extremely valuable exercise. About a year is spent in meetings and in correspondence, considering what we are doing and why, what still needs to be done, and how we should go about it. Present and future environmental factors that should affect our decision making are considered, among the most important being the current fashions in service provision and how they need to be accommodated if successful contracts are to be concluded with the purchasers of services. Most important, an extensive consultation exercise is undertaken with all stakeholders, deafblind people, families, staff, volunteers, government, purchasers, and so forth to identify need and how that need can be turned into demand. Each time that this consultation process has been carried out, the overwhelming response from families is for services, services, and more services. Inevitably, members who have children of school age feel that more should be done for this group, and this point has been given some attention. For instance, the concept of Intervention has been adopted from Canada, and it has been promoted in both the classroom and the home.

It has become very clear that, unlike the situation when the Association was established, families with a severely disabled child wish to have a seamless array of services for their child and for the family that will enable them to continue to have the sort of life they always wanted. Years ago, families who did not abandon their disabled children, often against the advice of the medical profession, were forced into a sort of disability subculture. They became social pariahs within their communities and were forced to devote all their spare time and energy to fighting for services that were simply not available. There are still many deafblind children and adults who are not getting appropriate services, but there have been many improvements on what was available forty years ago. It is very hard for those tired and ageing pioneers, who had to fight so hard for a school place for their sons and daughters, to witness the much greater variety of services now available to younger families who can appear to be passive non-contributors while they themselves are still fighting for a good residential place for their adult offspring.

It is also true and right, however, that expectations have increased, and the need and demand for support, services, and opportunities remains. Perhaps the gap between expectations and provision for many people is still as great.

Support

Unlike some countries, for example, those of Scandinavia where there is a culture of state provision of services for disabled people, the United Kingdom has always had a unique mix of statutory, private, and voluntary services for people with disabilities. Often, services are pioneered within the voluntary, or charitable, sector and then taken within basic state provision. There has always remained a substantial voluntary element within U.K. provision, however, and this is currently growing with the universal move towards privatization. Thus, the debates of years ago about whether, having pioneered services, Sense should let them go over to the state, which had the resources to ensure their healthy expansion and development, have now changed, since support organisations like Sense are regarded mainly as essential partners in the panoply of provision.

While there are many justifiable systems for the provision of support and services, there are some universal aspects of society that are true as much for disabled people and their families as for the able-bodied population. Each individual is a part of a family, which is part of a community, which is part of a nation, which is part of the world. Thus:

- *each deafblind person* is part of a family with immediate and more distant members, which is part of
- *a community support system*, consisting of friends, a local branch, local services, other support and social groups, and so on, which is within
- *a nation*, with a national government ultimately responsible for the care and welfare of the person and with national organizations like Sense with a critical role at that level, which is within
- *the world of disability*, specifically our international networks, such as Deafblind International or the European Deafblind Network, from which so much is learnt. The importance of this connection with organizations, services, and families overseas is often neglected in the tumult of the moment. But it has resulted in profound impacts in both directions, made possible by all the linkages expressed above, but particularly by the existence of a strong national organization, able both to give and to receive to the fullest.

For many years, the only training available to teachers of deafblind children was in the United States, at Perkins School for the Blind and Boston College, both in Massachusetts. They formed a vital professional link for the United Kingdom during the slow emergence of the profession nationally. Similarly, the recent acquisition of the concept of Intervention from Canada has caused a revolution in the provision of services at many levels. On the other hand, as the largest, and perhaps the first, deafblind parents' organization, Sense has been able to support the growth of parents' organizations in other countries, notably Canada and Australia.

In looking at the above continuum of support and services, we must effectively establish that there is no real dichotomy between disability and the rest of life. 'No man is an Island,' wrote John Donne in the seventeenth century. Nobody is truly independent – we all are absolutely dependent on others in all aspects of our lives. Even those who are within the norm of independence will have abnormal bouts of dependence at certain times, such is fate. We depend on farmers to feed us, tailors to dress us, miners to warm us, teachers to educate us, performers to entertain us, bosses to employ us, partners to love us. In this light, the support required by a disabled person and his/her family is but a slight, specific extension to that array of support we all demand.

The experience of the writers in meeting with families over almost twenty years in many different circumstances has been both positive and negative, and it has led to the identification of some truths.

- First, support and a support system must be seen as necessary by the family.
- Secondly, family members are the only people who can make any support work for them.
- Thirdly, the support that an organization and, indeed, that society in the way of services can provide may be vital, but it cannot meet all support needs, particularly in the realm of the spiritual strength that families with a multiply disabled child must have. An organization, its members, and its staff can, however, point out to willing listeners areas of need and how they might be addressed.

With reference to the continuum mentioned above, the first support needed by a disabled child and his/her family is that they themselves are operating well. Years ago, it was possible for the parents of even our most able children to be advised to leave their child behind in the hospital, since 'he would never be more than a vegetable.' Today, we are witnessing the birth and survival of many profoundly disabled children. Whatever the advice currently being given to their families, one has to believe that it is more sensitive than that often given in past decades. One has nothing but admiration, however, for those parents who, recognizing that the newly born disabled child may have a totally destructive effect on their family life, elect to give him/her up for adoption or care.

At the point of diagnosis, an organization like Sense can help individual family members in coming to terms with the situation. Some fathers have great difficulty in this respect, although in recent years it has been found that they adjust more readily to the news and are more ready to be involved in the care of the child. What often is neglected, understandably, is the effect on the siblings. One parent reported how she had not realized how much attention was being spent on her rubella daughter and, as a result, how neglected her two able-bodied sons had become. This situation was brought to her notice when she learnt that one of her sons had been caught stealing money, so that he could spend it on a school-friend; in her words, he was buying affection. A meeting of siblings was held at a Sense 'Weekend Away,' and it became apparent just how important, but neglected, an area this is. Regrettably, Sense has not yet found a strategic approach, but it is hoped that all staff and members, when advising families, are well aware of the importance of attention to brothers and sisters.

Again, the low incidence of deafblindness and the lack of recognition of it by service providers has meant that families usually require intensive help to convince their communities of their child's specific needs. Where there is a branch with some active members, be they parents or professionals, it is occasionally possible for this intensive advocacy to be provided by the organization, but usually it is the family itself that has to fight for access to the right services, advised by Sense's staff or members. The organization's forces are severely limited in this respect and often have to be prioritized for particular test cases, success in which will have a knock-on effect for others, or for cases of outstanding difficulty. As Sense grows in organizational strength, it is an avowed intention to have enough outreach staff to be able to support all families in their campaigning for services or benefits. Much is now being done, but there is still a long way to go. Peggy Freeman in *Good Sense* wrote about the early days: 'The Progress Reports revealed how great was the courage of the parents who struggled on; the cries for help are there in great number, but, sadly, we have no evidence of whether or how these cries were answered' (1996, 114). Of course, Sense's ability to respond is now much greater than it was then. It is a fervent hope that the day will come when Sense can respond effectively locally to every family's request for help.

Attitudes

It is of great interest to see how profoundly attitudes towards families with disabled children have changed since Sense was formed. Without question, many families in the 1950s experienced very negative reactions within society. Having a disabled child was held to be shameful, and such families often became outcasts within their communities. Margaret Brock has written about how people would turn away, so difficult was it for them to deal with the presence of a disabled child. It is interesting that Margaret has also written, 'But whatever our difficulties and frustrations, it is certainly true that we parents of disabled children are wonderfully privileged in that we meet only the best of people around us. All that is kind and helpful shows itself to us and it becomes easier to see a purpose in disabilities and to have faith in the future.' It was certainly a commonly held belief that a disabled person's life was of little value and not worth supporting economically. Many children were regarded as ineducable and were denied education, ending up in large institutions where they were kept warm, dry, fed, and clean. It is hard to imagine nowadays, when many minority interests are valued by powerful, well-placed people within our western society. It has been interesting to see how, in meetings with government ministers and officials, it is the parents in the party, once pariahs, who command the attention. Similarly, disabled people themselves are given centre stage in many public settings, whereas once they would have been put out of sight. It has been entirely pleasing to see how greatly valued Sense's children have become in the eyes of many members of the general public and how many people are willing to stand up to support the rights of this particular minority.

Growth of the Organization

Peggy Freeman writes in *Good Sense*:

In the early days, parent to parent contact was by meeting in small groups in each others' homes. Now 'At Homes' were introduced. These were generally hosted by parents who lived within an area and professionals were invited and attended. The Annual General Meeting which was obligatory from 1961 [when the organization was first registered as a charity] also provided a yearly opportunity for parents to get together from all areas. From the 'At Homes' grew Regions with small committees organising their own activities and this in turn concentrated parents' efforts on getting local provision and brought the special needs of their children to a wider audience of professionals. Day courses for parents were also introduced on a regional basis, or in places where a group of deafblind children were living. These courses were very popular and included talks by parents and professionals, with time for questions and, very importantly, time for parents to meet and chat with each other, feeling they had already met through the Progress Reports [which families regularly submitted to the newsletter]. These courses were to develop into weekend conferences and ultimately to the present Weekend Away.' (1996, 117)

The Weekend Away began in 1984 as an annual (now biennial) coming together of families, professionals, Sense staff, and volunteers. The intention behind it is to create a welcoming and relaxing atmosphere in which everyone can interact, learn from each other, socialize and generally contribute in whatever way to that part of our movement to which they relate. Creches, leisure clubs, baby-sitting and minding services are organized for disabled attendees and for the able-bodied children who attend. Many families are daunted by the prospect before their first attendance, but most usually fall into the swing of the event without difficulty and report how much they have gained from it in new learning and in new friendships.

Because our members are relatively few in number, we are not able to operate effectively on a local basis. In the early days, the first members operated as a national network, and then, as Peggy Freeman has stated, they established a small structure of regions, which provided a point of contact for the scattered membership: 'The setting up of formal Regions did indeed breathe new life into the Association. Each Region produced its own set of Progress Reports together with a report on the activities they had held' (1996, 119).

During the early 1980s, when the focus of the organization moved to the professional services that had been developed, the Regions were no longer an effective means of networking members. Many were satisfied with their involvement through services, and over the years different ways have been found of formalizing this involvement, mostly through consultation exercises in conjunction with our strategic and operational planning. In place of the Regions, with their vast geographical areas, branches were established as a formal but flexible means of allowing members to organize locally. Branches are voluntary groups that can cover any geographical or issue area and have formal constitutions and a contractual agreement with the U.K. organization. By issue area, we mean that a branch can be composed of those members who are connected by, for instance, a particular cause of deafblindness, rather than that they all live within the same locality. Thus, Usher UK, a group of people with Usher Syndrome and their families, is a U.K.-wide branch of Sense. Sense currently has some twenty branches throughout the country, established by families or a service professional who could see some value in providing a contact point and different activities for members on a geographical basis. These branches involve family members, volunteers, and professionals and are active to a greater or lesser degree, depending on the time, energy, and enthusiasm of those involved. They usually play a befriending, social, or fund-raising role, although influencing the local authority, and in recent years influencing Sense, to provide particular services has been the raison d'être of some branches.

Sense has always had one or more staff members devoting some time to supporting branches, enabling their development and assisting their networking. Branches are their own masters, however, and they will flourish or wither for many reasons – mostly the degree to which they continue to meet the needs of their members. It is clear that while a child's handicap is the reason for a member to join a branch and to gain positive help from it initially, it is rarely a reason for sustained interest. Continued involvement in branches comes about when there are other advantages, and these are usually social. Friendships are created between the members, which impels and encourages them to continue. Our Eastern Region continues to meet, some thirty years after its creation, with on the whole the same members as were present at the start. In contrast, the Scottish branch has disbanded, because it appears that the 'glue' provided by the members' relationships with our Scottish office provides them with all they need in this respect. This system of branches continues today, although we are currently looking at other ways we can provide families with the means of involvement, and hence support, that respond to their needs and the realities of their situations. A further development now taking place is the creation of a Family Network, which aims to enable every family, however isolated geographically, to have a sense of belonging to their organization,

Life goes in cycles, and certainly nothing stands still. It became clear to our overworked volunteers in the mid-1970s that an injection of new effort was needed, and so a full-time office with a general secretary was opened in Coventry in 1976. This was a very challenging time for the members, because it meant that responsibilities were being undertaken that could not be ignored or easily evaded. A course was set, which must lead to either success or failure. In retrospect, this was but a step towards what was seen as a realistic possibility – that the organization could professionalize and itself offer those services that simply were not emerging as a result of the Association's campaigning activities. Without a doubt, the demands and the possibilities were too much for volunteers to cope with, and almost certainly the organization would have died had it not fully professionalized itself with the opening of its first two services in 1980 and 1981. In the early days parents were the instigators and the workers. Of course, even then some professionals played an important role in supporting parents and their initiatives. As Sense employed staff and began to professionalize, the importance of the involvement of a wide network of committed 'outside' professionals did not diminish. In fact, the strength of the organization was perhaps in being able to mobilize many more people than were family members or its own staff.

The information provision and enabling role continues today as part of the task of the staff who work with families through the branch structure. The role of the first Sense staff was crucial in making the transition to becoming a service provision agency, however, and the interaction between family members and staff has been critical at times of organizational transition. Staff have had to be particularly sensitive to the effects on family members as priorities have shifted and the approach has become businesslike. They have had to work hard to maintain the family values of the original organization. In fact, the retention and reinforcement of the organization's value base has perhaps been a key factor in its present success.

In a way the roles of family members and professionals have reversed over Sense's forty years. Initially, parents were the leaders and professionals were their supporters and enablers. Today, professionals provide leadership and management, with some parents and family members playing a vital role through governance, for example, on Sense's Board of Trustees (called Council) and Family Forum and through involvement in key processes such as strategic planning.

It would be interesting at this point to compare Sense with a markedly different family-based organization in the United Kingdom, the National Deaf Children's Society (NDCS). This organization, with which we have been connected in many ways since our own formation, was founded during the Second World War and recently celebrated its 50th Anniversary. It had no need to become a service organization in order to survive. The much greater incidence of childhood deafness is recognized throughout the country, and relevant services have been in place for many years. Certainly, the NDCS have pioneered new services, most notably peripatetic teaching services for young deaf children, but they are now provided by the state in every Local Education Authority in the country. The NDCS has the 'benefit' of numbers and currently have over 150 local groups providing information, advice, and support. The groups themselves are well supported by the Society's regional and national offices, which enables the Society to attend to the individual needs of its members and thereby give them a powerful sense of ownership. The numbers within each locality means that, having singly or corporately identified areas of service need, branches of the national organization can effectively mobilize campaigning to press purchasers and providers to meet that need.

Unless there are a substantial number of members, the potency of a local branch is never likely to be sufficient to sustain intensive services or advocacy. But in a country the size of the United Kingdom, it is essential to provide a continuous awareness and advocacy activity if services are to be sustained and developed. In the smaller countries of Europe, for instance, the Netherlands, Switzerland, or the Nordic countries, where the general population numbers between, say, seven and fifteen million, it is possible for the national government to encompass the provision of services to groups large and small in a manageable way. This is not the case for a country like the United Kingdom with fifty-seven million people, where the responsibility for services is delegated to Local Authorities or to the National Health Service. The difficulty is that none of these services has strategic planning bodies at regional level. As a result, agencies like Sense must deal with over 100 authorities for the provision of health, education, and welfare services. On this basis, low-incidence disability needs will be entirely neglected unless enough noise is made. This fact was evident when the Department for Education and Employment (DfEE) made a major grant available for the development of deafblind educational services; for they would award it only to consortia of three or more LEAs. It was Sense that campaigned for this grant, and it was Sense that was commissioned by the

DfEE to coordinate the project during the three years of its existence, because no other body within government was capable of performing this function.

Not having a strong network of branches, Sense has had to create a professional structure to undertake services, campaigning, and advocacy below national level. This goal was achieved by the formation of seven Regions, four in England, and one each in Scotland, Wales, and Northern Ireland. These Regions are able to put pressure on both providers and purchasers to undertake or improve services for their deafblind users/constituents, but it is difficult, of course, to provide substantial individual help for every family. This was always the case, but it is even more so now, since growth has meant that Sense has become aware of many more families (or they have become aware of Sense!). Help can certainly be provided in those areas where Sense has contracted with a purchaser to provide a specific service to families, for instance, an Intervenor Scheme in Lincolnshire or the Respite Service at the Sense Scotland Family Centre in Glasgow. Otherwise, its most useful role is to campaign across the board for a service or a particular financial benefit, as was the case in the 1980s, when a successful campaign was fought for the extension of the Mobility Allowance. This is a state welfare benefit that is paid to people with a physical disability to compensate them in part for the additional costs of making themselves mobile. Sense persuaded the government of the severe mobility problems of deafblind people, and as a result, payment was extended as an automatic right to anyone with deafblindness. Sadly, this benefit is now under threat.

In recent years, Sense has attempted to close a major gap in its array of services by introducing a 'Person to Person' scheme, through which trained counsellors, all parents themselves of deafblind children, are available by telephone contact to family members with troubles they need to share and find answers to. This scheme has had its teething problems, but Sense is determined to find a way to support individual families more substantially, since the paid staff do not have the capacity to offer such a service at present.

Sense has found that the way to achieve services is to convince government at both national and local levels that real need exists.

1. First, one must persuade them to accept deafblindness as a disability category, and in order to do so, a definition is needed.
2. Then, it should be demonstrated why specific services are required. This is one of the biggest hurdles, since what marks out deafblind services as different is the need for high staff: client ratios, as near to one-to-one for as much of the waking day as possible.
3. A survey of need within the area covered by the authority is the next step.

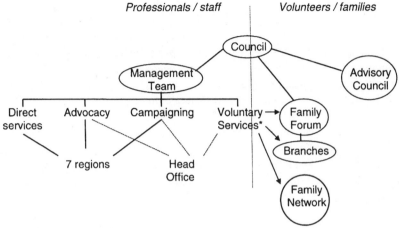

*Support provided to branches etc.

Figure 13.3   Sense Chart, Showing Organizational Relationships between Staff and Families

An authority may be reluctant to commission such a survey, because without doubt, once the needs survey has been undertaken, the inevitable outcome is pressure for services to meet those needs.

4. Subsequent steps will involve the mobilization of families as part of the campaign, discussions on what services to press for, substantial publicity on the existence of deafblind people and the services they need, and, nearly always, the establishing of 'deafblind' as a concept within that community.

Inevitably, when Sense became a service organization, families felt that they were less and less at the centre of the action, which, indeed, was true. One of the ways that was found to compensate was the creation of a Family Forum. Every branch sends representatives to this Forum, which meets on a regular basis to debate matters of concern to the branches and to families and considers existing or future services. The Forum has a permanent representative seat on Sense's governing council. It also holds its own weekend meetings and training days. Council members and staff are regularly invited to address the Forum on activities and performance.

Families are also well represented on the council. It was felt to be unwise to cement their involvement in the constitution or in by-laws, but it has long been policy for the council to be made up of at least one-third family members. In fact, in the past twenty years it has never been less than 50 per cent. As the organization grew, it seemed wise to try to strengthen the council with able business people, for instance, lawyers, or rich benefactors, 'the great and the good,' as they are often known. This was not a wise move. The family members and direct-service professionals, for so long the backbone of our Association, felt alienated and unable to establish a rapport with such people, who then felt out of place. Ways have had to be found to accommodate all the interests within the growing organization. Attendance at council meetings was found not to be the most practical way for council members to exercise their responsibilities, although it was legally essential. Thus, Council/Management Links were created, by means of which a council member is linked to a particular service or geographical region and develops a close relationship with it. This has worked extremely well, and is one of the ways in which parent members can have a regular rapport with different parts of the organization in a meaningful, practical way.

Difficulties

There are major difficulties that families and Sense, as a family organization, constantly must confront, mostly those relating to philosophies or to finance.

First, integration. The importance of having deafblindness identified as a distinct disability in its own right has long been recognized. A major challenge is to maintain this distinction within the philosophies of service provision in our country. Many of the services that are appropriate for congenitally deafblind children and adults appear to be suitable for other categories of disability, for example, multiple disability. As a result, many of the educational establishments serving deafblind children, through philosophy or practical necessity, integrate them within their multi-disabled provision. Many authorities have adopted policies of not financing children 'out-county,' that is, outside the services that they themselves provide. This means that there are rarely enough children to have a viable specific service within the authority, and some compromise must be reached. Families can overcome such policies if they fight hard enough, but it is usually a long and tough fight.

The same is increasingly true of adult services, especially residential situations, where one of the most fashionable criteria is providing on the basis of perceived 'friendship groups' rather than on the basis of specific service approaches. Readers will be well able to appreciate the difficulty this might impose where residents with very special communication needs live alongside those who can hear and speak.

Finance, too, is an area of challenge for us. Services for deafblind people are expensive because, of course, individuals need very high staff:client ratios. In a now perpetual climate of cuts, providers like Sense find that they have to work constantly to justify the higher costs that services for our group incur; for without such vigilance, some purchasers will inevitably choose cheaper options that do not begin to meet the needs of service users. No one can answer the proposition that the money needed to support one congenitally deafblind service user would support many more clients with less intensive needs, other than to state that all must be appropriately served.

Pluses and Minuses

Sense's quantum growth has dated from 1987. Until that time it was both a small parents' organization and a small service organization. The opening of the first residential project in Lincolnshire had certainly had its pluses and minuses. First, it represented the professionalization of the organization and a real commitment by Sense and by the nation to start doing right by its young deafblind adults. There were twelve places, and within a year all were taken. Fees were not cheap, and it took much pressure, and much huffing and puffing by the purchasing authorities to agree to pay. Because of the economic exigencies of the project, places had to be offered to suitable applicants on a 'First come, first served basis,' which nobody disagreed with, in principle. But the Association, still in many ways a club, had some growing to do to come to terms with the ramifications of this response.

1. First, there were only twelve places but more than 100 families who foresaw their children taking up one of the places -- hence, inevitable disappointment for many of the families.
2. Secondly, some of those who had worked hardest for this project had to contend with the reality that their children were considered unsuitable, a particularly galling situation for those families whose authorities had agreed to pay the fees.
3. Other families had children who were considered suitable but whose authorities would not pay.
4. Others, some founder members of the Association, saw places go to applicants whose families had never been members or contributed in any way.

Clearly, these outcomes had not been predicted by the committee for the Lincolnshire project, since no plans were under way for more homes. Many members left the Association and the then Midlands Region folded. It became clear that, having begun to offer services, Sense must continue on this route. We encouraged other organizations to provide similar projects, for example, the Royal National Institute for Deaf People (RNID) opened a unit in Bath, Henshaws Society for the Blind began one in Yorkshire, and a Scottish children's charity, Quarrier's, offered a building for a joint project in Glasgow. But these initiatives were not enough, and the opportunity came for additional services when Sense was offered a five-acre site in the centre of Birmingham, formerly a residential school for deaf children. This was the largest project Sense had undertaken, and within the space of three years, homes for a further thirty-six young deafblind adults were available, together with a Family Centre for the Midlands of England. Thereafter, new group homes were opened every year, and this process is ongoing, as every year more demands for places are made, particularly by school-leavers. As this chapter is being written, Sense is opening its first residential centres in the north of England, so that all of its regions are now offering a range of useful services.

As readers can appreciate, the introduction of new services had unexpected ramifications for the Association. Sense is not a business, in that a business exists as much as anything to make profits, but it is essential for everyone's good that Sense operate in a businesslike way. This attitude can have very unexpected effects, not least on individual families. Again, I quote from Peggy Freeman's history:

The Advisory Council meeting for 1991 was a lively one, when, for the first time the Advisory Council challenged Sense's management. [Note: The Advisory Council is an annual meeting for older members of Sense no longer active in the affairs of the organization]. Margaret Brock spoke on behalf of the parents in Sense who were concerned that now it was run on business lines and becoming depersonalised with a 'them and us' situation. It was suggested that there should be more contact and more should be known about the departments and the staff personally. Parents then joined in the discussion in a very positive way. Rodney defended by saying that Sense would not have funds today had it not been for the professional organisation, that the whole organisation was about families being put in touch with each other and there were three parents actually on the staff. He said that Sense was staffed by professionals who liked the family atmosphere and who were aware that families were the backbone of the whole organisation. However, an organisation did need people who could take an objective view. It was agreed to see how there could be more information about and contact with staff and copies of the internal newsletter would be made available to council members. (1996, 178)

This is a situation that will undoubtedly present on a permanent basis. Sense is still strongly a family-based organization in which both families and professionals feel at home.

As already noted, over half of the Sense council membership remain family members. Families are also involved in many voluntary capacities in the organization, although there are strict orders that there should be no pressure put on families for such involvement. In the early days, before there was any effective administration, most of the work was undertaken by family members, in addition to their own work and the heavy demands of a home with a disabled member. Some cracked under the burden, such that their only course was a total break with the Association for their own mental health. Once this situation was recognized, Sense determined that family members would never again find themselves under such pressure. In addition, many younger parents are only now seeking services, wishing to put any spare time they may have into their own 'devices and desires,' and good for them! There is absolutely no doubt that Sense is a professional operation and must be businesslike in its operations. As a family-based organization, Sense must examine every decision taken and determine if it is being taken for the good of 'the company' or for the good of its beneficiaries: deafblind children and adults. A good example might be where it would be appropriate to close a Sense day centre because it had become clear that the service users could be effectively retained in open employment with support from staff members, this being more stimulating and involving for the users and cheaper for the purchasing authorities. As a company, Sense might wish not to lose the business, but to protect the jobs of the staff, and might resist the change for this reason. As a charity with charitable objectives, Sense should forgo the business and do what is in the best interests of the service users.

In addition, as a service provider, Sense must also be clear that its principal duty is to the service user, not to his family. Usually, the needs of users and families coincide and there is no problem, but where they do not, there can be a very delicate course to steer. One instance will suffice. A disabled person in the United Kingdom has a disability pension that is his by right and which should be available to him wherever he may be. While he is a child and living at home in a poor household, that pension will become part of the general family income, such that the family will not be able to consider dispensing with it when the time comes for the disabled member to move into a home of his own. Thus, he might be kept in the family home in order to retain the income, arguably to his detriment. Or, when he does move, the family may refuse to sign over the pension. In such circumstances, Sense must act, first, in the interests of its beneficiary, the deafblind person. There is surely no situation of this nature that could not be resolved to the benefit of all concerned. Such resolution does not always happen and there may be an inevitable estrangement between the family and its organization, but this is rare. Unlike many professional organizations, which often seem frightened of parents, Sense relishes its involvement with families. There is a palpable sense of togetherness, often remarked upon, which could be lost but which it must work to maintain as it grows in professional sophistication. As long as Jessica Hills (a teacher who has been involved with Sense since the early 1960s) remains chairman, and the writers of this chapter remain in management, there is no doubt of the central role that families will continue to play in much of its work.

One of the major pluses in being both a family organization and a service-provider is that Sense is trusted by the families to do right by their children, even though hard work is necessary to retain that trust. Over the years, families have been frightened by the treatment that will be meted out to their disabled offspring in institutions run by the state or by private profit-minded individuals, and there has been, regrettably, a high proportion of abuse reported over the years. Sense itself as an employer is not going to be entirely free of such events, and, indeed, there have been one or two incidents over the years. It would be naïve to think that an organization with over 1,600 members of staff could winkle out a potential abuser, but being a family organization does place an enormous responsibility to minimize this sort of eventuality. Sense is confident that its policies and practices do mean that it is effective in this respect.

It is often said that being a service provider undermines one's ability to act as advocate and campaigner. Arguably, the reverse is true. In the late 1980s a young deafblind woman called Beverley Lewis starved to death while in the care of her mentally ill mother. Sense took up the case, not only in support of Beverley's family in their very real concerns about the adequacy of the services being provided both by the National Health Service and the Local Authority Social Services Department, but also because of the inadequacy of the law when it came to the protection of vulnerable adults. Had Beverley been a child (as indeed she was in everything except years), she would have had the advantage of an astonishing array of protective legislation. It was of great concern that when Sense sought allies among its fellow voluntary organizations, none of them was willing to take up arms against the relevant authorities through fear of losing the possibility of contracts with them. Sense's experience, however, was that the stance we took did not jeopardize in any way our ability to conclude contracts with these authorities. Similarly, it is felt that if an organization's own services are in any way lacking in quality, this will prevent them from applying pressure on other providers or wherever. Again, this has not proved to be the case. Nine times out of ten, the quality of one's services, and the organizational muscle that one acquires thus, is of substantial assistance in campaigning. Where Sense has been rightly criticized in the past for shortcomings in its own services, the organization's response to such criticism is the important issue, not whether the shortcoming exists. When it comes to campaigning, the additional benefit of being a family membership organization is the wealth of parent power that one can harness, which is often a winning element nowadays, since parents have become popular with both politicians and the media, in contrast to their position in the past.

Essential Elements

Without question, a family must first come to terms in whatever way they can with the reality of their new situation. This process can take a shorter or longer time, but attention must be given to the health of the family unit before any other considerations are dealt with. This must involve a willingness on the part of family members to want the best for their child and to seek it.

The family will need practical information, advice, and help, which will certainly come from a variety of local, regional, and national organizations, both state and voluntary. A battery of services, appropriate for all the ages that their child will pass through, should be in place or created to meet his/her need. This will be achieved by a cooperative effort of family, support organizations, and service purchasers and providers. The interaction will, on occasion, be more confrontational than cooperative, which is when the value of a very partial organization is particularly seen.

Finally, it is often in the smallest of ways, at a particularly critical moment, that the greatest of differences can be made: a day's respite care at a very difficult time; the right word spoken by the right person in the depths of despair, which reaches through all the emotional turmoil to the happiness at the centre of the individual; a small donation of money to buy a piece of equipment. Such items of support can be as important as whatever is provided when major life decisions are being made. But overall, it is the recognition by all those involved in family support that it is the right of the disabled member and his/her family to share in the benefits that so many of us take for granted and to work for a society in which they come as of right that will ultimately do most to meet their needs.

Conclusions and Statements

by Malcolm Matthews

As has already been noted, the development of any support system is rooted in the culture of that country. Sense's development occurred at particular points in the evolution of services in the United Kingdom and in a particular historical context. Some conclusions may be possible, but the reader must exercise caution in generalizing to other cultures and different times. The following statements arise mainly out of the previous text but follow a different order based not on priority but grouped in a way that I hope is easy to read.

- The combination of the drive, knowledge, and creativity of parents and the expertise and sustaining power of committed professionals is the key to the successful establishment and healthy growth of a family-led organization.
- It is important that professionals undertake an enabling role with a family organization or network.
- Many parents and family members will not want to be involved in running an organization.
- Great care should be taken to ensure that parents and family members who take on additional responsibilities to do with running services or an organization are not overburdened.
- The values of an organization are important and worth stating explicitly, for instance the importance of users (deafblind people), families, and professionals as partners.
- The value of parents and family members' being in contact with each other cannot be underestimated; contact and opportunities for sharing and friendship can be of significant mutual benefit.
- The need for practical information, practical advice, and practical help comes first, followed by the need for services.
- Services, services, and more services will be demanded – and are needed.
- Services and support are particularly required at times of transition, including at diagnosis, on entering school, on leaving school, and on moving from the family home.
- The value of specific support at critical moments should not be underestimated; a small grant, day's respite or even simply someone to listen can sometimes make all the difference.
- Often, it is how a service is provided that is of more significance than what is provided.
- Attitudes within society can be the greatest handicap for a family or individual.
- Exchanging and sharing information can be the basis of a family network.
- There are many different ways of structuring support groups and networks: geographically (e.g., a regional branch), according to disability (e.g., a national Usher group), by need (e.g., parents of younger multi-disabled children), by objective (e.g., the need for a legislative change or for a particular service, such as a family centre).
- Ideas for activities include social events, day courses with talks by parents or professionals, influencing government, and influencing service providers.

- Befriending is a valuable activity in itself, and perhaps friendship is a necessary condition for continued contribution to a family organization.
- Campaigning for specific services and for enabling legislation are appropriate initial objectives.
- Size may not be important, but a wide network of contacts is vital.
- Alliances with sympathetic professionals in a variety of organizations and fields are important.
- Involvement with other groups at a local level combined with regional or national (or even international) involvement around deafblindness may be appropriate for some families.
- Use should be made of international contacts. Others' concepts and ideas also should be tried, but they should be made appropriate; for instance, in the United Kingdom we are promoting the concept of Intervenors and providing intervention, but there are some differences in our models.
- Where services are provided by others, the most effective action might be to influence the providers to change their services.
- Campaigning and service provision can be combined.
- Provision of ongoing services cannot be the responsibility of parents' groups.
- Advocacy will always be a need for deafblind children and their families, since services are usually costly.
- Parents and people with disabilities are the most powerful advocates if they have access to information and support.
- Deafblindness is a low-incidence disability, so to become a priority for administrators provision must be planned for, based on a particular size of population. In a European or North American situation, perhaps, planning on the basis of a population around the five million mark is strategically viable. This may mean encouraging a group of authorities to share resources and plan together to provide services for deafblind children or providing a regional resource to cover more than one administrative district.
- Most professionals focus on one aspect of a child or person with disabilities; what is wanted is a group or an organization that can see the whole person, or even better, that can value the whole person.
- Planning and provision of services requires the involvement of or consultation with deafblind people or families.
- Running services must be businesslike, but business-led decisions must sometimes be resisted.
- Involvement of deafblind people and families in a service-providing organization helps with accountability and direction for the organization.
- Creating community awareness (including campaigning), advocacy, and ser-

vices all are required. They can be provided by separate bodies, but there are some advantages in one agency providing all three.

There now follow some specific conclusions and statements about starting an organization.

Starting

First, it is important to be clear about one's initial objectives. Most family support groups will have one or more of the following as aims.

1. Provision of mutual support by family members going through similar experiences or recently having had similar experiences. This support can be provided informally or through some people having specific roles. Sense provides training for a number of parents and others to develop listening and other appropriate skills. Information on those who completed the training is now available in a directory that can be used by professionals or directly by people looking for contacts. This approach is currently being evaluated.
2. Sharing information directly and by contact with professionals. A professional is more likely to be able to prepare and deliver a presentation on an area of parental interest to a group of people than is possible to an individual family.
3. Building confidence. Confidence building is a prerequisite for a group to develop the coordinated and determined approach necessary to influence service providers, funders, and government.
4. Influencing service provision.
5. Providing services.

A group is likely to be led by a family member or by a professional. If it is family member led, families likely will have greater involvement, become more involved, and have a sense of ownership. If a group is led by a professional, family members may miss out on receiving and giving support and accessing valuable information that other family members are able to share with them. Instead, support may be sought primarily from the professional. It can be difficult for parents to feel responsible for the group's achievements, and confidence building will be less if all family members need to do is turn up for the meetings. It may be difficult for some parents to be open and honest if a professional from whom they receive a service is involved in running a group.

At the same time, a professional who helps a group to form, establish itself, and meet its objectives can be a vital component of the group's success.

Sense started as an organization of parents involving professionals. This model is still valid, and Sense's branches continue as support groups of family members with professionals and volunteers also involved. One Sense member of staff, the Voluntary Services Officer, has the specific role of supporting such branches and groups. Specific responsibilities are as follows:

- Establishing appropriate communication strategies and monitoring their effectiveness
- Strategic promotion and development of new groups
- Meeting information needs in appropriate formats
- Facilitating groups to achieve their aims
- Promotion and development of the group profile
- Design, coordination, and evaluation of training in response to expressed need.

Influencing or Providing?

It has already been suggested that it is possible both to be a service provider and to influence others. Sense began providing services when in some areas influencing was not enough. In other areas Sense has not become a provider, for example, although our aims for school-age children have been of vital significance in the provision of deafblind education in schools, we do not run them. This is because there is a statutory right to education no matter the disabilities or abilities of a child and because both the state and the independent schools are providing for deafblind children, particularly in units designed to meet their specific needs. Sense's role has been

- to lead the push for recognition of multi-sensory impairment
- to campaign for government to have a policy on deafblind education
- to press for that policy to include the need for teachers to be trained specifically to work with multi-sensory impaired children   ·
- to push for resources to be available for training and networking and for a curriculum to be developed.

Sense has provided the structures and network to enable provision to happen nationally and locally, but not the provision itself.

Post-school provision was different, however, and in this area Sense needed to become a service provider to demonstrate what was possible. Its services aimed to be models of excellence, models to be followed by others, including the state. That was the original aim. In the United Kingdom the policy background has changed, and as already described, it has been government policy for some time that the state should be a purchaser of services, but not a provider. As a result, voluntary and private agencies continue to provide an increasing number of services, and Sense's provision continues to expand, as does its work influencing others – both the financers of services, that is, mainly the state, and also the other service providers.

For a support group or family-led group, direct provision can be a very real burden with no respite. Employment of staff quickly becomes a necessity, and the responsibilities of management and ensuring that the resources are in place can be great.

Choosing the Focus

Since one cannot focus on all areas of need at once, one must choose one's targets carefully. For a group of younger parents the aim may be influencing the education authorities and initiating or changing services in a particular state or locality. The focus then turns to the transition to school. Later on, the transition from school to what happens after may be the most important focus, depending on what already exists and on the statutory rights in different countries. This focus will change over time, particularly as the situations of the participants change. It is, of course, necessary to anticipate. Bringing about change often takes time, and it is frequently the case that it is not the pioneers themselves but those who come afterwards who benefit. Indeed, some of the original Sense parents who campaigned for provision have seen their children fail to receive quality provision, while those who followed have reaped the rewards.

Deciding on one's objects and targets is important. Having a vision is vital, but one must keep the targets realistic and not too numerous. If the aspirations are too wide ranging, the group will feel that it has failed, even if an objective analysis shows that a great deal has been achieved. Often for parents' groups the aims of mutual support and influencing others ought to be enough. Responsibility for direct-service provision can become all encompassing and can mean that the original objectives are dropped – fine, if this is what is wanted.

A small group can do little by itself. The key to success will usually be building up a wide network of contacts and marshalling the right support.

A Support System

The significant components of the initial support system in the United Kingdom have been

- Provision of information on deafblindness, specific conditions, access to support, and possible service responses
- Telephone advice to families, often provided by volunteers or staff with personal family experience of deafblindness
- Access to assessments that look at the whole person but include a focus on needs arising from dual sensory impairment and developmental possibilities and advice and information to the family and other professionals from the same practical perspective
- Support to individuals and their families in lobbying and arguing for resources and placements, since it is usually the case in the United Kingdom that if needs resulting from deafblindness are to be met, the resource requirements will be higher than an authority wishes to make available
- A short holiday for the deafblind family member in the long summer holiday period, which also provides respite for the other family members.

Of course, there are specific requirements according to the individual's circumstances, age, and needs. For example, if the person is of school age, then perhaps there are two key components: first, teachers who have had training relevant to deafblindness: secondly, the involvement of other individuals in the classroom, residential, or home setting to act in an intervention role. After school age the focus shifts to providing a home or support in the residence or home setting and access to meaningful activity, including continued developmental and educational opportunities. Whether making an economic contribution is included will depend on the cultural situation.

It is doubtful if there is an ideal support system in existence. Wants are always going to be greater than resources will allow. Providing a blueprint for a support system always seems to end up as a wish list or, alternatively, to have important omissions. Some documents have been written, however, that propose guidance for developing comprehensive service support systems. In the United Kingdom in 1989 the report *Breaking Through* (Deafblind Services Liaison Group 1989) proposed a series of recommendations for Local Authority social services departments in order to provide a comprehensive service to deafblind people. This document was a joint initiative of the Local Authority organizations and the national voluntary agencies working in the deafblind field. More recently in a document entitled *Deafblindness: Guidance for Good Practice for Authorities* (Deafblind Services Liaison Group 1996) the Deafblind Services Liaison Group has attempted to map the elements required in any local area for the needs of deafblind people to be met. It calls for a strategic approach to developing and providing services to deafblind people and makes the following recommendations.

1. Deafblind people should be identified.
2. There should be thorough and sensitive assessments of need.
3. Workers should be trained to deal with deafblindness.
4. Specialist services should be provided to meet assessed need.
5. Interpreters and guide-helps/communicator-guides/intervenors should be provided.
6. Service development should be backed by awareness raising, training, and adequate budgetary provision.
7. There should be regular monitoring of accessibility of local information services and the extent to which deafblind people can make use of them.
8. Deaf people have regular vision testing and blind people have regular hearing tests; any indication of the development of a secondary impairment should result in referral.
9. Authorities should work together to meet residential needs.
10. An individual education plan, rehabilitation plan or individual program plan should be prepared on a multi-disciplinary basis by a key worker for each deafblind person.
11. The contribution of technical assistance and equipment should be evaluated periodically for each individual.
12. An adapted physical environment shoud be provided.
13. There should be a total communication approach and developmental curriculum, including mobility needs.
14. A sensory curriculum that includes a tactile approach and the use of any residual vision and hearing should be provided.
15. Therapeutic support, including physiotherapy and speech therapy, should be available.

Creating Community Awareness

Bringing about change to gain a particular objective can involve action at a variety of different levels, with success depending on action at more than one level. For example, at national level an aim can be that reference to the specific needs of deafblind people is included in guidance or a code of practice. Action might involve building up a relationship with civil servants (government employees) in a department as well as lobbying the appropriate minister. National associations of local government or of their staff might be influenced to set up working groups to advise on good practice in relationship to deafblind people. At a more local level, local government can be influenced to include the needs of deafblind people in plans to make the financing of the implementation of the code of practice a priority. This action could be particularly effective if national guidance is making similar propositions. A local group might seek to influence both local government and the service provider.

Some specific examples might be helpful. The four main service-providing agencies in the United Kingdom for deafblind children and adults – that is, Sense, the Royal National Institute for the Blind, the Royal National Institute for the Deaf, and Deafblind UK – work together, particularly in lobbying over social service issues through a grouping called the Deafblind Services Liaison Group. The Group had developed an increasing concern about the lack of recognition of the needs of very elderly people who become deafblind. It was decided to press for the Social Services Inspectorate to undertake an inspection of Local Authority social services departments' work with elderly people who lose their hearing and sight. This action involved gaining some support from a key agency working with elderly people and having an initial discussion with the relevant officials in the Department of Health. Many more agencies working in the areas of both sensory impairment and the elderly were then contacted and asked to support the Group by joining the call for an inspection and writing to the department. This was followed up by a meeting with the relevant minister and making a formal request. The minister's response was that there would not be an inspection, but instead a working group was proposed:

• to produce initial guidance to local authorities
• to identify a number of authorities that would pilot new work in this area
• to produce a final publication.

Since then, Sense has been able to contribute to writing the guidance and to the pilot work within some local areas. The outcome was probably more effective than anticipated in terms of achieving some recognition of a need and some action at both national and local levels. The lobbying was probably effective, because, by the time the formal requests were submitted, the case had already been partly made and support marshalled. The officials were also in a position to prepare their proposal before the request was received by the minister.

In the United Kingdom, probably the production of two particular documents and the associated lobbying have been of especial importance. *Breaking Through* (Deafblind Services Liaison Group, 1989) has already been mentioned; this document provided the framework for a series of national and regional conferences, regional and local meetings, further documents and practical initiatives. Also published in 1989, and arguably of more importance, was the education policy produced by the national government, through the Department for Education and Employment (DfEE). Campaigning and lobbying had taken place over many years and culminated in a policy that reflected the aspirations of all concerned with the education of deafblind children. The DfEE Policy Statement advice included the following points.

1. By the time a deafblind child has reached the age of two, the planning of his/her education should have begun.
2. Local education authorities should make available services to families similar to those provided by the Sense Family Centres.
3. Preschool Advisory Teachers with expertise in working with deafblind children and their families should be provided.
4. Intervenors, working one-to-one with the deafblind child, should be appointed to enable the child to participate more fully in family life.
5. The teaching ratio for deafblind children should generally be one-to-one.

In seeking to maximize community awareness and achieve policy objectives, it is vital that they are considered in the light of other policy perspectives and knowledge of what is seen in the wider community as the right direction. Sometimes policy perspectives will be in accord. Thus, the policy to close long-stay mental retardation hospitals in the United Kingdom had a close fit with Sense's desire to develop small-scale homes in communities, and the arguments for resourcing homes concurred to some extent with government perspectives over good practice. Sometimes policy perspectives are in apparent opposition, and a clear argument should be prepared to establish a deafblind perspective. In the United Kingdom there have been concerns over the perspectives of the 'integration in education' lobby and over normalization. An uncritical approach to normalization might result, therefore, in limited opportunities for contact between deafblind people and in very limited opportunities for communication using specialized methods. An argument constructed within the framework of normalization theory and justifying specialist provision could be vital in establishing, maintaining, and developing specialist provision, and, indeed, just such a paper, *Principles for the Development of Residential Services for Deafblind People*, has played an important role in obtaining the support and finance for continued specialist residential provision.

Surveys identifying the numbers, ages, and circumstances of deafblind people in individual local government areas have been a necessary step in persuading many local governments to fund services. However, it has not always proved necessary to undertake such surveys before establishing services. Knowledge of the rough proportion of the population with dual sensory impairment in a few areas has facilitated estimation of the population in other, similar areas. The results of this approach have later proved to be remarkably accurate. Surveys will be costly if they are thorough. Where a survey has not been undertaken but an initial service has been established, it has often followed that many more deafblind children or adults have come forward once there is local knowledge of a service. The grapevine proves to be the most effective form of communication in a community!

Bringing about Change

There are a number of different routes to service provision for deafblind people and others. If one is not happy with the service provided locally, then there may be four or more possible routes to change:

1. Improving the local service that exists
2. Persuading others to provide a service
3. Providing a service oneself as a demonstration of what is required
4. Providing a service oneself in the long term.

Routes 1 and 2 may require the service provider to acquire additional resources and 3 and 4 will certainly require funds. Route 4 means funding on an ongoing basis. Persuading funders of the need for a different or specific service, therefore, is perhaps the primary and most important task, and the arguments should include being clear about what deafblindness is and the resultant needs, who has the needs, and what is different and special about deafblind services. The stages in lobbying or campaigning are as follows.

1. Proving deafblindness is a separate distinct disability with particular needs
2. Demonstrating why specific services are needed
3. Demonstrating the need of, for instance, a survey to identify people
4. Mobilizing families and others to press for provision
5. Publicizing the existence of deafblind people and the services they need
6. Eventually or if necessary, providing a pilot or demonstration service.

Whether seeking finance is the task or persuading others to provide, the most difficult aspect may be changing the mindset of the current funders or providers. Services are often provided to congenitally deafblind people by agencies for mentally retarded people. Either these services must recognize the extent and importance of sensory impairment as a reason for developmental delay and make very radical changes accordingly, or they must recognize that services focusing on intellectual impairment do not follow adequate approaches to meeting the needs of deafblind people. Similarly, services for blind and visually impaired people and services for deaf and hearing impaired people need to recognize their own inadequacies and the need for change if deafblind people's needs are to be met. However, services for these three client groups will always regard deafblind people as a minority group and an afterthought – hence the need always for recognition of the uniqueness and difference of deafblindness, the need always for radical change to services, and the need often for the development of new provision by new providers.

Providing services in the long term means raising revenue finance (or running costs) every year ad infinitum. Sense has managed with residential provision to cover the total costs of running such services from fees charged to local authorities or to the National Health Service. As a result, most fund-raising has been directed to the capital, start-up and development costs of new services. Once a residential service has been established and a good quality service is in place, there are no additional fund-raising costs on an annual basis. This approach has meant that growth is possible. Fund-raisers do not need to raise money to keep existing services going but can seek resources for new needs and exciting developments. They don't need to keep running in order to stand still!

Fund Raising for a Voluntary Organization

How do voluntary groups raise the money they need to do their work? In years gone by, when incomes were much lower, it was perfectly possible for charities to set up a service for disabled, elderly, or sick people and be able to pay for the service out of monies they raised. Often, this money was raised from rich people by way of an endowment, which would produce enough income each year to pay the charity's way. Of course, this is no longer the case. Since before the Second World War, it became clear that the government would have to become the chief purchaser of services or become a provider itself. These roles it took on when the Labour party set up the Welfare State in its postwar government. As a result, most of Sense's income is now fees for services, approximately 70 per cent of the total. But there are many activities for which Sense cannot bill anyone and that it thinks are very important, so it must look to the great British public. Such services include holiday projects, campaigning work, and our Regional Advisory Service, in which trained workers visit families at home and provide advice, information and counselling. This is how we go about raising this charitable (as opposed to statutory) income.

Sense has been fundraising professionally since the late 1970s, when it became a service provision organization. This fundraising was partially prompted by an appeal by a children's TV program, 'Magpie,' which raised sufficient funds to enable our Ealing Family Centre to be started as well as the purchase of the Manor House, our first Group Home. In subsequent years, fundraising continued, initially primarily capital fundraising, which came from charitable trusts and foundations for new residential work as Sense grew. In 1986 Sense opened the first of its charity shops in Kent, in order to produce some regular income that did not need to be spent on a specific purpose.

A Direct Marketing operation was established at about this time again in order to produce untied revenue income to meet the growing needs of Sense, as it developed an infrastructure and as it started to provide many more services. Direct Marketing means the creation of a cadre of supporters who regularly give Sense money, either through standing orders or through covenants, which is how tax is recovered in the United Kingdom. This operation also develops our income from legacies. The Fundraising Department has expanded to include a Corporate Fundraising Team plus other specialist fundraisers, and the strategy currently being followed is part of Sense's overall four-year strategic plan for the years 1995 to 1999.

When the strategic plan for fundraising was devised at the end of 1994, for the period 1995–99, a number of objectives were incorporated:

• to increase the different types of fundraising activity being employed, so that Sense would not have all of its eggs in too few baskets (there was previously far too much reliance on Direct Marketing and income from charitable trusts and foundations)
• to create income streams that would be more reliable than some of the activities previously employed
• to create a spread of activity, which would provide an increasing level of income, particularly revenue income for Sense's growing needs
• to reorganize so that fundraisers were sharing expertise within specialist teams.

Phase two of the strategy is concerned with a networking approach through individuals of influence and affluence who are well disposed towards Sense. These people are being identified, nurtured, and developed in order to create a network of 'Sense Friends' who are prepared to approach other individuals, companies, and trusts on Sense's behalf as well as get involved directly in fundraising and in support of fundraising, for example, through participation and organization of events.

The third phase of the current strategy is a promotional drive to increase the level of legacy income received by Sense. In the following section the organizational structure of Sense's fundraising is outlined, and the various fundraising activities currently taking place are explained.

The Fundraising and Communications Department covers all of Sense's charitable income generation other than shops, which are run by a separate Trading Department.

Direct Marketing

The Direct Marketing Team raises money from individual donors through mailshots and telephone work, and Sense has built up a database of over 50,000 individuals, who range from lapsed donors, that is, those who have not given for over two years, to donors who regularly give by deed of covenant and who have become legators, that is, those who have left a donation to Sense in their will. The Direct Marketing Team's job is to recruit new donors from cold lists that are bought from or exchanged with other charities on a reciprocal basis or by other methods, such as delivering packs through the household delivery service. Once individuals start to give, they are developed through a 'triggered' program of mailings, with the intention that they become regular donors giving increased donations and ultimately become committed givers and legators. Sense is starting to work more intensively with a number of its donors who offer the best potential for providing major gifts to the organization.

Targeted Appeals

The Targeted Appeals Team comprises three subteams.

The Capital Appeal Team
This team is responsible for mounting specific appeals for the start-up costs of new Sense centres. Generally speaking, this job is tackled by a 'Capital Fundraiser' recruiting and working with a volunteer committee in the locality of a new centre and fundraising through committee-run events and from companies and trusts.

The International Fundraiser
This is a relatively new post, dedicated to raising funds for the work of the Sense International Department. Sense is trying to establish an international committee, which will support its work in the same way that the Capital Appeals Committees work, but fundraising is also carried out through applications to charitable trusts and companies. Sponsored events, in particular, such as mountain treks, canoe adventures, and bicycle rides, all in exotic locations, are sources of income.

Appeals Committees Team
In 1996 this team was established to create a long-term base of support via per-

manent Appeals Committees in different locations. The committees operate in much the same way as the Capital Appeals Committees, the difference being they are raising money for Sense's ongoing revenue needs.

Field Revenue Team

This team has common characteristics in that all three subteams are raising money for untied revenue needs of Sense.

The Payroll Giving and Schools Team

This team's activities are split between two distinct jobs. First, promotion of Payroll Giving, in which the team of four canvassers secures regular donations from people in employment through a scheme whereby the money is regularly deducted from an employee's payroll by his company on behalf of Sense. Because this scheme was actually introduced by government, it benefits from attendant tax advantages to the beneficiary charity, since it receives the donation without deduction of income tax. The team also raises money via a program of Schools Fundraising, in which school children are encouraged to gain sponsorship for learning how to finger-spell with the deafblind manual alphabet. The operation also creates awareness of deafblindness and Sense's work with deafblind people.

Events Fundraising Team

This team is responsible for a range of events, including a program of 'sponsored workouts,' in which health and fitness clubs are targeted and the aerobics instructors are asked to organize a sponsored workout day for their members. The members are encouraged to gain sponsorship for taking part in a three-hour workout. The team also organizes sponsored runners for Sense in the London Marathon, and Sense has purchased a number of 'Golden Bonds,' which guarantee places for Sense runners. These places are then offered to runners for a minimum level of sponsorship.

This team is also responsible for larger-scale events, such as fundraising at some events organized by third parties. For example, the magazine *Investment Week* runs an exhibition and conference with an awards ceremony. Sense has secured the position of beneficiary charity, and the Events Team is responsible for organizing a fundraising raffle and casino at this event. In addition, the team will stage its own Sense event, such as the Sense City Ice-skate, in which teams from City companies gain sponsorship for competing against each other for the Sense Torvill and Dean Ice-skate Trophy and a prize. Other examples of Sense events are a piano concert, quizzes ranging from pub quizzes to more prestigious black-tie occasions, and fundraising lunches with celebrity guest speakers.

Community Fundraising Team
This team is responsible for developing other ways of fundraising from local communities and is currently running Sense's house-to-house fundraising program, in which each volunteer is persuaded to deliver envelopes to around fifty houses and then collect those envelopes with a donation enclosed. It is becoming increasingly difficult to raise money via this route, and Sense is allowing the operation to diminish. The team is therefore piloting new areas of fundraising, such as approaching university and college newspapers, church and youth groups, and other groups such as Rotarians, Lions, and Round Table.

Company Fundraising

The Company Fundraising Team is responsible for approaching companies for support in a variety of different ways. They include straightforward donations from community budgets held by companies and persuading a company to adopt Sense as a charity and to encourage their staff to fundraise on its behalf. The team also seeks 'cause-related marketing' opportunities, in which a company links promotional activity of its product or services to donations to Sense. There have been some notable major contributions via this route: £170,000 raised by the staff at the company N.F.C (National Freight Company) in 1995–96. The team is also responsible for 'selling' Sense into opportunities, such as being selected as the charity for the 1998 Chelsea Flower Show, a position that will raise £250,000 for Sense.

Trust Fundraising

Sense's Trust Team is responsible for raising revenue income from charitable trusts and foundations, and it will identify different parts of Sense's budgeted work as items for charitable trusts to fund. Much work is undertaken in researching the giving policy of trusts and foundations and the applications for funding are tailored to the needs of the trusts.

Sense's Charity Shops

Since establishing the first charity shop in 1986, Sense has invested each year in increasing the number of shops in its chain, and it now has more than forty-five shops divided among four shops regions. The shops operate by collecting second-hand clothing and goods which are distributed through a central warehouse, cleaned, and then redistributed to the various Sense shops. Sense shops are among the most profitable of charity retailers, and the operation has gone through a sustained growth in turnover in the eleven years of its existence. In 1998–99 it aims to net over £1 million in untied income.

Fundraising Professionalism

Sense's fundraising and shops operations subscribe to the idea of high standards and professionalism, and the staff employed undergo a thorough induction into Sense as well as work to agreed standards of good fundraising and retailing practice. They are highly conscious of the need to form a cohesive part of Sense's overall operations. Thus, the images and messages used by these operations are in tune with Sense's mission statement.

The Long, Slow Haul: Specialist Training in Deafblind Services

The small parents' group that was Sense in 1979 looked at the decades of campaigning for services they had undertaken, were forced to accept that the results were pitiful, and decided to start them themselves. Adult services were still non-existent, other than basic care within the wards of large mental retardation hospitals. Good children's services were confined to schooling and to a very small number of schools with a specialized unit. Training in the deafblind field for staff working with either children or adults was a dream. This was a time when a pioneer teacher had to sell up in order to finance a year's study at Boston College and Perkins School for the Blind in the United States, then the only training available. A decade and a half later, progress has been made, but there is still a long way to go.

In those days, few people understood the effects of their disabilities on deafblind and multi-sensory impaired (MSI) children. As a result, they had no educational 'category' with the magic 'definition' that causes services to happen. One of the major challenges was and is, of course, communication and its development in such children, another the low incidence of this group. In smaller countries, where the national government takes direct responsibility for educational planning, MSI children can be very well served.

Prerequisites for all services and the training of their staffs are as follows.

1. Strategic planning at regional level. The government's Department for Education and Employment (DfEE) recognized this when, in establishing a specific developmental program for deafblind education, it would accept only proposals from consortia of three or more Local Education Authorities (LEAs).
2. A high level of staff, specifically trained for all services.
3. Service environments controlled by specialist staff.

From 1979 until now, growth has been rendered more difficult because of fashionable philosophies and policies. Devolution of decision making to the lowest geographical tiers in the hierarchy of government, the generic approach in staffing, and the philosophy of integration, coupled with negative attitudes towards centralization, staff specialization, and special service provision all have provided barriers to the wider implementation of appropriate services, never mind the seemingly permanent policy in some authorities to achieve the lowest costs possible. Good services are costly and are simply not going to be provided within the general school service for every child and adult.

Children

If MSI children are to achieve their full potential, work must start from the moment of diagnosis. For this reason, Sense decided that its major contribution would be advisory teachers working with families with young children, with the eventual aim of having such a service, however provided, available ultimately to all, wherever they might live. At the same time, a campaign was begun to get the DfEE and LEAs to plan a national framework of schooling, supported by regional resource centres and adequate training courses. In the late 1980s this action led to a formal DfEE survey and report and thence to a £6+ million program. During the three years of the program, a substantial number of service initiatives coupled with training courses began and regrettably ended, in some cases, when the money dried up. But there has been a quantum increase in the number of specific services provided, as a recent survey has demonstrated.

There are two postgraduate courses for teachers of children with MSI at Birmingham and London universities. A new course, with a different emphasis, started in September 1996 in Manchester. The London course is not being offered this year. With the disappearance of finance specifically designated for MSI courses, the Birmingham course was no longer viable on a full-time basis, and so it was adapted for distance learning. There were forty students for the first and second years of this course and it is fully subscribed this year. It is offered at BPhil (Ed) and Masters levels. The healthy numbers applying suggest that the course is meeting the needs of teachers and that they feel it is worth studying for two years, largely in their own time, to achieve a qualification. In an intensive and expensive service, classroom assistants, or Intervenors, as they are becoming known, are invaluable team members. It is of great concern that they have little opportunity to develop their skills when they have such close and important contact. In-Service Training (INSET) courses are offered for this group, but all too frequently there is limited funding for their development, and they have no automatic right to training. Intervenors are also the only resource that some LEAs are able to provide for their MSI children within schools for children with severe learning difficulties (SLDs), and often only 'on the job' experience is considered adequate. Fortunately, the attendance at the courses offered by Sense West and the Royal National Institute for the Blind (RNIB) is increasing. An organization of Intervenors has recently been set up to offer more professional opportunities for its members to share skills and experiences and to campaign for professional recognition.

Overall, far too many MSI children are still within SLD schools with no specialist support. Sadly, there are few formal opportunities for training specifically within the Further Education (FE) range. Traditionally, local FE colleges have catered for students with mild learning difficulties. They are also beginning to address the needs of students with single sensory impairments, but the demands of those students who are multiply disabled have proved difficult to meet. Most colleges lack the pastoral atmosphere of schools or specialist FE provision. For the most part, their staff are increasingly sessionally/hourly employed, which makes continuity difficult. The curriculum requirements of this group of students are distinctive, requiring the kind of specialist teaching and support that in the past colleges have not been required to develop. Young MSI people have a right to access continuing education, but in order to do so they have to satisfy funding requirements of the agency that finances FE, the Further Education Funding Council (FEFC). Fortunately FEFC is applying its rules quite flexibly on the whole, but some students are finding difficulty in qualifying.

To date, the most successful forms of FE/Continuing Education have been found at specialist schools, for example, the Royal School for Deaf Children, Margate, RNIB Condover Hall, and the Royal School for the Deaf, Exeter, which are using their considerable expertise to meet the needs of these 'older' young people. They are doing this transitional curriculum in a separate way, but they have the advantage of all the back-up of school experience, medically qualified staff, and physical infrastructure.

Adults

As readers will know, deafblind or MSI adults are often considered within two groupings, congenital and acquired. Sense, being a parents' organization, has concentrated its efforts almost entirely on the former, and, indeed, residential and continuing education for this adult group has been its highest priority ever since it professionalized as an organization. It is no understatement to say that services for the group with acquired deafblindness are awful. For MSI people operating within the 'normal' range of functioning, much can be provided once the hurdle of communication difficulty has been negotiated. Provision of Communicator/ Guide support is essential in both the training and the work situations, however, and it is the financial cost attaching to this service, rather than a lack of specifically trained staff, that is the real difficulty. Sense and the other organizations involved in the Deaflblind Services Liaison Group have determined to put this situation right and are campaigning for the introduction of Communicator/Guide services in every local authority. Such a service is not at all expensive, given the numbers involved, and there has been recognizable growth in the number of such schemes, but it does not really address the needs of those who require intensive support in order to attend further/higher education or to work.

For the congenital group, although current practice in recruitment and training within the care field is heading along the continuum in a positive direction, we in the United Kingdom are far from achieving the professional status achieved within education. We are still clawing our way up from a historical perspective that viewed 'caring' as a vocation accompanied by poor pay, status, and conditions of service. Happily, we no longer see these services as being provided within large institutions, where the role was to attend to physical needs and nothing else, but some purchasers have still not come to terms with the ramifications (mostly financial) of providing a service that will meet all the needs of such a client, particularly the permanent educational input required. It is arguable that philosophically this battle has been largely won. A recent government document, the *Howe Report*, has gone some way to establishing a higher status culture for workers, but probably the strongest influence has been the demands from purchasers who are looking for quality services for their clients. It is the case, however, that very few staff would come to a specialist organization like Sense with appropriate knowledge and skill already in place, simply because there are few opportunities to develop these qualities. Sense has therefore adopted an approach of nurturing and 'growing its own' staff, providing an intensive induction training followed up by job-related training that takes them through Open Learning Modules related to their role. Topics such as communication, challenging behaviour, assessment, and individual planning are among the options. Without a doubt, any similar provider is in the same position when it comes to staff development.

Sense also offers an advanced modular program that covers management issues and higher-level practitioner skills. All modules cross-reference with National Vocational Qualifications (NVQs), which are also offered. NVQs are a range of training qualifications across many areas of work, providing staff with the means of having their attainments in one area recognized by employers in other areas. Sense's emphasis until 1998 has been on investing time and effort in developing specific, high-quality training materials that sit comfortably within the current network of vocational and professional qualifications. In 1998 the dearth of formal training led several agencies – Sense, the Guide Dogs for the Blind Association, Deafblind UK, the Council for the Advancement of Communication for Deaf People (CACDP) – to establish a working party to design a modular 'Diploma in Deafblind Studies' course, open to anyone meeting the criteria agreed upon with the granting university (to be determined). Temporarily titled 'Deafblind 98,' it has now been written. Current discussions will identify the university partner and establish implementation requirements, particularly course management.

It seems unlikely that Sense would be able to achieve service objectives within its specialist field by using generic training materials. It is clear that progress will continue to be slow, stop-start, and one step forward, one back, while service provision and staff development are left to the market-place, or rather to the anarchy of a host of non-strategic decision makers. Sense will continue to campaign on the many fronts described above, but an acceptance by DfEE and the Department of Health of the three prerequisites mentioned at the start of this article, followed up by action backed by resources would make so much difference. Certainly, Sense is not the only low-incidence, highly specialist disability area so placed.

Last Word

Inevitably, this joint contribution to an account of the creation and maintenance of a support system for families contains some overlapping and repetition. Additionally, it is extremely difficult to be absolutely logical in the development of this material, given the all-encompassing nature of the topic. We trust that we have avoided any major omissions, however, and we hope that, if nothing else, the message comes through loud and clear that appropriately meeting the needs of deafblind people and their families, no matter the country or community they live in, will be successful and effective only if a strong, partisan body exists to further their interests.

RESOURCES AND REFERENCES

Brock, Margaret (1976) *Christopher: A Silent Life*. London: Bedford Square Press
Deafblind Services Liaison Group (1989) *Breaking Through*. London: The Group
– (1996) *Deafblindness: Guidance for Good Practice for Authorities*. London: The Group
Freeman, Peggy MBE (1996) *Good Sense*. London: Sense
Hills, Jessica (1991) 'Outline of Sense's Views on the Development of Educational Provision for Deafblind Children.' In *Educational Provision for Deafblind Children: Proceedings of the Seminar*. London: Sense
Matthews, Malcolm (1993) *Principles for the Development of Residential Services for Deafblind People*. London: Sense
Policy Statement of 9 March 1989: *Educational Provision for Deafblind Children*. London: DfEE

14

Advocacy

STANLEY MUNROE

What Is Advocacy?

Human rights and personal choice are sometimes taken for granted. There are times when an individual's rights are not recognized or are ignored. *Advocacy* is necessary to protect those rights. *Webster's Dictionary* defines advocacy as 'the act of pleading for or supporting; an advocate (noun) as one who pleads the case for another, and to advocate (verb) as pleading in favor of or to defend by argument.' Advocacy can be further described as

- the process of empowering others to help themselves
- the process of support
- the facilitation of communication and/or action
- a united voice speaking for a cause
- a resource service
- the process of lobbying
- the education of individuals and populations who may be unaware of an issue.

Five examples of advocacy, in no particular order of importance, are described as follows:

Organizational Advocacy: The Red Cross, which advocates across a broad range of issues, including blood supply management, disaster relief programs, and elder support.

Organization or group committed to a special cause: MADD, Mothers Against Drunk Driving, which advocates or crusades against drinking and driving.

Professional advocacy: Paid professionals, such as lawyers or experts in a specialized field, may act on behalf of an individual client or group of clients to attain some form or redress or services, for example, worker's injuries or workplace sexual harassment.

Organizational advocacy directed towards individuals: An organization, such as the Canadian Deafblind and Rubella Association, that may advocate on behalf of specific individuals who are deafblind to obtain individual services.

Individual advocacy: Advocating for oneself or another person to acquire specific support, benefits, or changes; it can also include the individual's immediate or surrogate family who advocates for an individual who cannot do it alone.

The methods used for advocacy will often depend upon who, or which organization, is doing the advocacy and for what purpose or set of reasons. Advocacy takes several forms. The advocate may represent a professional or volunteer organization. The advocate may be a highly trained professional seeking changes in policy, a family member advocating on behalf of a child, or a friend or volunteer petitioning on behalf of another person who is unable to defend or represent him/herself.

Advocacy may focus on seeking means to

- alleviate a crisis
- access an existing program or facility
- correct a wrong
- break down barriers
- educate specific publics
- seek a change in legislation
- attempt to change or modify societal attitudes.

Advocacy for Congenitally and Early Acquired Deafblind Individuals

In many countries the law, in a form such as the Canadian Charter of Rights and Freedoms, guarantees specific rights. Such a law may state or entrench such rights. The Canadian Charter of Rights and Freedoms states, among other things, that no person shall be discriminated against because of a disability.[1] In other countries such guarantees may be embedded in precedents of Common Law. It is important to find out what guarantees exist for individuals with disabilities in your jurisdiction before you begin to advocate on their behalf.

The process of advocacy for those who are deafblind will incorporate many of the same methods used in advocacy for persons who face other challenging conditions. The initial motivation for the advocacy in the field of deafblindness is often to deal with a problem that either the individual who is deafblind cannot manage alone or that the parent or confidant of that individual cannot resolve without assistance. Such advocacy is usually directed towards improving the individuals' overall quality of life and recognizing the inherent barriers caused by the disability of deafblindness.

All persons who are deafblind have the right to a quality lifestyle and should not be discriminated against because of their disability. Achieving a certain quality of life, however, will often involve breaking down a considerable number of external barriers. It is in the crumbling of these barriers that the need for advocacy becomes apparent. The process of advocacy empowers the individual who is deafblind, through his or her advocate, to initiate or influence change.

Many of the problems or barriers connected with the disability of deafblindness are unique, but not insurmountable. They can be overcome through a carefully planned series of advocacy initiatives that involve education, community awareness, and a commitment to support the person who is deafblind to become a contributing member of society. While the processes involved in the actual advocacy for this disability may not be totally dissimilar from those that may take place for other disability groups, there also are significant differences.

Why Is Advocacy Different for Persons Who Are Deafblind?

While the basic rationale for advocacy and its various techniques may be similar for all disabilities, there are a number of critical issues that change the advocacy requirements for those who are deafblind. Let us consider them:

1. The 'uniqueness' of the disability
2. Deafblindness is a low-incidence disability
3. The lack of public awareness
4. The absence of a pool of community professional and semi-professional knowledge
5. The special educational needs.

All of the above points have been discussed in detail in other chapters of this text. There will not therefore be an in-depth review of them here. The following will allude to aspects of the problems that reflect on the advocacy process as they apply to individuals who are deafblind.

The 'Uniqueness' of the Disability

Deafblindness is a unique disability, which requires vastly different procedures for identification, education, development, and support of the deafblind individual if he or she is to enjoy the quality of life available to other citizens. For example, one of the aspects that sets these individuals apart is that, as their level of functioning improves, they require more, not less, support.

Deafblindness Is a Low-Incidence Disability.

The low incidence of the disability has various implications for the advocate. It is a positive fact, in that the number of individuals with such profound disabilities is small, and therefore positive responses to a request for support do not expose the agency or government to open-ended costs. This is an important point because, while the costs of support for the individual are high, the number of individuals is small. The advocate should know the approximate number of individuals with this disability in the jurisdiction served by the agency or government, information that can sometimes prove difficult to obtain for a variety of reasons.

Because of its low incidence, few people know about or understand the implications of deafblindness. Lack of awareness may result in premature mislabelling of young children who are deafblind by the medical community as mentally challenged or autistic. An incorrect label may make it harder for the advocate to know even approximately the number of deafblind requiring service in a given area.

Others may have been identified under the medical model, which names the treatments required and prioritizes problems by the urgency of those treatments. A child who satisfies the criteria to be identified as deafblind must be so identified regardless of medical problems. Deafblindness is a developmental, not a medical, problem.

Some persons identified as deafblind are sometimes placed in programs or institutions for the mentally or physically challenged and are thought to be well served.

Both government and agency bureaucracies may attempt to assimilate persons who are deafblind into organizations serving the visually, auditorally, physically, or mentally challenged. This approach does not allow for the specific support and services necessary to meet the needs of this 'unique' disability unless within the organization there is a clearly identified unit designed to meet the challenges of deafblindness.

Another consequence of the low incidence of deafblindness is the absence of a large pool of community knowledge in terms of trained specialists in the field and scientific knowledge about the disability and its causes, management, and prevention.

The Lack of Public Awareness

The lack of public awareness concerning the disability translates into problems for the advocate. There often is a serious deficiency in general information about this low-incidence, unique disability. Few members of the public will be against appropriate services for the individual who is deafblind, but this does not mean such services are supported. They are simply not thought about. This lack of public awareness may mean to the politician that improving services has a low, or no, priority.

Parents of children with other disabilities may say or think that the dollar cost per individual is unfair, not realizing that such costs will be higher if appropriate services are not provided. They may also feel that their child would make wonderful progress if only he or she had one-to-one support, not realizing there is a great difference between not being able to obtain non-distorted information and not being able to process it. Both of these ideas must be met head on by the advocate and defused before they become major issues. Where decisions to support dollar allocation are made at the local level, it is important for the advocate, and his or her agency, to prepare a carefully designed information package targeted at the decision makers, not at the general population.

The Absence of a Pool of Community Professional and
Semi-Professional Knowledge

Medical people and other professionals should be aware of the identification criteria so as not to mislabel persons who are deafblind. The advocate must be prepared to educate the medical practitioners, therapists, and community support people who visit the home or with whom the individual who is deafblind comes in contact. Once these community workers have been made aware of the role deafblindness plays in development, having these people give personal support, or write letters of support, is invaluable to the advocate in his or her efforts.

This lack of community awareness poses problems for the parents. Young parents need professionals who are informed and compassionate to offer them support and advice. Parents deserve the best advice, because their early understanding often determines how the child will be served best and will promote their understanding of the need for, and their ability to seek or provide, advocacy.

Sometimes existing policies can prevent the provision of appropriate support. Support for individuals with deafblindness may require changes in professional or agency policy. The advocate should identify such policies in a nonjudgmental manner and prepare the rationale for such changes.

Specific individuals working in government and social agencies responsible for funding programs for the disabled must be targeted by the advocate and made aware of the special needs of persons who are deafblind. Send them publications such as *Talking Sense, Intervention,* and *Deafblind Education* (now *DbI Renew*). Let them know about local, regional, national, and international conventions and workshops and support their attendance. The advocate should also invite them to visit a local support program with him or her. Remember that the official does not know what he or she is seeing. It will be necessary, in most cases, to explain why the clients in a local program are classified as deafblind as well as the strengths and weaknesses of the present program.

Special Educational Needs

In some educational jurisdictions there is no specific provision to meet the needs of the student who is deafblind. Education of a child who is deafblind must be individualized, pro-active, and extremely creative. Just as in other bureaucracies, the appropriate individuals within government or local agencies responsible for education must also be made aware of the needs of the individual who is deafblind and the strengths and weaknesses of the present approach. The use of examples of successful programs (these, by necessity, may have to be from outside your jurisdiction) and a suggested three or four steps towards achieving an appropriate program is an excellent way for the advocate to start. If practical, visits to successful programs by government officials should be suggested.

Differentiating between the needs of individuals with acquired deafblindness and those of individuals who are congenitally deafblind is essential, as is a ready and convincing explanation as to why the pooling of existing resources from services such as those designed to support the visually impaired and auditorily impaired are not adequate. It is usually recommended that consideration should be given to using an advocate who is not in the employ of the particular branch of government being approached, although, as pointed out later, the advocate will be educating its representatives to provide ongoing advocacy within the agency or branch of government. There are many examples of such employees advocating successfully for both individuals and groups of persons who are deafblind.

As can be seen from consideration of these five areas, advocacy content contains many unique elements. The main differences faced by advocates for individuals with deafblindness, regardless of their age, and to some greater or lesser extent faced by those advocating for other very low-incidence disabilities are a lack of understanding, few if any realistic expectations, and even fewer services existing to meet identified needs.

Advocacy for deafblind persons is on a continuum. The different purposes and procedures for the advocacy will be dependent on the age of the individual. At first, the advocacy will focus on needs of the parents, family, and young child. This advocacy will be designed to promote understanding of, and services to meet the needs of the infant, understanding by his or her parents of the disability, and the identification of reasonable expectations.

Advocacy will also be aimed at members of the immediate and extended family to promote the same types of understanding, thus laying the groundwork for each to become an effective support system and eventual advocates for the infant. Advocacy that is aimed at community support workers and program directors will be designed to promote acceptance, change policies where necessary, and develop needed support services. Often, at this stage, the advocate will find him or herself establishing new paths where none has gone before.

Next, the focus of the advocacy moves towards establishing support for education and the utilization of community resources by the young person who is deafblind. The advocate will have to identify clearly the specific needs of the student both in and out of school. It will be necessary to analyse existing services and identify both their strengths and their weaknesses. Care must be taken to avoid the pitfalls mentioned in the previous section; to continue family and community education through both individual interaction and the use of workshops; and to advocate just as intensely for appropriate programs and support for the out-of-school hours and holidays as for those needed for educational programs.

When the student with deafblindness becomes an adult, advocacy will continue to be necessary. Adult persons who are deafblind will need continued support to provide for post-secondary or 'continuing education,' to adapt training programs, to allow choice for accommodations, to provide necessary intervention support, to seek opportunities for employment, and to ensure appropriate medical and community support services. In addition, advocacy may change its focus and work to meet the needs of groups of individuals who are deafblind.

Just as the focus may change, the individuals doing the advocacy may change. Parents who may have performed a strong advocacy role in the child's early years may be advocating less in the adult's years because the parents may have died or the adult is living in another community, state, or province. It cannot be overestimated how important continued support through advocacy is for adult persons who are deafblind.

Advocacy from the Parents' Perspective

Parents of all children have goals or ideals for their offspring, usually relating to achieving a reasonable quality of life. This includes good health, adequate shelter, and an education that will result in a satisfying and productive adult life. Parents of children who are deafblind have the same wish for their son or daughter. Consequently, parents usually will become the first advocates for their child who is deafblind as soon as they realize that the community support system that works for other children will not meet the needs of their child.

It could be argued that the purpose of parent advocacy is to develop sufficient support to allow the parents to dream. Such 'dreams' often include the following for their children who are deafblind.

- That their child be accepted within their immediate family, their extended family, their neighbourhood, and their community.
- That their child be treated with respect and dignity by all.
- That society use all its efforts to ensure that their child will become a fully contributing member of society.
- That their child have an appropriate educational program and opportunity to have options of attending school either in their home community or at a facility specializing in deafblind education.
- That their child have an opportunity to receive appropriate support for a lifetime of formal and informal education, since learning never ceases.
- That their child have an opportunity to work with caring and understanding teams of professionals and experts trained in the appropriate field of deafblindness.
- That their child have the assurance of receiving the best medical care throughout his or her lifetime from a medical community that is understanding, caring, and willing to learn new things about their child.
- That respite care to assist the child and family be available on demand.
- That a social safety-net will exist for their child throughout his or her lifetime.
- That there is assurance that their child will be cared for, socially, emotionally, and economically throughout his or her life.
- That the services of trained Intervenors be available when needed throughout his or her life.
- That their child can exercise a choice of lifestyle; this would include, but not limited to, a reasonable level of choice concerning accommodation, recreational, spiritual and cultural activities, and personal relationships.
- That their child be suitably trained for employment or have a valued position as a volunteer in society that best fits his or her individual requirements.

Family Education and Awareness Training Needs

As an example of the type of support the advocate should be supplying, let us look at the needs of the family for education, training, and support. Deafblindness requires a major effort in re-educating everyone who will be involved in the life of a person who is deafblind. Having knowledgeable parents is a key step in the advocacy process. The first persons for whom training is critical are the parents or guardians of children who are identified as being deafblind. This process will include educating the parents themselves about deafblindness and providing them with sufficient knowledge to become the first 'expert' in their child's life. Education and training for parents concerning all aspects of the disability their child faces is a prerequisite for their having sufficient knowledge to act as an advocate for their infant, child, youth, or adult with deafblindness. Next, this education must extend to the remainder of the child's family, including siblings, grandparents, and others.

Following this step, the advocate must broaden the focus to the include the neighbourhood and ultimately the community. At this point, the advocate should ensure that the parents, if they are willing, are partners in the advocacy process and have become effective members of the advocacy team. Ultimately, it will become a family and community responsibility to assist in making a reality of the 'quality-of-life dream' established by the parents. It has been said that it takes a community to raise a child; the situation is no different for a child who is deafblind.

The support of knowledgeable persons in the community is the key. However, one cannot ignore, or overestimate, the role the parents have as advocates in the early years. They will become advocates (whether they wish to or not) and will play a major role in forming the perceptions of their child held by those outside their family circle, including medical personnel, emergency workers, and the workers in community services they wish to utilize. Parents who are unable to carry out community advocacy for whatever reason need a strong advocacy organization to provide them with support until they are able to assume the role. It is extremely discouraging when unenlightened medical and/ or educational professionals disregard the knowledge held by and the contributions available from parents. This attitude, which is all too prevalent, can be very difficult to ignore unless the parents have the active support of an advocate with specialized training in the field of deafblindness. Parents acting as educators or advocates are often threatening to professionals in the fields of medicine, education, and service delivery, which may cause negative reactions fuelled by professional insecurity. Not all professionals are secure enough to say 'I don't know' when presented with an area in which they possess little or no knowledge. Such reactions by professionals tend to destroy parents' confidence and fuel their insecurity in turn.

When parents choose not to take on the role of advocate (and some may not do so because of feelings of insecurity or guilt), they run the risk of having their child, as early as two or three years old, mislabelled as mentally challenged or developmentally delayed, and they will not have the knowledge or stature to question such labels. (Of course, a child who is deafblind is following a different, and longer, developmental path from that taken by his peers who do not face the same challenges. Such comparisons serve no useful purpose and merely provide some sense of security for the uninformed professional making them.) It is crucial that parents understand the disability, so that they have the confidence to advocate for appropriate services for their child.

Establishing an Ongoing Advocacy Process

Starting with the parent as advocate, the process will evolve as the child matures and various other persons enter the child's life. Advocacy will change as its goals change. It can be described as analogous to a wheel. The broad network of support persons serves as the spokes of the wheel. The child is at the hub and parents may be viewed as being both the grease that keeps the wheel smoothly turning and the cotter pin that prevents the unit from falling apart. At any one time the advocacy team may consist of parents, siblings, grandparents and other extended family members, community workers, medical personnel, social workers, psychologists, and educators. An independent advocate may be present on the team in addition to or supplementing the parents or other family members. Such a team may meet officially or simply exist to be called upon as needed by the deafblind person, the family, or a case manager. The team will be further strengthened by the inclusion of a representative of an advocacy organization. The individual with deafblindness must be included as an essential part of the team as soon as he or she is able to participate. The team is an evolving and dynamic support network.

Intervenors as Advocates

Woven tightly within advocacy and inseparable from education is the emphasis on the deafblind individual's receiving Intervention. Intervention, can arguably be a different form of advocacy, but so saying should not interfere with the clear meaning of intervention. Intervenors or persons who have worked as Intervenors can (and do) make exceptional advocates. Their experience helping a deafblind person to identify options, express wants and needs, and make independent choices makes them well qualified as advocates. This is not to suggest that the individual's Intervenor should also be his or her advocate; but that function should not necessarily be ruled out if it is the family's choice.

The advocacy role of Intervenors, whether they are a parent, a family member, a paid professional, or a volunteer will focus attention sharply on this fundamental need for intervention and the need for sufficient individualized support. It is in this situation that it is difficult to separate where intervention stops and advocacy begins or vice versa.

Different Forms of Advocacy

Individual Advocacy

Few individuals who are congenitally deafblind or who have early acquired deafblindness can advocate for themselves independently without support from other individuals, including family. For this reason little emphasis is placed on this form. Instead, in this section the focus is on other forms of advocacy, including the professional, political, and organizational forms.

Professional Advocacy

The role of the parents and family as advocates has already been outlined. The professional or agency-based advocate is useful in supporting the parents and family members as they advocate for their child. The professional advocate should empower families and eventually the person who is deafblind to advocate for themselves. Some of their duties include supporting the family as they make contact with government or community agencies and educational authorities; the writing, or assisting with the writing of proposals; and the gathering of necessary information for and the writing of Personal Plans. Strict confidentiality is an absolute must for the advocate.

Political Advocacy

The essential functions of a political advocate are to lobby the political and bureaucratic arms of government, to communicate awareness of the disability of deafblindness, and to identify and help to overcome potential problems that may arise. The purpose of this advocacy is to seek action at all levels of government in order to achieve services for all persons who are deafblind or to redress a specific problem that has arisen. The political advocate may take direction in terms of priorities and tasks from a non-profit organization, but final decisions as to appropriate action must rest with the person who is deafblind or his or her family. To function as an effective political advocate will require the individual to have good communication with that organization and to be aware of the needs of its members and client group. He or she must establish and nurture contacts at all levels of government and with private and corporate sponsors who may be called upon, from time to time, for both concrete and moral support. A strong and effective networking system must be established and maintained to ensure continued effectiveness of this process.

Organizational Advocacy

An organization will advocate to achieve certain standards or conditions for persons who are deafblind. This would ensure that persons who are deafblind achieve the best quality of life. The person who is deafblind should enjoy the same rights and freedoms as every other person. These rights are as follows:

• To have equality of opportunity to ensure that individual potential is realized
• To achieve independence and self-sufficiency through participating in the mainstream of society
• To have access to services that guarantee basic survival, personal, social, and vocational development and a sense of self-worth.

The advocacy role of the association would include the following aspects:

• Lobbying governments for services for persons who are deafblind, including intervention
• Early and continuing education, health, and psychiatric care
• Supported independent living requirements
• Recommending the need for developing service standards and greater coordination of services
• Special emphasis required to ensure employment opportunities and improved accessibility
• Explaining the need for a special definition of deafblindness
• Developing greater public awareness about the needs for persons who are deafblind
• Explaining the causes of and possible methods to prevent deafblindness
• Informing persons who are deafblind and their parents or guardians about the services available
• Explaining how to lobby or petition governments for services
• Ensuring that parents and professionals have the opportunity to work as a team in designing programs, in program delivery, and in the development of standards and guidelines.

Advocacy associations should act as a watchdog at all levels of government on behalf of persons who are deafblind, to ensure that they receive an equal opportunity to have the best quality of life. These associations should ensure that the services are appropriate, well conceived, well funded, and delivered according to recognized national and international standards.

The Process of Advocacy

Prerequisites to Begin Advocacy

If the advocacy is to be directed towards obtaining an individual service program for a person who is deafblind (e.g., year-round intervention program) or to seek services for a group of individuals (e.g., independent living facility for a group of young adults), a Personal Program, including parts 5 and 6 should be developed (see chapter 2).

Good Advocacy Practices

General Considerations

The following points should be incorporated into the advocacy approach you make to an agency or government body.

1. Make no apologies for the advocacy. Persons who are deafblind have the same rights as all citizens to a certain quality of life, and the advocate is simply attempting to gain services to ensure that these rights are fulfilled.
2. Focus on the benefits to the individual, the community, and to society as a whole when persons who are deafblind are provided with appropriate services. Supply as much background information as possible that is relevant to ensuring a positive outcome.
3. Identify the person in the target agency or organization who has the authority or power to make decisions or can influence the final decision. In other words, aim high in the funding organization.
4. Bring several key individuals to the meeting. Where appropriate, always include the person who is deafblind, accompanied by a Intervenor. Insist that the Intervenor communicate who is there and everything being said that would have relevance. The Intervenor is not a participant in the meeting when he or she is providing intervention. At the beginning of the meeting, as the Intervenor is being introduced, a short explanation of what he or she will be doing should be given. All meetings should be attended by a parent/guardian-appointed advocate and an independent professional in the field of deafblindness.

5. A group has impact and cannot easily be ignored. Be careful, however, not to have too large a group. A large group may make the official with whom you are meeting feel at a disadvantage, which may jeopardize present and possibly future results.

6. Assert as much influence as possible with the key individual to obtain a commitment and obtain this in writing. Remember, however, that in the eyes of the bureaucrat first meetings are usually to identify the problem, and follow-up meetings are usually held to explore specific, unresolved questions or to identify options available. A final meeting, to which superiors are often invited, is usually held to announce the solution.

7. Solutions are rarely negotiated at meetings. Usually they will be negotiated by the person you met with and educated and his superiors. This is particularly the case if you are attempting to establish a new program or to modify an existing program or set of regulations.

8. Create a record of each meeting and ensure that there is a follow-up schedule established for further meetings, correspondence, clarification, and so on, all of which focus on reaching the decision leading to the signing of the agreement to support the individual who is deafblind.

9. Once the 'right' decision is made, see if there is a way to acknowledge or publicly identify the contributions made by the funding agent and/or a particular bureaucrat. If it is their wish, involve them in the formulation of, or at least check with them on, the wording of any press release or public announcement. In other words, if possible, seek some form of recognition for the agency, corporation, individual, or private donor.

10. Be as assertive, courteous, competent, and persistent as possible. If at first you do not succeed, try again. Don't accept 'no' for an answer. Determine what went wrong, what new approach is necessary, and schedule a return engagement, always with the intent to obtain the 'right' decision. But keep in mind that the bureaucrat rarely expects to solve a problem or reach a decision at a public meeting.

Additional Useful Procedures or Tips

The following points will also be useful when an appeal is being made to a government or other agency by, or on behalf of, the individual who is deafblind.

Keep Records
Keep a diary containing the names of everyone you talk to or write to, record the date, name, title, agency, means of contact (complete address and telephone number), and advice or instructions received, as well as any follow-up action to be taken by you or by agency personnel.

Keep a file of all correspondence that you send and receive. If it is not self-evident, make sure to record the date and from whom a copy was received or to whom it was sent or given.

If possible, have the Intervenor assist the person who is deafblind to keep personal records of any meetings he or she participates in.

Preparing for the First Meeting

Contact all the people you wish to accompany you to the meeting, and make sure you know when they will be available (days, times, and dates) before you write or telephone to the agency.

Be sure you understand exactly what you are going to ask for. A request for 'more money for intervention' is too vague.

Have a Personal Plan prepared, including parts 5 and 6 (see chapters 2 and 10).

Indicate the number of hours that family members, volunteers, and paid Intervenors are spending with the individual who is deafblind. Be sure to indicate the value of these hours based upon the rate of pay that an Intervenor is receiving in your area.

Indicate the number of additional hours required and why, as well as how they will be used.

Identify any community resources that are being used and how. Include both the physical equipment used and the dollars that are being received.

Identify any community agencies to which you have appealed for funds and their response. Stress those from whom the response was positive. If the answer was 'no,' indicate why the request was refused.

Identify the consequences of the request's not being met. The worst thing that can happen is later to have some government official point out that you are receiving some assistance that you have not identified at this stage. Should such support be added during the advocacy process, be sure that all parties know of its existence immediately.

Summarize the most important points of (preparation) in written form for ready reference during the meeting. In some cases it is even advantageous to supply this summary to all those attending the meeting.

The written summary should be no more than *one page* in length. It should state the problem, show why existing services do not meet the need, and emphasize the important points made in the accompanying material. Attach the summary at the front of any additional material you are submitting.

Background Information

Identify the branch of government, public agency, or private agency you should be contacting for a meeting. Make the necessary enquiries to be sure that your request is going to be made to the correct funding source. Little else is as discouraging as to be told, after you have done all the work and presented a very good case, that 'Unfortunately, you should have approached this or that branch of the agency or government with your request.'

Identify the person in the organization whom you should be approaching. Usually, the initial telephone call should be made or the initial letter written to the head of the agency or the head of its local office.

If possible, maintain an approach to an individual who has the authority to say 'YES' to your request. Many organizations have layers of bureaucracy, and individuals who function on the lower level often have the power to say 'no' but no power to commit funds, that is, to say 'yes' to your request. Take the time necessary to identify who can do what. In many organizations your request will be referred to an individual at a lower level whose function is to screen all requests and to forward those that meet established criteria to a committee for further screening. You want to differentiate your request from the ordinary in this person's eyes.

This referral to a committee is often the first step. Comply with any instructions that you receive, either in writing or during a telephone conversation. BUT, in addition, write to the individual concerned requesting a face-to-face meeting.

Sometimes, you will be sent an official form to fill in and submit. Your goal is a face-to-face meeting. If you receive such a form, and you feel that you cannot present your case adequately by answering its questions or filling in boxes, in every appropriate place write 'Please see attached' and attach the Personal Program and any additional information you feel will help the reader understand the unique problems faced. Also attach the summary you have prepared (point (b) above).

Initial Formal Contact

Regardless whether the desired meeting is arranged by telephone or correspondence, the parents, person who is deafblind, or advocate should write a businesslike letter that

- thanks the individual for his or her time; be sure to spell the name correctly and identify the title correctly – if in doubt, contact the agency's receptionist for the information
- confirms the time, place, and date of the meeting
- identifies the purpose of the meeting
- identifies all individuals who will be attending the meeting; the meeting will start on a very poor note if political and/or expert individuals who the agency representative is not expecting to meet arrive – any initial advantage gained will be lost in the long run

- lists any accompanying information, not previously submitted, that will assist the individual with whom you are meeting to understand the request
- gives your address and telephone number for easy reference.

It is always a good idea to telephone the day before the meeting to ensure that the meeting will be held at the time and place agreed upon.

An Example

2 June 199–
Mr John Littlepower, Area Supervisor
Social Service Division 12
Government of Poorland

Dear Mr Littlepower:
Thank you for taking time to reply to the letter that I sent to the Director General of Social Services. We are looking forward to meeting with you in Conference Room 3A on Thursday, 11 June. My husband and I will be accompanied by Mr William Knowit, a consultant from the Ministry of Education's Deafblind Centre, Ms Sally Smooth from your Department of Social Services, as well as my son and his Intervenor. We would like the meeting to focus upon the steps that must be followed to obtain appropriate support for our son who is deafblind when he graduates from school next year. At present, it would appear to us that no such services exist. We have attached to this letter a proposed Personal Program designed for our son, a list of the support he is currently receiving and several letters from agencies and community programs stating that they have no existing programs for a young man who is both deaf and blind. You will note that several of the letters clearly show that these agencies do not even understand what his basic needs would be.
We look forward to meeting with you.

Mrs D. Termind
123 4th Ave.
Localville, Poorland
Home Telephone: 555 567 9000 Work: 555 111 2234

The First Meeting

First impressions are lasting. Do everything you can to ensure you make a good, business like impression. Arrive on time. It is usually wise to meet at some location close by and go to the meeting site as a group. There is nothing more disruptive than someone rushing in late. Identify who is going to speak for the group and make the main presentation. It usually should be the person who is deafblind, his or her advocate, or the parents, rather than a professional. The professional's role should be confined to a succinct description of deafblindness and its consequences for the individual in question. The professional should also be prepared to answer questions directed to him or her by the spokesperson for the group or the agency representatives present.

In most cases the underlying goal for this first meeting is to educate the agency representatives and elicit their support. The most important thing to keep in mind is that you are preparing the agency representative to speak on your behalf. The time you take in identifying exactly what information is to be conveyed to him or her is time is well spent. He or she is the person who will be answering questions raised by colleagues and superiors concerning your request when it is being discussed after you leave. The main thing to avoid is putting the agency representative in a position where he or she will have to say 'NO'!

If it appears that a negative response is likely, the spokesperson for the group should bring the meeting to a close by thanking the agency representative for his or her time, explaining that meeting with him or her has given the group much to think about, and, if possible, arranging a date for the next meeting after such consideration has taken place. If you force the agency representative to say 'no,' in most jurisdictions this answer will be defended all the way to the top, and even if you get it overturned at the political level there will be a lingering resentment at the agency level.

The client representatives should get together immediately after the initial meeting for five to ten minutes to discuss the next step and to compose a follow-up letter to be written by the deafblind person, his or her advocate, or the parents.

The Follow-up Letter

The letter is very important. It should accomplish the following:

1. Thank the agency representative for his or her time
2. List any items you feel have been agreed upon
3. List any items left to be discussed at a follow-up meeting
4. Request or confirm the date for a follow-up meeting as well as identifying its purpose and who will be accompanying the writer.

An Example

12 June 199–
Mr John Littlepower, Area Supervisor
Social Service Division 12
Government of Poorland

Dear Mr Littlepower:
My husband and I wish to take this opportunity to thank you for taking time to meet with us on Thursday, 11 June. We found the meeting most helpful. It is our understanding that we have agreed on the following:

- Deafblindness is a unique disability, which cannot be served by existing services to adults who are either blind or deaf.
- There are no appropriate services to meet my son's needs as a person with congenital deafblindness when he graduates from school in June next year.
- You will investigate services being received from our government by other persons who are congenitally deafblind.

It is agreed that your branch of government is the proper agency from which to seek support.

A second meeting will take place within the next three weeks to examine items not yet addressed and to hear the information that you have been able to obtain.

The type and amount of support to be made available was yet to be identified at the close of the meeting,

In addition, as the meeting closed, it was suggested by you that you may wish to invite other individuals from government services to attend the next meeting.

After discussion among those who attended on our son's behalf, we find ourselves in complete agreement with your suggestion. We request that you let us know their names and the areas of government these additional people represent prior to the meeting.

You also requested copies of the magazines *Talking Sense* and *Dbl Review* as well as the loan of *Programming and Support for Persons Who Are Congenitally Deafblind*. I will mail all of these items to you in a separate package when I mail this letter. We look forward to hearing from you about the date, time, and location of the next meeting as well as who will attend. We plan to have the same two people accompany my husband, my son and his Intervenor, and me.

Mrs D. Termind
123 4th Ave.
Localville, Poorland
Home Telephone: 555 567 9000 Work: 555 111 2234

Subsequent Meetings with 'Higher Authorities'

Subsequent meetings may be with the same agency or government representative, alone or with others of equal rank, or with the representative accompanied
by other individuals who have the power to say 'YES' to all or part of the
request. It will still usually remain, in the agency's eyes, the original representative's meeting, but the addition of more agency staff usually can be seen as
progress.

Before the meeting gets under way, always find out the names of any new
agency members (write them down, spelled correctly), their titles, and their
responsibilities. They will probably represent either another part of the agency
or the representative's superior. ALWAYS begin by thanking the agency representative for arranging the meeting and for his or her understanding and support. Involve him or her as much as possible in educating the new people about
deafblindness and why routine service provisions do not meet the needs of the
deafblind individual upon whose behalf the advocacy is being made.

In addition, the following points should be noted.

1. All other suggestions concerning the first meeting continue to hold true with
   any additional meetings with the same agency representative.
2. If the meeting includes a superior, or a representative from another part of
   the agency, write a separate letter thanking him or her using the format suggested above.
3. Remember that, in most cases, there is nothing that demands attention as
   much as a file, and your correspondence is building one. Telephone calls do
   not always have the same effect.

In many respects, the most important thing to remember is that the government
or agency representative you are meeting with wants to help you (no matter
how you may perceive it under the stress of the moment), and it is your job to
present facts and shape arguments that will assist him or her when meeting with
others.

In some agencies, decisions on fund allocation are made by a committee. It
will be the individual you have been talking to who will make the case for or

against support for your request. If your efforts at advocacy result in the request's being turned down, ask for another meeting and seek advice concerning how you can make another request that will be more successful. This is not the time to become discouraged or angry. Try to find out what arguments and approaches will be successful with this agency at this time. On many occasions the author has been told which approach will work best, when and how to bring the correct kind of political pressure, and/or the name of a specific person to whom the next attempt should be addressed. Above all, try to get any 'no' you receive turned into a 'maybe'!

Other Advocacy Techniques

If the objective is to get the message across and influence the bureaucracy or a funding agent, a number of other techniques are quite effective.

Lobbying through Letters

Letter writing is still a useful and constructive tool for calling attention to an individual situation or for seeking solutions to problems with a wider population of individuals with deafblindness. Letters can be written personally or through a form letter containing the standard information. The letters can be mailed, faxed, or sent through the Internet, providing the target audience has a fax number or electronic mail address. The more messages the better is the best advice. Letters should be courteous, legible, (preferably typed), and brief. They should be well organized, outlining the purpose, describing the issue, and presenting the recommended solution. The letter must be signed, a return mailing address included, and a response requested.

Preparing Briefs

A brief, which is a more detailed written description of an issue, can be a very effective tool for presenting an argument. Although it takes more time, it will demonstrate to the target audience the commitment for the cause presented. Briefs usually outline the purpose, describe in more detail the background issues or problems that should be addressed, outline a series of recommended options, determine the range of outcomes the various options can achieve, and present a desirable solution. Often governments ask for briefs regarding new policies, and organizations should take the opportunity to present their cases for consideration. Briefs are often used by organizations to present issues in a well-organized format.

Lobbying Elected Officials

Never underestimate the effectiveness of lobbying elected officials at whatever level of government they represent. Since they are elected to represent their constituents, they should know and understand the issues at hand in their particular area of influence. Don't forget that the issue presented does not necessarily stop with that elected official. He or she has a wide range of contacts at all levels of government and can broaden the influence if the issue is presented appropriately. Before taking a particular issue to an elected official, determine what his or her sphere of influence is. The influence that each level of government has over each individual who is deafblind should also be well understood. For example, if one is advocating for an individually based service program for an individual person who is deafblind, contacting a local or state representative would be more useful and effective than contacting a federal representative. If the intent is to get a municipal zoning bylaw changed to make it easier for a group independent-living facility to be established, then one would contact an elected municipal official rather than a state official. In some countries, contacting federal elected officials about deafblindness might be effective only for constitutional items, matters of employment equity, immigration, and so on. The differences of federal, state or regional, and municipal or county responsibilities vary widely among countries.

When lobbying elected officials, provide them with as much background information as possible (briefs, copies of letters written, and news articles). Invite them to a meeting of your advocacy organization. Invite them to speak at a public function. They will usually ask you, either directly or indirectly, for a prepared speech or particular points that reflect well on them. If the elected official you are lobbying is a member of a sitting government, it is sometimes wise also to inform the opposition party of the issue and approaches you have made to the elected governing party officials. Approaches to avoid include going to the opposition first or putting a government minister in the position of not being able to answer a question. Any short-term gains will probably be more than offset by the long-term consequences.

Using the Media

Advocates, be they individual or group, should recognize that using any and all forms of the media, TV, radio, and print can be an effective way of advocating. If lack of public awareness is an issue, change can be made through the media. The media must be educated first, however, after which media personnel can become effective partners to extend the message.

The media can be effective alternatives or additional means to put pressure on elected officials and government bureaucrats if personal advocacy did not gain a positive response or if you cannot obtain a meeting. An aware public then can become effective supplementary advocates.

Advocates and advocacy organizations should prepare news releases, letters to the editor, and public service announcements. Encourage public speaking and interviews on high-profile or local talk shows. Place advertisements in newspapers and magazines in an attempt to use the media to get the messages across.

Summary

1. Undeniably, persons who are deafblind have the same rights as every other person to a certain quality of life.
2. Individuals who are deafblind must not to be discriminated against through having a disability, according to the laws of most countries and the human rights guidelines of the United Nations.
3. Advocacy is the only way to develop a level playing field, equal for all citizens, regardless of disability and of the country in which they reside.
4. Advocacy for persons who are deafblind is different from that for other disabilities because of critical issues such as the uniqueness of the disability, its low incidence, special education needs, absence of a pool of community professional and semi-professional knowledge, and lack of public understanding.
5. Parents usually are the first advocates for their children who are deafblind. The purpose of this advocacy is to ensure that their children achieve quality of-life goals not unlike those desired by parents for any infant or child.
6. Education is a key step in any advocacy process. From the family perspective, education about deafblindness starts first in the home with the parents and family. This education and awareness then extends to the broader family network, to the neighbourhood, and eventually embraces the entire community.
7. Woven tightly within advocacy and inseparable from education is the emphasis on Intervention. Intervention is a form of advocacy and Intervenors can make exceptional advocates.
8. Advocacy can take the form of individual advocacy (i.e., parents or individuals interceding on behalf of an individual), political advocacy (i.e., lobbying political and bureaucratic arms of governments on behalf of an individual or group), and organizational advocacy (i.e., involving an organization striving to achieve certain programs or standards for groups of individuals).

9. Good advocacy practices include not making any apologies; being courteous, assertive, competent, and persistent; focusing on individual and community benefits; and identifying the key individuals who have influence and can make decisions.

10. When an appeal to a government agency is being made on behalf of an individual who is deafblind, the following tips may be useful: keep good records, prepare well for the first meeting, create a favourable first impression with a first meeting, and send a follow-up letter summarizing items agreed to and outstanding issues to be dealt with at later meetings.

11. Additional advocacy techniques include lobbying through letters, preparation of briefs, lobbying elected politicians, and utilizing the media.

NOTE

1 The Canadian Charter of Rights and Freedoms. Part 1 of the Canada Constitution Act, 1982. Section 15(1) states: 'Every individual is equal before and under the law and has the right to equal protection, without discrimination based on race, nationality, or ethnic origin, colour, religion, sex, age or mental or physical disability.'

REFERENCE

Merriam-Webster's Collegiate Dictionary, Tenth Edition Copyright © 1994 by Merriam-Webster, Inc. Merriam-Webster OnLine at http://www.m-w.com/home.htm

15

Physiotherapy for the Multiply Challenged Deafblind Individual

SHEILA EISLER

Introduction

Physiotherapy for multiply challenged individuals of all ages who are classified as deafblind is of a non-traditional nature. It is made all the more demanding because of the impairment of the two distance senses. Clients with sight and hearing are able to see actions carried out and the expression on the instructor's face and can clearly hear instructions. Those individuals who lack the full use of the distance senses, however, rely on tactile cues, taste, smell, and to a lesser extent any residual vision and/or hearing. For example, when you want a deafblind child to bend a knee, you (or the Intervenor) verbalize and also place a hand on the limb in the direction of movement. In addition, begin to establish a sign or gesture for that movement in order to build a vocabulary for future communication during therapy sessions. In the author's opinion, charisma, ability to read body language, ability to establish a bond, and an encouraging, positive attitude all are qualities required for treating deafblind individuals of any age.

The therapist forms part of the interdisciplinary team support for the deafblind individual. He or she has a duty to provide clearly written objectives; to ensure that those working with the individual can perform the exercises correctly; and to suggest to the parents and Intervenors activities that will incorporate the exercises in these daily activities. In the author's experience, no matter how poor a prognosis may appear on first examination, most deafblind persons have potential for improvement. This potential should be tapped to its fullest extent. In addition, they should have access to a full range of services available to those with other disabilities. There is strength in the continuation of physiotherapy from preschool, through kindergarten, to graduation, and into adult life. Teamwork is essential among medical personnel, physiotherapists, educators, family members, caregivers, and all others who are involved with the deafblind individual. Sufficient time should be allotted for each physiotherapy session to permit the therapist both to work with the client and to demonstrate how routine activities in the client's life can be utilized to ensure that benefits from the session are forthcoming. Visits to infants or children who are deafblind should be booked as equivalent to two sessions.

People who are involved with a young adult graduating from educational programs should be encouraged to visit and observe any physiotherapy program in which the young adult is participating prior to graduation. The parents and Intervenors should be present for periodic evaluation of the young adult's treatment program with reference to ongoing goals. This will help to ensure a smooth transition into an adult physiotherapy program. Many multiply challenged deafblind individuals will continue to need regular physiotherapy throughout their adult lives.

The individuals with deafblindness whom the author has treated have had different degrees of sight and hearing losses in addition to physical handicaps of varying severity. The aims in treating infants, children, youth, and adults – to make them as functionally independent as possible and to improve their quality of life – are the same for all.

On occasion, the author has accompanied a deafblind individual to consultations as part of the team to contribute to the decision-making process. Many multiply challenged deafblind individuals have numerous medical conditions that must be considered.

Physiotherapy should still be part of the program during periods of hospitalization for treatment or confinement to the home for periods of recuperation, though in a more passive form. The physiotherapist can always be involved in positive reinforcement of the caregivers and in advising on any physical actions that may be undertaken to ensure that non-affected body systems do not atrophy or suffer owing to lack of activity.

Programming

Medical and Other Problems

The majority of deafblind individuals whom the author has treated have **cerebral palsy**, which varies from mild to severe. Other conditions seen are **spina bifida** and **hydrocephalus**, deformities of the spine and limbs, which may be congenital or acquired, and degenerative neurological diseases. The most common symptoms seen are as follows:

• Deformities of the spine
• Posture with developing spinal deformities

- Deformities of the *peripheral joints*
- *Spasticity* of one or more limbs
- *Flaccidity* or *hypotonia* in varying degrees
- Generalized weakness
- 'Non-functional movements,' such as head rolling, arm waving, and rocking
- No concept of space, themselves, or themselves related to space
- Poor balance and coordination.

Non-Medical Considerations

The author feels that physiotherapy should not be a separate entity, but should be an integrated part of the Personal Plan. As such, elements of the therapy program will be seen in all activities. All individuals who interact with the deaf-blind person must be aware of the goals and objectives of the physiotherapy program and educational program and how they may be carried out during daily activities. Children who were receiving physiotherapy prior to admission to school should automatically receive physiotherapy as part of their Personal Plan until such time it is no longer needed.

Program Goals

The main goals of the physiotherapy program are as follows:

a) To teach *body image*
b) To teach *spatial awareness*
c) To teach an understanding of movement
d) To teach an understanding of exercise
e) To increase mobility
f) To increase strength and endurance
g) To improve standing and walking posture
h) To teach a good heel/toe gait
i) To improve coordination
j) To improve balance reactions
k) To improve fine finger and gross hand manipulation.

Any or all of these goals may be found in each individual's physiotherapy program, depending on the specific problems that have been identified.

Initial Approach

When a client with deafblindness is referred, the first task of the therapist is to get to know him or her, and to begin to establish a bond. The physiotherapist must gain acceptance to the level of the individual's cooperating passively with him or her. If the individual does not trust and have confidence in the therapist, his or her full potential will not be achieved. This bonding is important, since the deafblind client will be naturally suspicious. Approach him or her slowly. Establish a special touch for recognition, thus beginning to build a routine to promote interaction and communication.

When specialized equipment, for example, braces, is to be utilized in helping a deafblind client towards independence, certain procedures must be followed. This routine is important in order that the deafblind individual does not perceive such equipment as a threat and a limitation to whatever mobility and freedom they already possess. For example, where a brace may be directly placed on a sighted individual, with a deafblind person this procedure must never be hurried. The brace should be introduced slowly, and the individual should be allowed to handle it and become familiar with it. Work on body awareness and image to ensure a better understanding of where the brace is going and what it will do once it is in place. One or more whole physiotherapy sessions may be utilized for this purpose. It is important to promote understanding of the benefits of the braces by letting the deafblind person stand independently and then feel the support given by standing in the brace. It is imperative that all caregivers involved with the individual understand the correct fitting of the brace, have knowledge on how it works, and be involved in inspections for pressure sores.

Assessment

Once the confidence of the client has been gained, assessment can begin. This step must not be hurried. It must be remembered that the distance senses of sight and hearing are impaired. The physiotherapist must use his or her eyes and ears to note reactions as assessments are carried out, in addition to the tactile sense, which is much more important in the assessment of these individuals.

Prioritizing Problems
Which disabilities create the most problems? There are often multiple problems to be identified.

Body Image
Lack of the functional use of vision and hearing limits the formation concepts of body parts and how they function. There is often little or no *spatial aware-ness*, and this must be taught throughout daily activities. Young children who are deafblind have often been 'cocooned in a safe world of inactivity,' and the

problems resulting from this mistaken approach must be addressed and overcome. Awareness of body parts, the directions in which they will move, and
how such movements apply to movements in and through space must be taught.
One should not assume that, because an individual can respond correctly to a
request to raise his or her arm when lying on a mat, this ability will transfer to
raising the arm when standing. Simple movements, such as lifting a foot when it
is bare, may not transfer to lifting the foot once a shoe is put on. The knowledge
of body image, understanding of space, and where one is in space is something
that must be continually assessed and promoted as growth and development
takes place.

Posture

Posture can be poor because of an established spinal deformity, leg length dis-
crepancy, or *pelvic rotation*, any of which will produce an apparent shortening
of one leg. It may also be poor because of a developing deformity or hypotonia
of the muscles caused by inactivity. In addition, without sight, the deafblind
individual cannot 'see' and model others' good posture. Thus an *anterior
head position* and *protracted shoulder girdle* may often be observed in these
individuals.

Joint Range of Movement and Muscle Power

These capacities are usually poor, because of inactivity. Tightness of muscle
tendons is often noted, particularly of the *Achilles tendons*. This may have
resulted from poor positioning during infancy.

Gait

Gait is evaluated once the individual is ambulatory.

Balance

It is important to establish good balance and stability. The establishment of
head and neck control is essential for focusing the eyes and learning to use
residual vision.

Perception

Perception is often very poor and needs to be stimulated for efficient use in
daily activities. Occasionally, a child may present with hypersensitivity and tactile defensiveness. To reduce this problem always alert the child before attempting to manipulate him or her. Rubbing the problem areas (mainly feet and
hands), with firm pressure is helpful.

Spasticity
Spasticity must be reduced in order to facilitate smooth movements of the limbs. Some spasticity in the lower limbs, however, can often be used to advantage for stability in standing and walking.

Non-Functional Movements
These movements must be replaced by socially acceptable actions that will provide the stimulation sought (see chapters 5 and 6 for a full discussion of this point).

Implementing the Program

Physiotherapy should be started as early as possible for infants and children who are deafblind to prevent the development of deformities. Physiotherapists who carry out home visits should schedule their appointments to allow for 'getting to know you' periods during each visit until the client indicates that it is no longer necessary. The deafblind individual will need time, and maybe many visits, to become familiar with the therapist. Physiotherapy should not be started until the individual is comfortable and relaxed.

It is imperative that family and non-family Intervenors watch and participate during the physiotherapy sessions. In addition to having clinical responsibilities, the physiotherapist will take on the role of instructor for those present and must ensure that procedures are taught correctly. This will allow the observers to carry out the procedures and maintain continuity between visits by the physiotherapist. At the end of the physiotherapy session 'good-byes' take place, indicating the end of exercises, maybe with an established routine or a cuddle, while the therapist discusses specific parts of the program with the caregivers.

Helpful Hints for Working with Infants

The author would like to see children first when they are babies, thereby eliminating certain problems later on. The following is a list of 'helpful hints,' prepared by the author for people working with very young children.

Positioning
This factor is very important, since many deformities develop through incorrect positioning of the baby, such as *plantar-flexed feet* and *laterally rotated hips*. When the baby is lying, the head should be in a neutral position and the legs should be together. There should be no weight pressing the feet down creating

plantar flexion of the feet and tightness of the Achilles tendons. Change the baby's position frequently. Proper positioning is also important for maximizing the child's ability to use residual vision and hearing.

Passive Movements

All joints should be taken through their full range of movement at least twice a day. This will prevent tightening of ligaments and will develop the baby's concept of space and position in space. Deafblind infants and young children do not naturally go through the range of movements during their daily activities. Care should be taken to ensure that activities promote this range of movement throughout the day through the use of appropriate intervention techniques.

Fine Finger and Gross Hand Manipulation

Important for any infant and more so for the deafblind child whose method of communication will be signing, emphasis should be placed on developing hand movements from the basics. Hand movements are necessary for gross hand function, which ultimately leads to efficient fine finger manipulation. Encourage the baby to grasp objects by initially curling your fingers and hands around the baby's fingers and hands and exerting a small amount of pressure. Progress to objects of varying sizes and textures. Activities throughout the day, such as dressing, washing, eating, exploring and playing with objects, '*father play*,' are some of the most effective ways to promote development in this area. All such activities should be enjoyable and should promote communication between the Intervenor and the infant.

Non-Functional Movements

If the baby exhibits movements such as head shaking or excessive rocking, replace them with a more socially acceptable activity using appropriate intervention techniques. If non-functional movements happen during a therapy session, gentle pressure or touch may still the movement. If you do this, be sure that the child consciously participates in the remainder of the session. Often, when such an approach is taken, the child may shut out the world for minutes or even longer periods.

Programming for Children, Youth, and Adults

A physiotherapy program must be prepared to meet individual needs. Begin by exercising all muscle groups. Take care to stimulate all senses emphasizing the use of residual vision and hearing. Remember that the deafblind individual is often very suspicious and apprehensive of any additions to, or changes in, routines. For this reason, it is important to begin very slowly and progress at the individual's own pace. Sometimes there may be swift progress, which then may plateau for a period. Communicate through vocal and tactile cues and sign language. Be sure that your body language is relaxed and conveys success and pleasure when any attempt is made to communicate.

Exercises are broken down into basic components initially and are started in the form of passive movements, with the physiotherapist supporting and carrying the limb through a range of movement. Many repetitions are essential to reinforce each movement, and it is good practice to allow individuals to initiate exercises to enhance this reinforcement. It is important not to move on too quickly, since doing so will produce confusion or frighten the child and could result in resistance. By supported repetition, the infant, child, or youth with deafblindness learns to carry out the movement independently. Encouragement is given by tapping or applying pressure to areas you want moved. Remember that you are working on motoric memory rather than visual memory.

Begin with small movements in a stable, secure position, and then, as confidence is gained, widen the range of movement and change positions. Start with exercises on the floor in a stable position. Progress to exercises performed while seated on a chair. Then progress to exercises done while standing with a wall or Intervenor for support. Finally, proceed to doing exercises while standing independently. Another example of exercise progression is from rolling, to sitting, to kneeling, to crawling, and finally to standing. The deafblind child may 'jump' one of these stages, and progress is encouraged, but it is important to go back and teach each phase through the use of age-appropriate activities of daily living. Occasionally, full potential may be reach in a particular area. When more progress is not expected, goals should be modified and directed at the prevention of regression.

Tolerance for activity is often low, and it is sometimes advisable to adopt a 'little and often' routine. Therapy sessions should incorporate a 'work time, relax time' approach. It is vital to overall success that therapy sessions include 'hands-on' people. They should watch when the therapist is working so that they can continue exercises by incorporating the movements in ongoing routine activities. In addition, they can be provided with a list of exercises with a description as to how to carry them out and suggestions as to how they may be incorporated in daily routines. This list can then accompany the deafblind individual to be used by people who were unable to attend the therapy sessions. The list should include photographs of the therapist and the individual carrying out individual exercises. Photos of the exercises being incorporated into daily activities will also greatly enhance the usefulness of the list. This approach will maintain continuity and help to reduce the chances of regression due to breaks, holidays, or major changes in daily routine.

Exercises should be functional and directed towards achieving independence, for instance, hand exercises will improve hand function for eating and performing life skills. Exercises should also be enjoyable in order to motivate the individual to do them.

Physiotherapy programs for deafblind individuals require a long-term approach extending over many years. Lack of interest and boredom must be avoided by varying the format, the equipment used, the methods of presentation, and a positive response from the therapist to work well done. During the week, where applicable, it is recommended that the physiotherapy program be varied to include exercises on a mat, or a bench, hand exercises at a table, and standing, in addition to instruction in the correct method for climbing and descending stairs.

Hydrotherapy and Swimming Pools

Access to a *hydrotherapy* pool is very advantageous. Warm water relaxes and will aid in gaining range of movement. It also is invaluable for teaching balance and gait. In addition, the properties of the water can be used to provide resistance for muscle strengthening. Use of a regular pool for swimming and 'play exercises' will help to enhance the child's confidence and to improve cardiovascular development and spatial orientation. A multiply challenged deafblind individual who is limited in range of movement often displays improvement when manipulated in a swimming pool. Understanding of movement through space is often promoted in this environment because the resistance of the water provides a more tangible cue than that of air. The water provides additional motivation to explore and play as well as to reach, stretch, and rotate his or her limbs, and water play can lead to the development of further recreational pursuits.

Practical Applications of Physiotherapy Exercises

Over the last sixteen years the author has developed many ways of promoting significant progress through physiotherapy. When she carries out an exercise program, her personal rule is 'Give the minimum support required to gain maximum output.' This may be total support or as little as a gentle tap in the direction of movement. All the exercises will begin with the therapist doing them coactively with the deafblind individual. As the individual moves from the awareness stage to the acquisition stage, the therapist and the individual will do the exercises co-operatively. When the routine is established and the child understands what the desired outcome is, the therapist will gradually reach the stage where he or she provides only an undifferentiated prompt to support the child in the activity. The ability to generalize the particular exercise and to assimilate it into a general level of response will be achieved by incorporating the exercise into the daily routines. The individual follows life-skills and recreational activities he or she enjoys, at the same time moving through the Reaction Sequence as the therapist moves in parallel through the Presentation Sequence. (see chapter 2).

Be generous with praise and encouragement. To see a smile of pleasure when success is achieved and progress is made is the physiotherapist's greatest reward. The following are examples of how exercise can be woven into activities, which will disguise hard work through the promotion of enjoyment.

Spasticity

Spasticity can be reduced by rocking, shaking, or stroking the affected area. Stroking with an ice cube wrapped in a tissue is sometimes very effective.

Improvement of Muscle Power

Encourage the child to push his or her legs straight against resistance from a flexed leg position. To improve muscle power in the upper limbs, have the child lying across your knees (you are on the floor sitting on your heels) and encourage him or her to push up on extended arms. Progress to modified push-ups and then wheelbarrows, with the child 'walking' on his or her hands while you hold the hips and legs.

Balance

Balance is improved by having the child sit cross-legged on the floor, in four-point kneeling, sitting in a chair, or by standing and then gently pushing him or her in all directions. Wobble boards, tricycles, wagons, skate and scooter boards, roller and ice skates, float boards, trampolines, stationary bikes, swings, slides, merry-go-rounds, teeter totters, gliders, and spring-mounted animals all provide fun activities to improve balance. Horseback riding has proved a favourite both of individuals who are deafblind and of the person providing intervention during the activity

Coordination and Control

Slow, smooth movements are essential for achieving coordination and control. Work towards these goals by alternate straight-arm raising and lowering and alternate knee bending and straightening. Initially, these exercises will carried out passively. Progress by decreasing tactile cues until the exercise is done independently upon request. Next, incorporate these exercises into games like 'follow the leader.' The therapist is the leader, while the Intervenor and deaf-blind child are the followers. Once the game is understood, switch roles. Through the use of vibrating floors and musical instruments that emit vibrations, such as drums, pianos, and guitars, encourage the child to incorporate these exercises into rhythmic movements. Playing toy soldiers, ballerina, or gymnast, complete with appropriate costumes, can also make these exercises more fun for the children.

Hand Exercises

1. Therapy Putty
   a) Roll in both hands to make a ball.
   b) Roll out on a table with one hand, then the other, to make a sausage.
   c) Pinch the ends with tip of thumb and index finger and curl around and squeeze ends together to form a 'doughnut.'
   d) Flatten the putty to make a 'cookie,' using alternate hands.
   e) Make 'patterns' in the cookie with the tip of thumb and tip of each finger in turn.
   f) Make containers by flattening the putty ball and then using fingers and thumb to shape a bowl, cup, glass, box, and so on.
   Exercises done with therapy putty usually have many practical applications and can be promoted much better with deafblind individuals when they are incorporated into daily living-skills or recreational activities. Making pizza, cookies, biscuits, pie, and other dough-based food items will promote the same exercises and also provide a tangible reward for the effort. Having the child make his or her own play dough or therapy putty will help to maintain interest in finger and hand exercises. This also allows the therapist to control the consistency of the 'putty' to match the level of functioning strength of the hand and fingers. As always, the therapist or Intervenor must use these activities to promote the use of any residual senses, communication skills, integration of sensory input, perceptual and conceptual development, as well as the physical exercise involved. Adding corn meal, rice, pasta, white dry beans or anything else you fancy to your dough of flour, salt, food colouring, water, and a special scent promotes variety and increases motivation to do finger and hand exercises. There are a number of commercial toys on the market that use putty or dough-like material and they often include cookie cutters and other pieces of equipment that can be

used for cutting, shaping, weaving, squashing, and building, while at the same time further promoting finger and hand exercises. Activities such as pottery, jewellery making, weaving, knitting, woodworking, and hand and machine sewing represent some of the many hobbies that incorporate hand and finger exercises while they provide recreational activities for the deaf-blind individual. Shopping trips to purchase supplies for such activities promote the application of finger, hand, and other exercises during real-life experiences.

2. Tap the fingertips of each finger in turn.
3. Make a fist and knock the knuckles on the table.
4. Tap the back of the hands and fingers on the table.
5. 'Sweep' the table with the palms from centre, out, and back.
6. Fingertips and wrists down, fingers straight and bent at the knuckles, tap the table (*lumbrical action*).
7. Turn the hands over to touch the table with the backs of the hands, then back to touch the palms to the table (*pronation* and *supination*) for receiving things.

Suggested activities, items 2 to 7, can be made more appealing by adding texture and noise to the activities and by varying the surface of the table, which may be accomplished by placing a piece of velvet, silk, or corduroy material, or fur under the hand. Rug samples, bubble packing, sandpaper, or other textured materials also may be used. The use of keyboards and other percussion or stringed instruments also will add variety to the exercises.

8. Tap the fingertips of both hands together.
9. Tap the heels of the hands together.
10. Interlace the fingers then place them 'quietly' together (palms touching).
11. Pick up buttons and small objects with the tips of the thumb and each finger in turn.
12. Use an elastic band for strengthening the finger and thumb flexor muscles. Place the tip of the thumb into the band and pull to stretch it with a finger. Repeat with each finger in turn.
13. Make a fist, then spread the fingers and palms flat on the table.
14. Curl the fingers of the right hand over the fingers of the left hand and try to pull them apart.

Once the following exercises are introduced and the fundamentals have been taught, they can be incorporated into a variety of routines and become part of a recreational program. Shopping for exercise clothing and using a variety of school or community gym facilities can provide motivation for practising exercises. Having the deafblind individual help to plan and carry out an exercise class for others will provide further opportunity to practise and better develop these skills. Projects like this will also allow Intervenors and other team members to work towards the achievement of a number of objectives found in the individual's Personal Plan. These exercises can also be practised in therapy and swimming pools. The application of imagination can go a long way towards taking the drudgery out of the repetition required to persevere with the needed therapy exercises.

Lying

1. Feet up and down.
2. Alternate knee bending and straightening, slowly with control and against resistance.
3. Alternate straight leg raising, toes pointing upward.
4. Sit-ups.
5. Alternate straight-arm raising above the head.
6. Both arms straight above the head and down with control.
7. Curl up in a ball, then stretch in all directions.

Crook Lying
a) Lift alternate feet up and down, keeping the heels down. Lift both feet up and down, keeping the heels down.
b) Lift the bottom to make a bridge.
c) Keeping the knees and feet together, drop knees from side to side.

Prone Lying
a) Push-ups.
b) Hands behind the back, lift the head and shoulders.
c) Tuck the toes under and lift the knees to make a bridge.
d) Alternate straight-leg raising, keeping the pelvis down.

Side Lying
Lift the top leg up in the air and down (keep the leg straight). Turn over and repeat with other leg.

Four-Point Kneeling

Gently push in all directions to improve balance reactions and strengthen the arms and legs.

Crawling

Use of obstacle courses will make all aspects of this exercise more fun. Paths can be varied through the use of equipment that will provide opportunities to go through, around, under, and over them. Paths between obstacles can be indicated through the use of mats and other tactile material.

Sitting on the Floor

Lift the bottom with the hands and move backward, forward, sideways, and in a circle.

High Sitting

1. Alternate and together, move feet up and down.
2. Mark time, lifting alternate knees.
3. Straighten alternate knees.
4. Straighten both knees with the toes pointing upward.
5. Lift bottom, pushing on the hands.

Standing

1. Start with the back to wall – head up, shoulders back, legs straight, arms by the sides, and feet together; step away from the wall and maintain this good posture.
2. Stand on one leg, then on the other.
3. Squats done slowly, with control.
4. Crouch down as small as possible, then jump up.
5. Arm swinging, backward and forward.
6. Raise alternate knees.

Gait

Begin gait training by having the child stand in the circle of your arms and carry out modified 'squats' until the feeling of transferring weight through the legs is established. Then, giving lots of support, progress to a heel/toe gait in order to establish the correct gait pattern from the onset. Bad habits formed in early stages of walking are very difficult to break! As confidence is gained, reduce the amount of support until the individual is walking independently.

Conclusion

In conclusion, working with infants, children, youths, and adults with deaf-blindness is enormously satisfying and challenging. The physiotherapist must understand the challenges posed by the loss of the effective use of the two distance senses. He or she must use this knowledge, combined with patience and imagination, to modify assessment techniques and the resulting treatments.

All deafblind individuals should have access to an assessment by a physiotherapist. If one is not available, every attempt should be made to have the family doctor make arrangements for access to an appropriate assessment. When the assessment indicates that treatment is necessary, a routine of frequent physiotherapy sessions should be established and the physiotherapist should become a member of the support team. Where it is needed, physiotherapy should viewed as an essential part of the individual's Personal Plan.

Summary

1. Physiotherapy is not isolated to one age group, but should be available to all age groups from babies to adults.
2. There must be empathy and a bond between the therapist and the individual.
3. The therapist must have a positive attitude and use generous praise, to ensure that maximum potential is reached in the individual being treated.
4. There must be teamwork between all who work with the individual who is deafblind, with the aim of gaining functional independence and improvement of his or her quality of life.
5. During the initial meeting and throughout the time the individual is receiving physiotherapy, never rush when treating individuals who are deafblind.
6. Integration of the program into school and home life is important. The program must be geared to the level of function of the individual and the ability to take part in school and home activities.
7. Therapists who carry out home visits should arrange to schedule their appointments for longer periods to allow for 'getting to know you' and 'good bye' routines, which are very necessary.
8. When you are carrying out an assessment, it is necessary to use your eyes and ears to note reactions.
9. Physiotherapy should be carried out for the whole child, and should not be limited to one area, such as a limb.
10. Security and stability will result in an increased confidence of the individual.

11. Start exercises with passive movements in a small range and gradually progress to independent movement and a widening of the range.
12. Repetition is used to reinforce the exercises in the individual's mind.
13. Functional exercises result in the individual's being more independent, for instance, hand exercises for eating and keyboarding.
14. Make the exercises interesting, varied, and fun to prevent boredom and loss of motivation.
15. Use the minimal support required to gain maximum output by the individual.

16

Intervenor, Teacher, and Consultant Training

MARGOT McGRATH-HARDING, WILLIAM THOMPSON, and JOHN M. McINNES

Introduction

It has been established in previous chapters of this text that deafblindness is a unique disability. As a unique disability, it requires individuals with a specific set of identifiable skills and a unique set of knowledge to work towards the amelioration of the problems associated with deafblindness. In this chapter we shall address the specifics of these requirements as they apply to Intervenors, teachers, and consultants.

Intervenor Training

by Margot McGrath-Harding

Introduction

Currently, there are two major avenues for the training of Intervenors: in house and academically based. An in-house training program is designed for those employed by a specific agency, family, or program. While this leads to the Intervenor's being very well trained for one particular situation, it does little to promote a more global understanding of deafblindness or intervention. Intervenors develop only limited transferable skills that allow them to take advantage of other opportunities. Given few resources to draw from, Intervenors can feel inadequately prepared for the physical and emotional demands of the job. While formalized training programs offer greater possibilities for a broader background and understanding of philosophies and theories of intervention, they are unable to provide a depth of experience that on the job training allows.

Not many sighted hearing people get up each morning wondering who, of the many colleagues they know, will be working with them that day. Few would stay in situations where they are expected to play a major role in job training new staff every few months. Not many could live with that lack of comfort in the familiar and routine. For many people who are deafblind it is a way of life. The attrition rate of Intervenors has long been a concern for deafblind people and those who work with them. There is little consistency in the provision and quality of intervention when deafblind individuals are forced constantly to adjust to and become familiar with new staff. Employers find recruitment and hiring of new staff an extraordinarily time-consuming process. When that time and energy is redirected into a broadly based staff training program, it is likely to decrease the repetitive nature of staff recruitment. A comprehensive Intervenor training program, although also time consuming, is still one of the best investments that can be made. A model that comprises opportunities before hiring for both general and specific information, time for observation of theory in action, and finally, a chance to experience hands-on work will help to ensure employees are taken on who will have a solid basic understanding of the job. An integral basic element of the entire process is ample opportunity for reflection and feedback. The agency/program will benefit, since it will have a more satisfied staff who feel qualified in performing their assigned tasks. This job satisfaction will be reflected in the quality of the work demonstrated and the length of commitment to the job. Ultimately, the greatest and primary beneficiary is the person with deafblindness who is now able to depend on the predictable and familiar.

The Interview Process

Few people would have difficulty describing what a bus driver, a store clerk, a doctor, or a bank teller does. Asking what an Intervenor does is likely to produce universally blank faces. Deafblindness as a disability is not commonly known to the majority of the population; the process of intervention is even less familiar. People are not accustomed to seeing Intervenors on a daily basis or acquainted with what the actual 'work' entails. How can the standard interview process/techniques be adapted to meet this challenging situation? It is inconceivable, and grossly unfair to all involved, that a person would be hired for such a complex and demanding job immediately following standard interview procedures.

Good intervention is not something that can be tested and compared against universal standards, as in words per minutes typed correctly. The ability to do the job cannot be accurately assessed through discussion. Unlike the situation for the majority of occupations, what would normally be considered part of an after-hiring training program must start during the interview stage. The interview process should address the need for information for both the applicant and the employer, opportunities for observation, and finally, some experience with hands-on work. The initial step of the interview process should be a significant amount of time devoted to informing applicants about the disability of deafblindness, the process of intervention, and the role of the Intervenor. The information shared during this phase will contribute valuable information to the process of making an informed decision for both the applicant and the persons doing the hiring. A comprehensive model will also call on the involvement of a number of people: the deafblind person, the employer (often one and the same), the applicant, and experienced Intervenors. It is fundamentally understood that the person with deafblindness will be as fully involved in the selection process as he/she is capable. This participation may range from directing and involvement in the entire process, expressing a preference from among a number of applicants, or involvement through the use of an advocate. Observation and hands-on time will provide a concrete opportunity for the deafblind person's participation. Hands-on experience is the single most significant contributing factor to the applicant's understanding of what intervention is all about. Explanation and education can provide only a limited understanding. It is unfortunate when the hands-on experience happens too late in the process, and what results is a disaster for the person who is deafblind, the job applicant, and the administrator. A comprehensive interview process should build in both opportunities for the applicant to integrate the information with what he/she observed and time to reflect on these experiences during the process. This can be a time of self-discovery for the prospective Intervenor, who may be faced with acknowledging personal limitations. Addressing this issue in a sensitive way by allowing timely and supportive opportunities to withdraw from the process is ideal.

Each person, regardless of abilities, is unique. His/her likes/dislikes, personalities, and hopes are owned by him/her alone. Each intervention process is unique, because of the specific communication needs of the deafblind individual, the skills of the Intervenor, the assignment of and required level of intervention specific to that situation. In all instances, however, there are underlying tenets that are shared. Each deafblind person deserves the respect and support of those who work with him/her. Each has a right to a quality of intervention that meets his/her individual needs. Each situation calls on the Intervenor to respect the underlying philosophy of intervention, keeping the needs of the deafblind person foremost in mind and actions and 'doing with, not for.' Although it is expected that each staff training program will be reflective of the needs of the specific deafblind person, program, or organization, some aspects should be common to all. Programs share common broad requirements of Intervenors. They need employees who have a basic understanding of intervention and who possess at least the beginnings of communication skills and the practical abilities to work with people who are deafblind. As these common needs are addressed in a staff training process, the unique features of each situation will also be satisfied. Staff training programs should vary tremendously from situation to situation. A residential facility should incorporate aspects that may prove unnecessary for a community-based service-providing agency. A family seeking an Intervenor in the home for a child with deafblindness will focus on areas that may not apply to a person living independently. In larger organizations, corporate policies and procedures need to be included. It is vital that the unique characteristics of each locale be addressed when the training program is developed. Tailoring in this manner will produce a program that will incorporate the goals and objectives of the program and the specific needs of the client and will reflect the philosophy of intervention that is practised in the situation.

Information

The initial meeting of the applicant and interviewer combines some components of a standard job interview and serves as an information session. If the applicant is familiar with intervention, it is an opportunity to discuss background and previous experiences. For the inexperienced, it is important to discover his/her understanding of deafblindness and intervention. An introduction to the disability, the philosophy of intervention, and some basic information regarding the specific situation is important at this point. Protecting the confidentiality of the person with deafblindness must always be primary in the minds of the interviewer. Although the applicant requires some degree of general information to understand more clearly the demands and responsibilities of the job, it must be remembered that he/she is not yet in the position of employee and as such should never be privy to personal information.

For those who are inexperienced, it is easy to feel overwhelmed with information at the first meeting. Alternating information sessions with observation and hands-on work would allow the applicant time to digest information, integrate it with what is observed, and build on it as some limited hands-on activity is practised. In family situations it is important that the applicant begin to have an understanding of the integration of the Intervenor and family roles. Subsequent information sessions would provide applicants with an opportunity to discuss what they have observed/experienced and to learn about specific policies and procedures of the agency or program.

For an academically based program, the information stage begins with the intake process. Presenting information on deafblindness and intervention should be the starting point, since applicants often have little awareness of deafblindness and intervention. Group information sessions are an efficient model when large numbers are involved. A maximum of twenty-five people in a group will allow presenters to encourage participation of all attending and to promote peer interaction. Presenters can make observations and gather information from this process that will be valuable when admissions are determined.

The in-depth information is delivered in the classroom. Courses to be offered should be determined through the activities of a development/advisory committee. Many will be reflective of the length and focus of the overall program, but there are those that should be considered standard to all programs. A course that serves as an introduction to the field of intervention should be among the first courses offered. In addition to the lecture material, field trips will provide the students with an opportunity to meet people with deafblindness and observe intervention.

Communication courses should be considered essential from the outset. It should be anticipated that communication courses would continue throughout the program. Communication courses are natural opportunities for the involvement of people with deafblindness as instructors or lab leaders. Learning a new language from a native user is by far the most advantageous way.

It is important that emphasis be put on all methods of communication including *large-print* notes and *two-hand manual alphabet* as well as *Adapted American Sign Language (AASL)* and *Signing Exact English* (SEE). Technical skill alone will not ensure effective communication. Communication courses should incorporate theories of communication and communication at all levels from the informal gestural to formal language. Course content that addresses concept development and work with minimal language will broaden the students' ability to communicate effectively with any number of persons with deafblindness.

If the program focus encompasses the areas of both congenital and acquired deafblindness, students may be in danger of confusing distinct communication systems. Learning AASL has all the demands of acquiring any new language; asking the student to learn SEE simultaneously can be overwhelming. Staggering language acquisition will allow the students a greater chance of success. It is possible to spend one semester learning basic AASL for communicating with those who acquired deafblindness, while learning theories of communication for those with congenital deafblindness. Communication courses commonly require a high level of student feedback. Varying course delivery with group work, lab activities, video texts, reviews, and arrangements for student/teacher consultation will give ample opportunity for student success.

Grade one Braille should also be considered an essential communication course in a program that is training Intervenors for people with acquired deafblindness. Experience has shown that *grade two Braille*, while useful for students, is less of a mandatory consideration for those entering the field. Skill in grade two Braille lends itself well to post-employment training or professional development.

For programs that include skills related to work with people with acquired deafblindness, it is important to build in content relating to Deaf culture and Deaf history. The majority of people who are adventitiously deafblind are also culturally deaf. To be unaware of the culture, its values, traditions, history, and richness is to do a disservice to the clients whom the students will eventually work with. The subject can be addressed by either offering stand-alone courses or ensuring that it is reflected throughout all courses in the program.

Student Intervenors must acquire comfort in guiding techniques for a diverse group of clients in a variety of areas. Public facilities in the local area often lend themselves well to the practical aspect of this course. Basic sighted guide can be practised in stairways, local streets, stores, bus routes, and subways in the community. Initially, the student being guided should be under occluders. As the students become more proficient in guiding and communication techniques there are opportunities to mask both vision and hearing simultaneously. This will present more realistic experiences of the complexities of travel. A familiarity with route descriptions and environmental modifications would be an asset for any Intervenor. It is important, however, to respect the boundaries between the role of the Intervenor and that of the *orientation and mobility* specialist.

In the past few years there has been an increasing number of people with deafblindness who are also considered medically fragile. Intervenors are often called upon to be skilled in medication delivery, wheelchair transfers, diapering of adults, and suctioning. An understanding of basic anatomy and physiology, emphasizing vision, hearing, and the central nervous system, would provide Intervenors with support in these areas. It would also offer an opportunity for the students to become familiar with the significant causes and syndromes associated with deafblindness.

The final course that may be considered essential is one that deals with the skills of daily living. This is a natural pairing with information on assistive devices. Students should have an understanding of some of the hi-tech equipment in use, for instance, computer programs and interfaces, should be somewhat more familiar with what might be called medium tech, for instance, *TTY*, *silent page systems*, and *FM systems*. Low- or no-tech assistive devices should become very familiar to the students, for instance, hi marks, sock tuckers, Braille markers, and marking systems.

Many courses, although not considered essential, can certainly be considered highly recommended. They should in no way be considered 'soft' courses; all can play some valuable part in ensuring that Intervenors are fully equipped for the task. They are not mandatory, however, in ensuring that Intervenors have developed 'entry level' skills. One such course is Interpersonal Skills. Intervenors who are not working in a team situation are rare. Schools, group homes, agencies, and private homes require Intervenors to consult and work with an assortment of professionals who are also concerned with the deafblind person. Conflict is a common occurrence in any working group, and the resolution requires much thought and skill. A variety of general education courses contribute to broadly based learning. Courses in English, psychology, and sociology have tremendous relevance to the field of intervention and may prove useful to the students if pursuing further education.

Observation Time

The requirement of observation time demands a great deal from all involved, particularly those who are being asked to commit a significant amount of unpaid time for what is little more than a very lengthy job interview. In addition, donating their time is not guaranteed to pay off in a job, and they may discover along the way that they do not want the job at all! Fulfilling the requirement of this observation time, however, will, if nothing else, demonstrate their motivation and commitment to the job and build in a valuable 'out' for all parties.

The use of well-trained, experienced Intervenors for observation will ensure that applicants are exposed to an example of high-quality intervention. This provides them with opportunities to integrate what they have heard in the information session. It will also give them experiences to model when they are involved in hands-on work. The subtle facilitation skills required in good intervention can be invisible to those without experience. An additional person available to interpret processes and point out examples of different aspects of intervention that otherwise may go unnoticed is of value. Ultimately, the observation time will provide applicants with an opportunity to acquire a more concrete understanding of intervention and help them to discover if this is a job they will continue to pursue. Students in formal training programs who have the opportunity of a variety of field trips will have some limited early exposure to a diversity of intervention situations. Each field placement will provide a different experience and will require observation time at the outset. Upon completing the observation time it would be beneficial to provide applicants with an opportunity to reflect on and discuss what they observed. This can be a valuable time for the interviewer to assess growth in understanding and gauge attitudinal changes. There is a natural break at this stage to allow any of those involved to withdraw from the process.

Hands-on Work

For those involved in the hiring process it is expected at this stage that the applicant is able to articulate some basic explanation of deafblindness and the process of intervention. It is the ability to transfer these concepts into action that guarantees the quality of the intervention. Hands-on experience gives the applicant an opportunity to move one step closer to being actively involved as the facilitator of intervention. There are many people who, though unable to articulate the theories and concepts associated with intervention well, are highly successful Intervenors. Conversely, there are those who can speak eloquently on the subject but are unable to facilitate the most basic of activities. It is important to continue to view this as another valuable opportunity for each person involved, not as a 'test' for the applicant. Applicants will be able to experience concretely some hands-on intervention, assess their own comfort level, and allow them to reflect again on continuing in the training process.

Over the last decades much has been learned about the necessity of bonding between the Intervenor and the congenitally deafblind person to produce the most successful working arrangement. Although it is unrealistic to expect an instant bond between the applicant and the deafblind person in such an artificial situation, interactions can be indicative of a future relationship. For the person with acquired deafblindness, the information that hands-on time provides is an invaluable element in making an informed hiring decision.

There are always instances when a specific combination of Intervenor and deafblind person is not successful. When it is obvious that a combination does not work, there is nothing that can be done to make it work. This does not necessarily mean that the Intervenor should, without delay, start to think of another profession any more than one would think that the deafblind person will never successfully work with any Intervenor. It simply means that the particular combination was not successful. In team situations, this problem can often be circumvented when key Intervenors are assigned to clients. In 1:1 situations it is far more difficult. There is often no alternative other than that the Intervenor should not be hired. It is an unfortunate situation requiring a great deal of sensitivity. If the Intervenor has a good grasp of the philosophy and practice of intervention, it is easier to depersonalize the situation.

At the completion of the hands-on experience one would expect the applicant to have spent anywhere from five to twenty-five hours immersed in deafblindness and intervention. Ideally, there has been ample opportunity to observe, reflect, discuss, question, and experience. The applicant, interviewer, and person with deafblindness have been provided with enough information to make a well-informed decision that will likely be successful. In-depth on-the-job training now begins for the new employee.

For students in an Intervenor training program hands-on experience often takes the form of practicums or field placements. Many find it the most significant course offered in the program. It certainly should be the most significant in terms of time. Following the continuum established, placement will follow time spent in observation and time spent in the classroom. It is important that placement sites be well prepared for the level of student assigned. A first placement will allow a student considerable observation time, moving eventually to primarily one-to-one work. Entering a final placement, students will move more quickly into solo work. Through their involvement, placement sites play an active role in the success and continued relevance of the program. In addition to ensuring that the student is prepared to enter placement, it is vital that the program support the needs of the personnel and placement site. Supervisory workshops offer an ideal forum to provide some assistance to those supervisors who lack experience or who would like an opportunity to share information among colleagues.

Field placement courses are common in disciplines related to community/ social services. Often a seminar course is required in tandem with the practicum. This course allows students time each week to meet with a facilitator in smaller groups to share field experiences. For those involved in their first placement, it is an invaluable time to sort through their observations and integrate them with what they have previously learned in the classroom. Students often take advantage of this time for peer support in celebrations and challenges.

One could use the analogy that the ideal intervention team is a completed picture puzzle, the pieces being the deafblind person, the Intervenor, and the intervention process. Missing pieces may be crucial to a full understanding of the picture. As you assemble the puzzle, you may have hints as to what the picture will finally be, but for an appreciation of the full scheme all pieces are essential. It must also be noted that when one puzzle is completed, one cannot assume that the next puzzle contains the same pieces or results in the same picture. The experiences a person has in any situation may be of help in another situation; some skills are transferable and training time can be reduced. It cannot stressed enough that experience with one person who is deafblind does not mean experience with all. One must respect the uniqueness of the individual. Training will be essential, no matter how experienced the Intervenor.

Post-Employment Training

Staff training following hiring is essentially a continuation of pre-employment training. It is important at this point to encourage the Intervenor to become more familiar with the personal information needed to perform the job safely. Is there medical information that he/she should be aware of? What are the emergency preparations? Detailed information about vision, hearing, and health issues is essential. It is necessary to expand on the theories and philosophy of intervention, relating it to the specific situation. How is the philosophy reflected in the toileting routine, in the eating routine, on the paper route, in the different classes at high school or university or in the seniors' craft class? What are the routines that the Intervenor is normally involved with and how are they accomplished?

Tangible skills, such as the particular communication skills used by the deaf-blind person, need to be learned. Some can be acquired through observing other Intervenors and actually working one to one. Some need a more formal, instructional situation. New staff need to be familiar with agency/program policies, the nuts and bolts of hiring, job descriptions, pay rates, vacation allowances, and benefits. Familiarization tours and opportunities to meet other staff should be included.

For deafblind people, who are not easily able to articulate their routines, one of the more successful ideas is to keep an updated series of binders holding detailed information. One binder could contain medical information, clinical reports on vision, and hearing and health concerns. It would be essential also to include anecdotal reports from staff. Often a doctor's office assessment bears little resemblance to what is experienced on a day-to-day basis. Frequently, 'no light perception' on an eye chart is seen at home as picking up a cheesy at 12 inches. 'Profound sensorineural' hearing loss on an audiogram can be experienced as responding to country music with a heavy bass beat. This is important information for all staff to know. Another binder can contain home routines: morning, bathing, toileting, eating, and relaxing. Routines listed step by step are invaluable references for both new and experienced staff. Routines are not always static: a new bath toy has been discovered or that dreaded broccoli is now on the 'likes' list. Staff should be sure to devote time during each shift to becoming familiar with any changes. Routines outside the home can be addressed in another binder. Which leisure activities are favourites and which are not? School practices, job routines – all can be documented. Encouraging new staff to spend significant time reading information will help them in the transition to becoming experienced Intervenors.

It would be a grave mistake to view staff training as complete when staff are comfortable and capable on the job. Ongoing professional development allows staff to expand their skills and knowledge of the field. Sponsoring or participating in related workshops can be beneficial to staff. There should be opportunities to build on communication skills, first aid knowledge, and other skill-based areas. In addition, there exist a number of non-skill-based workshops in team building, interpersonal skills, or crisis intervention that would be of value to any Intervenor. One instrument that can facilitate and support the Intervenor in the field is the *Intervenor Self-Evaluation Guide*. This guide contains general information about intervention and specific guidelines that the Intervenor can use to evaluate his or her knowledge and functioning. It also provides a useful instrument to facilitate discussion between the Intervenor and the individual with deafblindness, his or her advocate, the family, or, where the Intervenor is employed by an agency or facility, as part of an agreed-upon standard of performance. It has been used successfully in these ways for many years.

Academically Based Training Programs

It must be stated at the outset that developing, implementing, and supporting a formal training program for Intervenors is unquestionably a costly proposition. There are costs in the development phase, travel for the development committee and underwriting the cost of Intervenors for committee members and community participants. Implementation costs, such as the purchase of Braillers and other program equipment, is a significant though one-time expense. Ongoing expenses include the provision of Intervenors for staff during class time and for related meetings. There are areas, however, where the population of people with deafblindness, the understanding of intervention, the demand for Intervenors, the emergence of intervention as a profession, and a funding body can support the development of a formal training program for Intervenors. Ideally, the initiative should come from the community, but in all cases the program must reflect the needs as expressed by the community of consumers and service providers.

Intervenor training programs can provide a pool of Intervenors who have an in-depth understanding of the philosophy of intervention, a variety of skills that are transferable among a number of Intervenor situations, and a global awareness of deafblindness. The high proportion of skill-based courses lends itself well to the community college venue. The skills and experiences students acquire will facilitate an easy entry into the working world. They will significantly reduce, not eliminate, the amount of on-the-job training needed and will provide staff who have a solid understanding of the demands and expectations of the job. An academic and skill-based education, however, can never replace what is gained through hands-on experience. Therefore, Intervenors who have completed a formal Intervenor training program should always be considered 'entry level' Intervenors.

There is considerable flexibility possible in the development of an Intervenor program. Length of program, area of concentration, and courses offered all are areas that should be addressed during the developmental phase. Allowing ample development time, minimally one year, will pay off in producing a program that is relevant and accountable to the local community. It is important that each program be reflective of the needs of the local community. What is a successful program in one part of the country may be totally inappropriate in another area. There are certain constants, however, that should be inherent in any Intervenor program. It is of primary importance that the consumers be involved in every aspect of its development and implementation. A development committee composed of people with deafblindness, family members, Intervenors, employers, and program administration is one of the first steps in the process. Ideally, community meetings will take place in a number of locations to ensure that all members of the community have had an opportunity to provide input. It is then the responsibility of the development team to take this information and design the program. Information from community meetings and the development committee should determine its focus. Will the program concentrate on skills needed by Intervenors working with people who are congenitally deafblind or on those needed when they are working with those who have acquired deafblindness, or will it address both? This may answer the question of the length of the program: providing a theoretical, skill-based and practical education in both areas would be difficult in under two years.

Regardless of the length and focus of the program, it is not difficult to follow the model of information, observation, and hands-on experience. Information will be contained in a variety of formal classes. Observation and hands-on work will be addressed in the provision of field placements or practicums. This is an invaluable opportunity for developing Intervenors to put into practice what they have learned in the classroom and for people who are deafblind to be actively involved in the education of Intervenors. The value of ongoing community involvement cannot be understated. The development committee now becomes a program advisory committee, which meets on a regular basis to share information and advise the administration on program issues.

As it is in the field of intervention, student attrition is always a concern. In order to reduce failures or withdrawals significantly, a comprehensive intake process is essential. A language screening that assesses basic spelling, synonyms, antonyms, precise skills, and concept explanation provides valuable information to the interviewing committee. Experience to date has shown that previous formal education has little impact on student success. Applicants with university education and those who have not completed high school are equally successful.

Staffing is a primary contributing factor to the success of the program. It is hoped that all program staff can be recruited from the field of experienced Intervenors and deafblind people who possess the qualifications mandated by the administration. Staff who are inexperienced in adult education can take advantage of courses dealing with the preparation, delivery, and evaluation of college curricula.

Family Situations

The employment of an Intervenor in a private home creates a special situation. Even when it is the ideal situation for the person who is deafblind and his/her family, there are still significant drawbacks, not the least of which is the lack of privacy. Having a person who is not a true member of the family so intimately involved with daily life in the home will affect all family members. Anticipating these difficulties will allow family members and Intervenors to develop strategies to minimize the impact. Clarity around rules and expectations of the house is imperative.

Families often find the first stumbling block is discovering where to recruit the person who has the unique skills and attitude to become an Intervenor. Many have had success starting with advertisements in local papers, colleges, universities, and employment centres. If significant information is started, for instance, age of person, hours, pay, and a short job description, the number of inappropriate applications will be reduced. Word-of-mouth methods should not be overlooked. Many successful pairings have resulted from the friend-of-a-friend situation. All applicants should be expected to submit a detailed curriculum vitae. After the submitted résumés have been examined, three to five people will probably be invited for an interview. As the addition of an Intervenor to the home effects all members of the family, some experienced families have encouraged all members to read the résumés and participate in the selection process.

An extensive interview/training process can be modified to suit the needs of the home intervention situation. It is vital that, in addition to the person with deafblindness, the family members be comfortable with the Intervenor. Because of this factor, the interview should take place in the home with parent(s)/guardians and the person with deafblindness participating. It is best that the interview process, though following an information, observation, hands-on model, be in a somewhat more informal atmosphere, since that will be the eventual working atmosphere in the home.

The initial interview in the home will provide the applicant with an opportunity to meet other family members, in addition to the person with whom they will be working. As already stated, provision of an introduction to deafblindness, intervention, and general job-related information is important at this point. Clarity around the demands of the interview process should be stressed. This first meeting presents opportunities for parents to observe the comfort of the applicant with their child. After completing the personal interviews, those interviewing should feel prepared to invite one of the applicants to continue the process.

The next stage is arranging for the applicant to observe an experienced Intervenor in the school or day program or the present Intervenor in the home. This stage will naturally lead into some hands-on time as the culmination of the interview process. Applicants should complete this process with a very clear understanding of the tasks the job entails. It is hoped that both applicant and parents and/or deafblind person will have a clear idea as to the suitability of the applicant. In-depth, detailed training will continue after the Intervenor is officially hired.

Family Members as Intervenors

Much has been learned about the benefits of early identification and provision of intervention. The unfamiliarity of deafblindness to the general population, however, extends also to the medical profession and those involved in supporting families. Some families who live in major urban centres are fortunate to have access to information, services, and support. For families without these advantages, medical examinations and referrals prevent a timely diagnosis and referral for appropriate services. It is at this very early point in a child's life that, through necessity, the parents first develop their role as advocate.

Resources for parents are integrally related to the provision of early intervention. Most often, the first Intervenor in the life of a deafblind child is the parent. The needs of this new child are so far reaching and complex that parents often feel inadequately prepared to meet them. In addition, many parents are unable to access support or services, owing to distance or lack of knowledge. Discovering the type of services available, where they exist, and how they can be accessed can be an overwhelming task. Enquiries should start at the local level; agencies/programs involved with disabled children, particularly blind children, may be a valuable place to begin. Many locales have a diversity of parent support groups, which not only provide much needed support to new parents but are often the best informed regarding accessing services.

Parents who are faced with all the issues related to a new child who has a disability must also very quickly become familiar with the process of intervention, how it is accomplished, and what their role is. Ideally, this support is provided on a regular and ongoing basis through bi-weekly visits by a consultant who is a highly trained specialist. New parents usually are unaware of specific techniques that may be helpful in the daily life of their child. Methods to promote language development, sensory stimulation, gross and fine motor skills, concept development, and daily living skills can be taught, primarily through demonstration, to the parents at a rate that keeps pace with the development of the child. These techniques should be accompanied by an understanding of the rationale for them, the expected result, and the anticipated next step. Developing a cue, often a distinguishing feature, that the parent will use to identify him/herself should not be suggested in isolation. Embedding it in the overall development of language and communication and relating it to the next step of a sign will assist parents in a more broadly based understanding of the significance. Parents continue to need support as the child develops and achieves milestones and as challenges arise.

Although all family members are often called upon to act in the role of Intervenor, it must always be remembered that their primary role is that of a sibling, parent, or relative. Giving too much responsibility for intervention to family members risks straining relationships. Certainly in day-to-day family life intervention happens on an ongoing basis among all members. In discussions with families about training of family members as Intervenors it has become clear that there is little formal training. Familiarity with routines, communication, preferences in all aspects of life develops from the experiences of daily life. All families have an awareness of individual idiosyncrasies; this situation is no different for families who have members with a disability. Consistency and structure are vital to the life of the person who is deafblind. Therefore, it is important that there be clear and current information among family members concerning the needs and routines of the deafblind member of the family.

Teacher Training

by William Thompson

Introduction

It is now accepted worldwide that deafblindness is a unique disability (McInnes 1993). Deafblindness is not only a unique disability but also a low-incidence disability, which creates a number of problems. Dr Thomas Clark of the University of Utah (now retired), has identified one problem resulting form this low incidence that is often overlooked or whose importance is not recognized. There is no pool of community knowledge available to those parents or professionals who are involved with those who are congenitally and early adventitiously deafblind.

Partly because of thè fact that this unique population is so widely dispersed and partly because of the lack of locally trained staff to meet the 'very specialized instructional needs' (Heubner et al. 1996), there is a definite need to provide a central location for specialized staff training.

Training

The residential school would provide the ideal setting for the training of specialist teachers, Intervenors, and other staff necessary for the education of students who are deafblind. Certification requirements for teachers vary from jurisdiction to jurisdiction. At one time educators believe that a 'general special education' background qualified a person to teach children who were deafblind. This is definitely an assumption that falls far short of meeting the program needs of this special population.

There are many approaches to educating teachers to become specialists in the area of deafblind education. In some parts of the world universities and colleges offer courses as part of a specialist certification program or as specific program concentrating on the area of deafblindness. Other programs are offered as concurrent (on the job) training or as summer courses leading to certification. Regardless of the route taken to this specialization, there are certain topics that must be covered to prepare a teacher for certification as a Specialist Teacher of the Deafblind.

These topics are outlined below, within a three-part structure. It is assumed that an individual will have certification as a teacher and have three years' experience teaching in regular or special classrooms prior to enrolling in a program leading to certification as Specialist Teacher of the Deafblind. It is also assumed that throughout each part of the program the enrolee will work with a variety of infants, children, youth, and adults with deafblindness for a minimum of of eighty hours of supervised practicum per session.

Part I

The Child with Deafblindness

• Define, include simulations, provide opportunities for hands-on interaction with children who are deafblind

- Characteristics, the child in the family, preschool and educational options and supports, other support agencies

Causes of Deafblindness

- Congenital and adventitious causes, including Rubella Syndrome, other common syndromes, other causes
- Prevention

History of Deafblind Education

Growth and Development

- Review of 'normal' growth and development: physical, cognitive, communicative, social-emotional, with stress on the role of the distance senses
- Accompanying complications on normal developmental patterns caused by deafblindness
- Testing and evaluation procedures: use and abuse

Programming Elements

- Goals of deafblind programming
- Basic assumptions
- The 'Total Communication Approach'
- The team approach
- Intervention
- Techniques for developing communication, perception, cognition, motor development, life skills, orientation and mobility, social and emotional development
- Precision teaching: objectives, long- and short-term goals, activity-based programming, daily planning and record keeping, communications with the family
- Identification and development of individual learning styles

Manual Communication

- Introduction to various communication modes: SEE, ASL, Adaptive Communication
- Part One of signing course (beginner level)

Assistive Devices

- Introduction to what is available and how to use it appropriately, for example, hearing aids, FM systems, optical aids.

Family dynamics

Part II

The Five Senses

- Review
- Sensory integration, assimilation, and perception

The Eye

- Anatomy, disease of, function of
- Corrective procedures
- Visual assessment: formal and informal
- Remediation, visual aids and devices

Specialized Techniques to Promote the Use of Residual Vision

The Ear

- Anatomy, causes of hearing loss, function of
- Audiograms
- Hearing assessment: formal and informal
- Remediation, hearing aids and devices
- Auditory training

Specialized Techniques to Promote the Use of Residual Hearing

Tactile Discrimination

Sensory Integration

Programming

- Demonstrate the ability to design individual pupil programming

- Writing a Personal Program Plan
- Manual communication
- Part Two of signing course (intermediate level)

The Grieving Cycle

Part III

Prior to enrolling in this part, the participant must have at least one year's experience working with children who are deafblind.

Functional Assessment of Infants and Children Who Are Deafblind

- Preparing the case history
- The hands-on team assessment
- Assessment report writing, including suggestions and recommendations for programming in the school and non-school settings

Workshop Design and Implementation

- Preparation and delivery of a workshop on a subject related to deafblindness

Interview and Consultative Techniques

Develop the Skills and Knowledge to Participate in or to Chair Professional and Parent Case Conferences

Assistive devices

- Completion of a familiarization course
- Alphabetic Braille
- Introduction to reading and writing using alphabetic Braille (grade one Braille)

Consultant Training

by John M. McInnes

Introduction

The position of consultant is one of the most important and demanding positions in the field of deáfblind services. The consultant is called upon to combine the knowledge and hands-on skills of the Intervenor, the in-depth knowledge and experience of a specialist teacher of the deafblind, and the knowledge and skills of a family support worker. Simply being given a title such as consultant or area support worker does not equip one to fulfil the role, nor does training and experience of an Intervenor or teacher, in and of itself, prepare one adequately to be a consultant. Regardless of the title, the individual must have appropriate training and experience in the fields of intervention, deafblindness, group dynamics, and family support.

Sources of Recruitment

Candidates for the position of consultant may be drawn from the ranks of specialist teachers of the deafblind, resident or classroom workers, or Intervenors. Each of these disciplines represents an area in the field of deafblindness where extensive knowledge and experience may be gained. This extensive exposure is essential as a foundation upon which to build the skills and acquire the knowledge necessary to become an effective consultant. One cannot take a course that will equip him or her to become a consultant. Rather, one must gather and assimilate knowledge from several fields.

Areas of Knowledge Required

The consultant must have the following.

a) An in-depth knowledge of the role, function, and training of the Intervenor.
b) Extensive experience in working with infants, children, youth, and adults with deafblindness. Where an individual does not have experience in working with all four groups, experience in at least two of these four areas is essential.
c) Training as a specialist teacher of the deafblind. Where the consultant's background lies in one of the other areas such as social work, formal training as an Intervenor, or as a residence worker, he or she should be given the opportunity to audit teacher-training courses.

d) Training in social work with particular emphasis on family dynamics, the grieving cycle, the dysfunctional family, and the structure of the social service delivery system, as found in the area in which he or she are working. Where the consultant's background lies in teaching or as an Intervenor, he or she must take or audit courses in the above-mentioned areas of social work training.

e) Formal training as an Intervenor. Where the consultant comes from other backgrounds, training in the theory and practice of intervention and the training of Intervenors, at least in the two groups of clients upon which he or she will concentrate, is necessary.

f) Training in the structure and function of the educational system.

g) Training in the techniques and methods of educating and counselling parents and professionals.

h) Training in the techniques, methods, and responsibilities of team building and leadership, both in general and as it applies to the position of a consultant working out of a area or regional centre.

The one area that cannot be lacking is experience in working with individuals who are deafblind. If a prospective consultant does not have extensive experience in working with at least two of infants, children, youth, and adults with deafblindness, then he or she should not be considered for the position. Experience of the type needed is not something that can be gained on the job in the depth necessary after a person has been appointed and is working as a consultant.

The training required in the areas of educational structure, roles and reporting relationships of staff, union and professional working agreements, and so forth will be from a different perspective from that learned in teacher training. The consultant will be an outsider, an educator, a consensus builder, a specialist, and a team leader. Special skills will be required to function in this role and will require a depth of knowledge and skills that is different from those learned solely in teacher training, Intervenor training, or social work courses. It is extremely unlikely that one will find too many candidates for the position of consultant who have all of the necessary background, training, and experience. Each prospective consultant should have his/her background, knowledge, training, and experience assessed. The individual's shortcomings should be identified. Once identified, a specific personal plan should be drawn up by the prospective consultant to overcome his or her identified shortcomings.

Such a plan may include auditing or taking appropriate courses, individual study, consultation with experienced consultants, and working as a team member. Where there is a resource centre and a number of consultants with varying backgrounds, members of the consultant staff should be used to present courses in the area of their specialty to the group. This approach has many advantages and should be pursued.

A formal peer review presentation, where the consultant presents his or her observations, proposed Personal Plan, and proposed course of action for its implementation to a group of centre consultants for comments and suggestions, provides an excellent vehicle for growth. This approach is also valuable as an ongoing practice wherein working consultants make a presentation to their peers two or three times a year. Ongoing training, promoted through the case review process, will result from the discussion among centre staff or, where practical, by having an outside expert in a specific area attend the review and add a new perspective.

In any case, to be effective, training for the consultant should be viewed as an ongoing process, and not as something that has taken place before the consultant is hired.

The Consultant's Role

I'd rather see a sermon
than hear one any
day. I'd rather one
should walk with me
than merely show the
way ...
I can soon learn how to do it
if you'll let me see it
done. I can watch your hands
in action, but your tongue too
fast may run. And the
lectures you deliver may be
wise and true, but I'd
rather get my lesson by
observing what you do.   Edgar A. Guest (Dalton 1948)

This poem by Guest should be the guide that every consultant follows. The consultant fulfills many important functions but social visiting and 'tea drinking' is not one of them. The nature of the disability of deafblindness, its low incidence, and the lack of in-depth knowledge in most members of the local lay and professional community make his or her role unique in many aspects, such as the following:

- placing an emphasis on parent, community professional, and community worker education
- making extended bi-weekly visits to home, educational, and professional settings
- demonstrating the techniques required for program implementation
- interacting in a consultative and advocacy capacity with professionals therapists, community agencies, and so forth
- gathering information for, designing, and implementing a Personal Plan and evaluating progress in terms of identified objectives
- making initial evaluations leading to the decision as to whether the infant, child, or youth is to be identified as deafblind and formative evaluations over extended periods to facilitate programming
- acting as a team leader to coordinate services and support
- providing parent counselling in appropriate areas
- being a speaker at community service clubs and other organizations
- acting as the family consultant and supporting the family and client over an extended period, usually several years
- Assisting the parent to avoid becoming a 'hostess-secretary' rather than a caring parent and supporting Intervenor.

Even with all of the above taken into consideration, however, the bureaucrats overseeing the program must remember that the consultant is not *Super Person*; ongoing support and training is essential. With the advent of real-time communication using the internet, the number of on-site visits may be somewhat reduced from the suggested minimum of once every two weeks. Under no circumstances, even when scheduled weekly or bi-weekly interaction over the internet is taking place, should a consultant's on-site visits be fewer than once per month. When the internet option is adopted, the consultant *must be given special training* to use the internet-interactive approach as an effective tool.

Caseload

In most cases the consultant must not have a caseload of over eight to ten family units if he or she is to provide adequate support to the individual who is deafblind, the family, and the community and act as case manager in addition to being part of an assessment team from time to time. Factors such as the age of the client and his or her level of functioning, the distance and time required for travel, the amount of paperwork required by the particular organization, and the depth of the consultation required all will work to reduce the number of family units the consultant has as a caseload below ten.

Where the consultant is fortunate enough to be able to return to the resource centre each day and be home each night, and where the client is a preschooler, it is anticipated that the consultant would spend approximately two to four hours consulting with the parent and demonstrating appropriate techniques to be used with the infant. Where the family unit contains a student attending a preschool or school program, it is expected that approximately two hours or more will be spent consulting with the parents and two hours consulting with the educational staff. Regardless of the client placement, an additional hour for each hour spent in consultation should be allowed for making notes concerning the visit, writing reports, reviewing or writing the Personal Plan, and other tasks directly related to the family unit.

It will also often be necessary to make return visits to the home to consult with family members who are absent during the visit. In fact, it is often better to plan for such a second 'home visit' to take place during the early evening for the family of an infant who is deafblind.

Consultants who must travel considerable distances and are not able to return to the centre each day should plan their week's visits in a chain or loop. As they travel out from and gradually back to the resource centre they will require time for the travel, consultation, and other tasks listed in the previous paragraph.

In addition to the tasks directly related to the family unit, time must be allowed for the consultant to prepare workshops, to act as a partner in an initial evaluation team, make community presentations, and to consult with his or her peers. As ongoing training and peer review are important aspects of the consultant's job, at least one day every two weeks should be set aside for such activity.

Consultants who are denied sufficient time to carry out all aspects of their role will soon burn out trying. They will begin to see the essential relationship that must exist between themselves, the family unit, the community program staff, and medical and other professionals they are expected to support eroded and eventually destroyed. When the consultant begins to see parents turning to agencies that have been established to support infants, children, and youth with other disabilities, they will know that an understanding of the uniqueness of the disability of deafblindness has been lost and that, in most cases, a basis for future failure of the infant, child, or youth is being established.

Consulting is a job that cannot be half done. Either it will be done correctly or the time spent making occasional visits and giving the workshops will be wasted.

Summary

1. Working with individuals who are deafblind requires specific knowledge and background experience.

2. There are two major avenues for training Intervenors: in house and academically based.
3. In-house training provides a greater background of experience over a limited range.
4. Academic training provides a broader knowledge and understanding.
5. Owing to the fact the responsibilities of the Intervenor are not widely understood, a comprehensive interview process, which includes an overview of the disability, observation of an Intervenor, and hands-on experience is necessary.
6. Technical skill alone does not ensure adequate communication.
7. Staff training following hiring is essentially a continuation of pre-employment training.
8. An academically based Intervenor training program can provide future Intervenors with an in-depth understanding of the philosophy of intervention, a variety of skills, a global awareness of deafblindness, as well as the ability to work with individuals of various ages.
9. The Intervenor with little or no previous training and experience who is hired to work in the home obtains an ongoing training geared to equip him or her to work with a particular individual.
10. Intervenors working in, and out of, the home should have a written contract that clearly spells out responsibilities, hours of work, working conditions, and so on.
11. An interview for an Intervenor who will work out of the home should contain the same three elements as the college-based or centre-based interview: background knowledge, observation of an Intervenor at work, and hands-on experience.
12. The residential school with a separate deafblind unit provides an excellent setting for training teachers.
13. Training, leading to certification as a specialist teacher of the deafblind, is extensive and consists of both theory and practice.
14. Residential school staff training consists of both initial and ongoing training.
15. Consultants may be drawn from a variety of backgrounds, but regardless of background, specialized training is necessary to ensure competence in educational theory, areas of social work, group dynamics, and counselling of families.
16. Case conferences, with or without outside experts, are an excellent way to upgrade knowledge and skills continually.
17. The consultant's caseload will be influenced by age of the client and his or her level of functioning, the distance and time required for travel, the amount of paperwork required, and the depth of the consultation required.

REFERENCES

Heubner, Kathleen Mary, Jeanne Glidden Prickett, Elga Joffee, and Theresa Rafalowski Welch (1966) 'A Self Study and In-Service Training Program for Individuals Who Work with People Who Are Deafblind.' In *Rehabilitation and Education for Blindness and Neural Impairment* (Winter). Washington, DC: Heldref Publications

McInnes, John M. (1993) 'Educational Services: Reaction.' In *Proceedings of the National Symposium on Children and Youth Who Are Deafblind*, ed. John W. Reiman and Pattie A. Johnson. Monmouth, OR: Teaching Research Publications

Morrison, James Dalton (1948) *Masterpieces of Religious Verse.* 1st ed. Poem #1144. New York: Harper

17

Final Thoughts

BRYNDIS VIGLUNDSDOTTIR

Having read the splendid contributions written by experts from all over the world and presented in this book, I am keenly aware that there will hardly be a great deal I can contribute to its volume or value. While the purpose of this contribution is not that of a book review, it is tempting to say a few words about some of the areas covered in previous chapters.

Anyone connected with people who are deafblind or impaired people in general will benefit from reading the book and contemplating the philosophy of respect for the clients, in this particular instance, deafblind persons, and looking closely at the tender, yet structured, approaches and methods discussed. At times the book becomes a clear textbook and will be of great value for those educating people working with people who are handicapped, whether they are deafblind or otherwise disabled.

There is, for example, a splendid chapter on the philosophy and the tactics of being an advocate and providing services at the same time. This could result in conflicts, but in the chapter the author discusses a highly effective, structured, and positive approach to the task.

Throughout this book the authors advocate the just and needed services to people who are deafblind and discuss the environment needed to provide the services and to enjoy the services. Many splendid guides in various situations describe and discuss different modes of residence and educational environment. Many authorities are called upon to substantiate opinions and attitudes, and all of this is needed. It is certainly very important to have sound and thorough knowledge and be supported by learned scholars.

But I suggest that, when it comes to the daily intervention, the daily grit, at home with the family, in the schools, or in a group home, the learned approach must be carried and supported by a vision, attitudes, and caring understanding towards the human beings. These components will move all concerned forward on the path towards a still better world for people who are deafblind.

The spirit of this book, the context of which is gathered from around the world, demonstrates that 'man does not live from bread alone.' It also demonstrates that the Beatles erred when they sang: 'All You Need is Love.' In truth a combination of bread and love is needed. And that is what this book is about.

The authors do not diminish the intricacy, problems if you like, involved in teaching/working with people who are deafblind. But the discussions are open, honest, and offer guidelines and ideas regarding various approaches and programs. It is the task of this book to focus on the realities and needs of people who are deafblind. Yet I am constantly reminded of 'these other people with disabilities,' the other children of this world who we see on our television screens on the evening news. This is stated – not to diminish the importance and need of the best services for deafblind persons but rather to attempt to sensitize us to the realities of the conditions in which a great many of the human beings of this world live. In the final analysis there is but one family, The Family of Man. We all belong to that family, whether we are refugees in Zaire, orphans in Croatia, or a deafblind senior citizen in Iceland.

A conversation I had in 1986 with Naomi Gazit, an elderly lady in Israel, comes to mind. During the very difficult times of the Holocaust when children were being smuggled out of Europe and put on shore in Palestine, she was there with her helpers to comfort the children and give them shelter. Thus, she established one kibbutz after the other, working, comforting, advocating, believing in the value of the children she was serving. She had children of her own and told her daughter that in her later years she sometimes wondered if they felt neglected. 'No, mama, we always thought and were sure that the more children you were comforting and holding in your arms the more you loved us, too. Your love seemed to grow with every shipload of children!'

Again, the subject of these 'other people with disabilities' is introduced here – not to suggest that the advocacy and services to the deafblind persons are not of the utmost importance – rather to advocate the observation that we are all one family and there are some, far too many, that have no or very ineffective advocates. But it is also my observation that when the lot of one group of people within a society or culture improves, it is usually easier to obtain improvements for the next group. It should suffice to mention the societal changes across the lines in the wake of the French Revolution and more recently the effect of the revolution of the 1970s, 'The Revolution of the Flower Children,' when conditions of and attitudes towards minority groups of all kinds were examined and improvements demanded. Improvements began to take place and spread like a wave across the boundaries of gender, colour, and every imaginable human condition.

Therefore the value of this book should be manifold. It should and can have a great value for those who are working at improving the quality of life of people with various disabilities. These disabilities may be caused by sickness and the disabling conditions of old age, the disabling effects of psychiatric sickness, learning disabilities among schoolchildren attending the public schools – the groups are there and the same approaches, the same holistic support as advocated for in this book are, in fact, needed and will be highly effective in all these situations. The value of this book is also that it advocates professional integrity and cooperation, warns against acting as experts in the field of deafblindness, while the expertise is indeed only fractional and leads to fractional approaches and results. The emphasis must be on 'doing the correct thing correctly'! Or, as John McInnes says in chapter 1 of this book: 'Deafblindness is a unique disability that requires a specialized level of knowledge.'

A fair amount of the book focuses on children, and it is noted that some authors label adult deafblind persons as children. Infancy and early childhood are of immense importance, since these are the formative years. When essential parts of the senses, such as sight or hearing, are impaired, the experiences are only in fractions, bits. If sight and hearing are totally lacking, there is a serious gap, a void of experiences. If the child who is deafblind also has an intellectual impairment, the road towards language acquisition and maturity leading to a life of quality becomes all the more difficult to travel. This book emphasizes all through, in strong terms, that providing partial services will only result in partial experiences, partial or no understanding of language and situations that lead to 'compartmental' life, life without the experience of being a whole, thinking, participating person.

I was pleased to see that the reader is challenged to question previous diagnoses, and one shudders at the thought of how many deafblind persons must, through the years, have been misdiagnosed and therefore suffered unduly. The approach must rather be to attempt to establish communication and through communication meet each individual at his/her level.

This same fundamental rule seems to be appropriate in regard to all human beings. We simply like to be met at our interest level. If we stumble upon the interest level of those who will not reveal it on their own, there is hopefully a basis for further connection, the interest in communicating with you will grow and the quality of experiences improve. I am tempted to share a story from my teaching days in Boston.

We had worked together without evident interest or results much longer than was acceptable. The boy, whom we will call Alfur, seemed apathetic, more or less only tolerating us in our efforts. He loved ice cream, so we would go to the corner store to pick up cones and try to 'make language happen' in connection. One afternoon in the spring, walking back to the classroom, Alfur ran ahead and stood by the vine that grew along the walkway, jumping up and down. He was also trying to reach for something. At a closer look, he was all excited about the spiders, that make their habitat on the vine leaves. In no time did he learn the sign for spider, used it too, and there is no need to say the classroom got a fair supply of spiders, which provided a wealth of language/communication opportunities. They also resulted in trust. Alfur had experienced that being together was in fact fun; he became interested in 'hearing, seeing, experiencing' more. Had we only caught on to these spiders sooner! Time for the deafblind youngsters is so immensely important. And when we are considering doing the right thing in the right way, it has to be what is of interest to our client and done in such a way that he/she can follow what is happening.

Many interesting and helpful examples of programs are presented in the book. Although they may not be totally applicable in all the countries where this book will be read, owing to differences in culture there are basic elements that are pan-human and therefore of value. My observation and opinion are that it is important that the methods used for assessing other people and gathering information about the same people prior to establishing the program for the individual in question should be fair, culturally appropriate, and professionally sound.

There should also be a warning about plans! While planning is certainly of value, most important, we must not become the slaves of plans. That may extinguish the fire of the creativity of the moment often so sorely lacking in the flora of experiences of people who are deafblind. I am not advocating that we will function well as teachers or intervenors on the spur of the moment – far from it. In other words, I believe professionals, teachers in particular, must not put their trust in inspiration for their professionalism. Here is a precarious road, which emphasizes that the skills to work with human beings must be composed of professional know-how, the art of being human with other human beings, and love of life, so intense that you have to share it with others. If this is our professional manifest, we may at times have to deviate from previously written everyday plans. Having a carefully researched and contemplated plan certainly allows freedom to deviate from it if need be!

This chain of thought calls attention to the need for well-informed, well-educated, well-'composed' people who are working in various categories with people who are deafblind. Let us remember that deafblind people are, at least in their early years, totally at the mercy of their co-workers. A thorough plan, a program, is necessary and most useful. But in no instance does it guarantee the appropriate implementation or personal growth of the person for whom it was written. The ideals and approaches in educating intervenors and teachers of people who are deafblind advocated for and described in this book are a splendid model to strive for in the services to people who are deafblind and their families.

It is of great value to identify some of the skills essential to intervenors. Identifying the skills calls for identifying the nature of the task at hand and the job situations. This proves to be a difficult task and could probably never be done thoroughly! The intervenors work in as many different situations as the people who are deafblind and to be intervened with are. But there are many universal components in the idea of intervening. A great many common situations and aspects are identified, and therefore the guide for training intervenors presented here is of great value. Once more we are talking about what is essential to us all, mutual friendship, love and concern, and information on and discussions of important and non-important issues alike. It is only when we enjoy these factors that our life is fulfilled.

The plans presented in this book are, on the whole, educationally ambitious and socially integrating. The contributors to this book hardly discuss or exhibit concern for providing funds. Yet the reality is that funding is very important and may often cause the gap between ideals presented through good plans and the execution of the plans. Whereas this may be of different importance in different cultures, funds will have to be available in one way or the other.

Another thought to share: Did we have plans written for our life span? How would it have altered our development if someone had decided what stage of development we should have reached at a certain post in our chronological age? Might we have been hampered? Would it have improved the quality of our schooling? Might we want to look at plans for deafblind persons in this context? The issues discussed in various chapters of the book on the quality of life for people who are deafblind are, in fact, such issues as we want for ourselves. It is mentioned that persons who are deafblind must enjoy respect, their privacy should not be invaded, their independence must be regarded, and so on. The fact that there is a need to discuss this in a book underlines the problem at hand. We all want these areas to be safe for ourselves. But let us consider the very terminology of referring to adult people who are deafblind as 'children.' I am not implying that the privacy of children should be invaded or their decisions not respected within the limits that their experience allows them to make decisions. I am merely saying that maybe we need to look closely at our very attitudes when working with people who are deafblind. This is true in regard to all other groups of people with disabilities and, for that matter, to their families.

Our ability to develop and later function as mature human beings grows through or by emotional and intellectual relations in early childhood. The early experiences and bonding cannot be overemphasized for further intellectual development and emotional growth. This puts the deafblind infant at a disadvantage and must be a sharp reminder to those concerned to strive towards vigorous assistance to the parents. The authors of this book are keenly aware of this truth, as the program guides and suggestions presented witness.

We are all learning new skills all our lives. The amount of knowledge we acquire is different in each case, our mode of learning is different, and the depth of our knowledge is also vastly different at different stages of our life. But in all instances will the results of our efforts be influenced by our environment, the encouragement of our peers, teachers, and those who love us. The deafblind person has in the beginning to learn almost everything through another person – whatever the new skill is. This makes his/her acquisition of knowledge all the more complicated than it is for us. When working with people who are deafblind, we must offer such knowledge and skills as we are asked for or we suspect that the person we are working with might be interested in – and we must deliver with joy.

I am reminded of an incident from my childhood and would like to share it. I was eight years old and had recently learned to knit a complicated version of a heel. My sister, who was three years older than I and did not yet possess this enviable skill, asked me to teach her. Being eager to do so, I started to show her. I neither knew nor understood that it would be helpful to divide the procedure into steps and teach clearly each step at a time, demonstrate, and explain. She did not understand, she did not learn, she became frustrated and disappointed, and I, the teacher, became very impatient, thinking she was not very clever, and told her so in no uncertain terms. Then my sister taught me a lesson never forgotten. She told me I must not be impatient because she could not learn at once. Impatience confused her even more, she said. And I also must be glad, happy to be teaching and sharing something I knew but she did not yet know and wanted to learn.

How very true! And how often I have wished teachers of this world were extraordinarily happy people, glad to be able to share and pass on knowledge to other people! If this is my wish for the teachers of seeing and hearing children, how much more intense the wish for teachers who work with persons who are deafblind and so totally dependent on the disposition of the adults they encounter. Maybe this joy of sharing knowledge would be more overwhelming if we believed and kept clear in our mind that underneath the silence of deafness and behind the darkness of blindness there is the core of the human being, the mind, the soul, where there is the need and longing to learn, know, ask questions, be answered, to wholly participate in life. The deafblind person may not yet know about this longing, but you know it is there because he/she is a human being.

For effective teaching I believe we need to have sound didactic knowledge and to possess the art of sharing knowledge. This could be likened to playing a violin. You could know all there is to know about the methods of playing but the violin must be well tuned to sound right and you must touch it correctly to convey the music the composer had in mind.

It has been observed that human beings of all cultures play. Play is a learned activity, an activity of interaction of peers. The daily life of deafblind children is dominated by the process of learning the daily living skills and the language related to these actions. They need to learn what other children learn through being alive, awake, seeing, and hearing, and thus they experience and understand their environment. It proves extremely difficult to incorporate play, true children's play with all its adventures, thrill, and flow of ideas, into the daily life of deafblind children. When children are engaged in true play they are at their best sharing thoughts, ideas, and interacting. The lack of this experience is one of the aspects I regret about the reality of deafblindness in childhood. The lack of true play, including play on words, affects the entire life span, and play is extremely difficult to teach.

What possibilities have deafblind children for playing? Their waking hours are usually either highly scheduled or void. I do not have the answer to these complicated issues but am only sharing concern and wishes that we might find a way.

This is related to the need to be sensitive towards understanding the reasons for challenging behaviours. What alternatives can we offer? What skills could we introduce? What might we offer of interest and therefore of value? We might add: of value to whom? May I remind us of Alfur and his spiders!

The highly sensitive and controversial issue of sex and sexuality is honestly discussed with due respect and sensitivity towards all concerned. Previous attitudes did not regard sex and people who are deafblind as being compatible. This change of attitude is another example of how the waves of benefit spread from one group to the next as discussed before. A sex liberation has truly occurred! If adult people who are deafblind are indeed regarded as adults, they will be supported to be responsible for their own decisions and actions. Are we not advocating for this in our approaches and interactions with other people, be they children or adults? Why is it so difficult to truly adopt this attitude towards people with special needs?

The chapter on the family and the family viewpoint could not be more powerful and thought provoking. It emphasizes the need for parents as active partners in the lifelong process of securing the best possible quality of life for their offspring who is deafblind as well as for the other members of the family. It should be noted that everything said in this book pertaining to families of persons who are deafblind, who are supporting their family members with special needs and trying to survive as a family at the same time, could and needs to be said for families of people coping with various other impairments, too. Once again this does not diminish the need for support, psychological, financial, and universally professional help and advice, and mutual respect, when the family is that of a person who is deafblind. It only calls attention to the belief that the same principles are at hand although the name of the disabling condition is different. It is even true when the disabled person is your aged parent who used to be a supportive pillar of society but towards the end of his/her life span loses the power of thinking, loses the magic of communication, is unable to comprehend the environment, and becomes functionally severely impaired.

Different authors have been publishing their writings on this issue. Many professionals have understood the value of partnership with parents. This goes for all children and parents and the families of people with special needs. Different cultures are at very different stations in this respect. The chapter referred to in this book is of value for all advocates of a parent/professional partnership. Here is a powerful discussion and plea on behalf of parents, grandparents, and siblings of all persons with special needs. It discusses the everyday life span realities of the core family and the extended family. This is a reading of value to all aware, human beings. When closely examined, the needs are the same for all of us, whether we are deafblind children, ninety-year-old persons suffering from dementia, or, for that matter, busy executives. The basic needs are the same, those of enjoying love, security, and recognition. When these qualities in life are absent, the lack is manifested in isolation and loneliness, the degree of which depends upon various factors. In the final analysis there is but one person, All Human Beings.

The broad spectrum presented in this book and the quality of the writing is a testimony to the sincere interest of a group of deeply concerned and able persons affiliated with people who are deafblind in various situations. What is 'common' in all the situations is an impaired ability to communicate. Therefore the item probably most often mentioned in this book is COMMUNICATION. As for services to people who are deafblind, communication has to be the core. Whatever is done centres around communication, and in the final analysis the services are performed through and for communication.

Let us consider how this magical concept is explained. According to Webster, the verb *communicate* means: to make known, impart; to give or interchange thoughts, feelings, information or the like, by writing, speaking, and so on. One of the definitions of communication reads: any connective passage or channel.

It is noted in this book that the more services a person enjoys, the more acute the need for improved and increased services becomes. One of the unique aspects of deafblindness is that it does not disappear with increased communicative skills and possibilities. The consequences of deafblindness become more acute once the deafblind person has experienced the beauty of mental interaction – communication – and his/her soul craves more and ever deeper levels of communication. A deafblind person will only have this communion directly with another human being. Therefore, it is true beyond description that the need for intervention is never 'on a diminished level' when communication is referred to.

Communication is always an adventure. Seeing, hearing, motivated, nurtured, stimulated, and naturally curious children take the initiative and make communication happen. When a child is deafblind, the situation is quite different and calls for a great deal of guidance and coaching in order for him/her to enjoy any degree of communication and acquire communicative skills.

The intricate procedure of communication and building communication cannot be overemphasized. And the art of conveying and receiving ideas and messages truthfully and completely is for everyone a difficult task, let alone when the person concerned is deafblind. The task is awe inspiring and has to challenge everyone concerned with deafblind persons.

Let us reflect for a minute on how a 'normal, hearing, seeing, alert' baby begins to communicate, learn language, and be a member of the Family of Man. Language and other human experiences happen in close contact in an integrated, natural approach, and thus the baby identifies with this very pleasant group, Family of Man. This is when bonding is happening, and bonding is the very basis for the spiritual, emotional, and intellectual growth. If this is so with the hearing, seeing, alert baby, how much sharper the need for this approach when we are working with and for a youngster who is deafblind.

I have often thought of the story of the creation in the Old Testament. The Lord was speaking, communicating with the surroundings she/he was creating. It is reported that the Lord said: Let there be light; let the earth put forth vegetation, and so on. *The Lord needed to talk* in order to create. And having created man, *he breathed into his nostrils the breath of life and man became a living being*. (Gen. 2.5). And they started communicating. *It was at the point of communicating that man became 'a living being.'* What a beautiful report!

Never must it be thought that I believe the absence of communication is an indication of not being 'a living being.' The account of the creation of man is to me a powerful reminder that man was given the ability to communicate and was intended for communication with his fellow men. Every human being was given the wonderful seed of communication, planted into his/her innermost core. All the more serious our responsibility to help this seed to grow, nurture communication to grow and bloom.

The authors of this book advise and reminds us that in our efforts towards working with and for the people who are deafblind we must tread lightly, though surely, and have before us a guiding light, that of love and professionalism.

18

Resources

JOHN M. McINNES

The following is not a detailed list of all programs and resources available. Rather, it is intended to provide access points for parents and professionals to begin to find services or information that will meet their particular need and to encourage and facilitate communication among individuals and organizations. The editor wishes to thank Rodney Clark, Mike Collins, Bob Segrave, Sharon Barry-Grassick, Elin Ostli, Lois O'Neill, C.C. Davis, and the individuals in all of the relevant organizations listed for their assistance in obtaining and compiling the following information. Program descriptions have been written and checked by representatives of the relevant organizations.

National Programs

Argentina

Instituto Helen Keller
av. Velez Sarsfield 2100, Bg. Postal 4, Ciudad Universitaria, 5000 Cordoba
tel: 51 60 50 46   fax: 011 54 51 60 50 46

Australia

Australian DeafBlind Council
P.O. Box 267, Clifton Hill, Vic. 3068
tel: +61 39 482 1155   fax: +61 39 486 2092   TTY +61 39 489 3091
email: dba@internex.net.au
The purpose of the ADBC is to be a national council representing people who are deafblind, their support networks, and organizations working in the field. Membership is open to individuals who are deafblind, their families, and other

support people and organizations serving people who are deafblind and other interested people.

Note: The DBA of Victoria (which is a state organization) acts as secretariat for the ADBC (which is the national organization).

Carronbank School for Deaf-Blind Children
7 Allen Street, P.O. Box 311, Glen Waverley, Vic 3150
tel: (03) 9561 2536   fax: (03) 9560 3262
Carronbank school for vision/hearing impaired students is administered by the Directorate of School Education for students across the State of Victoria. Programs range from early intervention to preparation for work/adult placements.

The Deaf-Blind Association – Victoria
P.O. Box 267, Clifton Hill, Vic. 3068
tel: 03 9482 1155   TTY: 03 9489 3091   fax: 03 9486 2092
email: dba@internex.net.au
The Deaf-Blind Association provides support to deafblind people and their families. This includes community support, respite, long-term accommodation, recreation, independent living training, and specialized information. The Association provides staff training for other organizations and is a natural referral point for people with Usher Syndrome.

NSW DeafBlind Association – DBA (NSW) Inc.
P.O. Box 1295, Strathfield NSW 2135
tel: 02 9334 3333   TTY: 02 9334 3260   fax: 02 9747 5993
email: 100363. 600@compuserve.com
The DeafBlind Association (NSW) Inc. is a peak body for people who are DeafBlind in NSW. It provides advocacy, support, and social networking services to people who are DeafBlind. Once a month – hopefully more often in the future – the Hand Over Hand Club meets on a variety of activities decided by the members. There is a monthly newsletter – *Rainbow News.*

The Forsight Foundation for the Deaf/Blind
220A North Rocks Rd, North Rocks, NSW 215
P.O. Box 240, Carlingford, NSW, Australia 2118
tel: (02) 9630 5599 (International: +61 2 9630 5599)   fax: (02) 9630 6888 (International: +61 2 9630 6888)
The Forsight Foundation for the Deaf-Blind provides accommodation, support, and training for people who are deafblind with multiple disabilities (e.g., epi-

lepsy, paraplegia, cerebral palsy, and intellectual impairment). Currently (1998) it supports a research project into Congenital Rubella Syndrome and is seeking contacts.

The Royal New South Wales Institute for Deaf and Blind Children
361–365 North Rocks Road, North Rocks, NSW 2151,
tel: (02) 9871 1233   fax: (02) 9871 2196

Renwick College
361–65 North Rocks Road, North Rocks, NSW 2151
TTY: 02 9872 0303   fax: 02 9873 161   email: rcms@CC.newcastle.edu.au
A centre for research and professional studies in the education of children with sensory impairments. The college is administered by the Royal Institute for Deaf and Blind students and is affiliated with the University of Newcastle. People with appropriate qualifications may apply for admission to the following degrees programs: Master of Special Education (Sensory Disability), Master of Education, Doctor of Philosophy, and Graduate Certificate of Education (Sensory Disability). Enquiries through the Assistant Registrar, Faculty of Education, University of Newcastle, Callaghan, NSW 2308, Australia.

Western Australia Deaf-Blind Association (Inc.)
151 Guildford Road, Maylands, WA 6051
tel: (08) 9272 1122   fax: (08) 9271 3129   TTY (08) 9370 3524
email: grassick@iinet.net.au
The WA Deaf-Blind Association (WADBA) is a support and advocy service which strives to enable individuals with the unique disability of deafblindness to meet their aspirations and needs and to participate in the community. WADBA conducts individual needs assessments, links individuals into existing services where possible, and works in collaboration with other agencies to establish services where inadequate or no services exist specific to the needs of individuals who are deafblind. In addition to a small but growing resource library, information is available through a quarterly newsletter distributed to members, clients and service providers. WADBA provides training and assistance in developing individual communication programs as well as deafblind awareness and community education.

Queensland Deafblind Association (QDBA)
P.O. Box 165, St Lucia, Queensland 4067
tel: (07) 3365 1504   fax: (07) 3831 4507
email: g.mathiesen@mailbox.uq.edu.au

The Deafblind Association of South Australia
President: John Crawford. tel: (home) (08) 8344 4978
Secretary: Pauline Locke. tel: (work) (08) 8266 8552
The aims of the South Australian Deafblind Association are as follows:
To advocate and lobby for better services for people with Deafblindness
To inform and promote awareness of Deafblindness and the special needs of a person with deafblindness
To assist in the education of teachers and healthcare workers, to be able to teach Deafblind children and adults
To encourage people with Deafblindness to advocate for themselves at all levels of policy, planning, and service delivery
To seek changes in laws and policies to assist people with this disability
To lobby for more effective early detection of Deafblindness and for more timely assistance, especially with education
To be involved in ongoing research to examine the extent of consumer participation in service planning and provision, documenting any difficulties by consumers and service providers.

Austria

Osterreichisches Hilfswerk für Taubblinde
1100 Wien, Humboldtplaz 7
tel: 602 0812–0   fax: 602 08 12–17 email: oehtb@netway.at
web page: http://www.oehtb.at/oehtb
The supporting organization, which started out as a parents' association, was established in 1981 by parents of deafblind children, their teachers, and friends. The program's aims are to support integration during everyday life, provide occupational therapy, workplaces, leisure and recreational of activities, transportation, specialized support, and domiciles for deafblind people. The association has thirteen living-communities, Accompanied Domiciles (apartments), for a self-reliant life. The association also has two information centres. One provides information and help regarding early care for multiply sensory disabled children, advisory services for parents, therapy, and home visits. The other concentrates on information and help for adults.

Belgium

KMPI Spermalie
Snaggaardstraat 9, 8000 Brugge
tel: 50 340 341   fax: 50 337 306   email: Spermalie@lnnet.be

Provides day and residential educational services to students who are deafblind. The program offers both a functional and an academic curriculum, diagnostic and transitional placements, extensive evaluation services and transition as well as day and residential services for deaf-blind adults in a residential setting (Klavervier); home teaching for children and adults; and the Secretariat Anna Temmerman Association to look after the interests of children and adults in Flanders.

Brazil

Fundacion Municipal Anne Sullivan
Av Conde de Porto Alegre 820, Caetano do Sul, CEP-09561–000
tel: 11 453 0588/412 1568   fax: 11 453 0588

Bulgaria

Research Institute for Education
Cul. Tzakia 125 Fl. 5, 1113 Sofia
tel: 2 737 1380   fax: 2 722 321

Canada

Canadian Deafblind and Rubella Association (National)
C/o W. Ross Macdonald School
350 Brant Avenue, Brantford, ON N3T 3J9
tel: 519 754 0729   fax: 519 754 5400   email: cdbra.nat@sympatico.ca
web page: www.cdbra.ca
The CDBRA supports and assists persons who are deafblind and their families across Canada by promoting recognition of deafblindness as a unique disability; by developing programs and services to meet the needs of the individual with deafblindness; by advocating for the rights of persons who are deafblind and their families with governments and other agencies; and by promoting quality lifelong intervention as a right of all persons with deafblindness.

Canadian Deafblind and Rubella Association (Ontario Chapter)
350 Brant Avenue, Brantford, ON N3T 3J9
tel: 519 754 4394   fax: 519 754 0397
Is committed to ensuring that persons who are congenitally or early adventitiously deafblind are provided with the resources and services that will meet their individual needs; assists individuals who are deafblind, their families,

Intervenors, professionals, and community personnel with issues related to advocacy, support, education, and training; and administers adult programs and summer programs based on the philosophy of Intervention.

Canadian Deafblind and Rubella Association (N.B. & P.E.I.)
34 Island View Drive, Fredricton, NB E3C 3V8
tel: 506 452 1544

Canadian Deafblind and Rubella Association (Saskatchewan Chapter)
83 Tucker Crescent, Saskatoon, SK S7H 3H7
tel: 306 374 0022   fax: 306 374 0004
Provides group homes for deafblind children, youth, and adults, which operate with twenty-four hours of intervention service. The programs are community based and focus on the inclusion of individuals with deafblindness with their environments. This organization advocates provincially for the rights of persons with deafblindness.

Canadian National Institute for the Blind, Deafblind Services
1929 Bayview Avenue, Toronto, ON M4G 3E8
Toronto tel: 416 480 7417   TTY: 416 480 8645   fax: 416 480 7699
Hamilton tel: 905 528 8558   TTY: 905 528 9914
London tel: 519 685 8300   TTY: 519 685 8426
Ottawa tel: 613 563 4021   TTY: 613 567 2937
Sudbury tel: 705 675 2458   fax: 675 6635
Provides services and support to those individuals eighteen years of age and older, congenitally and adventitiously deaf-blind. The core services provided are intervention, case management, counselling, orientation and mobility, technical aides and devices, rehabilitation, communication skills training, literacy, volunteer program, and consultation.

Canadian National Society of the Deaf-Blind
Box 405, 422 Willowdale Avenue, Willowdale, ON M2N 5B1
tel/TTY: 416 445 4482   fax: 416 445 4559
e-mail: Reachingout@titan.tcn.net   web page: www.cnsdb.ca
The CNSDB is a national consumer-run society advocating for deafblind Canadians. Any adult Canadian who is deafblind may join as a full member to participate actively or simply to share the many benefits of membership. Others who support the goals of the CNSDB are invited to become associate members. The CNSDB publishes a quarterly *Newsletter*, which is distributed to all members.

Centre Dominique Tremblay
775 St Viateur, Charlesbourg est, Québec, QC G2L 2S2
Provides services home based or centre based for a population of deafblind persons of all ages, whether the person is congenitally deafblind or early adventitiously deafblind. Programs are individually designed to fit the needs of each person.

Centre Champagnat
5017 St Hubert, Montréal, PQ H2J 2X9
Provides educational services for deafblind adults.

Centre Jules-Leger, Faculté d'Education, Université d'Ottawa
Centre Jules-Leger 281 rue Lanark, Ottawa, ON K1Z 6R8
tel: 613 521 4000
The residential school program provides personal programs of instruction for school-aged children and youth. Specialist teachers and intervenors design and implement a twenty-four-hour, five-day-a-week program, in cooperation with the child's parents. The resource program provides support for infants, children, youth, and their families from the time of identification and support for children attending their local schools. The level of service support is determined on an individualized basis.

DBR Housing Society
6060 Christina Road, Richmond, BC V7C 2R8
tel: 604 277 9207

Ecole Gadbois
8777 24 E. Avenue, Montreal, QC H1Z 3Z8
Provides special classes for deafblind children.

George Brown College of Applied Arts and Technology Intervenor Program
P.O. Box 1015, Stn B, Toronto, ON M5T 2T9
Voice and TTY: 416 415 2357   fax: 416 415 2565
email: reid@gbrownc.on.ca
This is a two-year, diploma-granting program that educates students to work with both those who are congenitally deafblind and those with acquired deafblindness. Students study a variety of communication methods, including Adapted American Sign Language (AASL), Signed Exact English (SEE), and Braille. Practical courses address the skills needed in Orientation and Mobility, Assistive Devices, and Working with Medically Fragile Persons. More general

education courses involve English, Interpersonal Skills, Anatomy and Physiology, Values and Ethics, Sociology, and Psychology. Graduates have been successful in finding employment in the field within Canada and internationally. Many have found the skills transferable to related professions.

Group Home for Deafblind Persons (Brantford) Inc.
P.O. Box 27012, RPO Stanley, Brantford, ON N3S 7T8
tel: 519 752 6450   fax: 519 752 9045
An apartment accommodation (in a six-unit apartment building) housing nine adults who are congenitally and early adventitiously deafblind. This setting was chosen to provide a lifestyle of supported independent living for each adult with deafblindness to allow each one to achieve an optimal level of independence through the appropriate use of intervention and thus be able to make maximum use of existing community resources while being a participating member of society.

Independent Living Residences for the Deafblind in Ontario
169 Stephenson Crescent, Richmond Hill, ON L4C 5T3
tel: 905 770 4948   fax: 905 770 0598
Provides intervention and programs for individuals who are congenitally or early adventitiously deafblind to allow them to live in a community-based setting and to develop the skills necessary to reach an optimum level of independence through the utilization of Intervenors.

Intervenor for Deafblind Persons Program
c/o Medicine Hat College; 299 College Drive SE, Medicine Hat, SK T1A 3Y6
tel: 403 529 3910 (Wendy Johnson); 403 504 3611 (Teri King)
fax: 403 504 3510   email: wjohnson@acd.mhc.ab.ca; tking@acd.mhc.ab.ca
A two-year diploma program that prepares students to work with individuals who are either congenitally or adventitiously deafblind in residential, educational, and community based settings. Graduates of this program will have studied a variety of specialized communication methods such as Adapted American Sign Language, Signing Exact English, Large Print Notes, Finger-spelling, 2-Hand Manual, and Braille; specialized practical skills, such as sighted guide techniques, knowledge of technical aids and assistive and augmentative devices; as well as general theoretical courses, such as Lifespan Development, Interpersonal Skills, Current Issues in Sociology, Fundamentals of Reading and Writing, Observational and Functional Assessment Skills, and Anatomy and Physiology. Students are required to complete extensive practica throughout the four western provinces and the United States.

Intervention Manitoba
Suite 201, 1100 Concordia Avenue, Winnipeg, MN R2K 4B8
tel: 204 949 3730   fax: 204 949 3732
Provides Supported Independent Living Programs (day, residential, and Intervention Services) to individuals who are deafblind.

Institute Raymond-Dewar, Programme de la surdicecité
3600 rue Berri, Montréal, QC
tel: 514 284 2581   fax: 514 284 0699
Provides services home based or centre based for a population of deafblind persons of all ages, whether the person is congenitally deafblind or early adventitiously deafblind. Programs are individually designed to fit the needs of each person. Support is often given in collaboration with other rehabilitation centres, schools, or hospitals.

Manitoba Chapter – Outreach Program: CDBRA
Suite 201, 1100 Concordia Avenue, Winnipeg, MN R2K 4B8
tel: 204 949 3730   fax: 204 949 3732
Provides assessments, training programs, seminars, and consultative services.

Provincial Outreach Program for Deafblind Children (British Columbia)
103 Seacote Road, Richmond, BC V7A 4B2
tel: 604 668 7810   fax: 604 668 7812
email: Joyce_Olson@richmond.sd38.bc.ca
homepage: http://www.sd38.bc.ca/POP Listserv for intervenors at
DB_Intervenor@listserv.sd38.bc.ca
Provides consultation, in-service, and resources to school districts within British Columbia that support students with deafblindness (ages four years nine months to nineteen years) in their home schools. Also offers an Intervenor Training Program through part-time studies, in affiliation with George Brown College in Toronto.

Rotary Cheshire Homes, Inc.
422 Willowdale Avenue, Suite #101, Willowdale, ON M2N 5B1
tel: 416 730 9501,   TTY: 416 730 9578,   fax: 416 730 1350,
email: rcheshire@onramp.ca
Operates a sixteen-unit apartment building specifically built to accommodate adults who are deafblind and wish to live independently but need and want Intervention Services for access to their neighbourhood, community services, recreational facilities, news, information, and educational opportunities. The twenty-four-hour on-site Intervention service provides access to visual and

auditory information to enable each individual to make informed decisions for freedom of choice and independence. RCH is a private non-profit organization dedicated to serving the needs of persons who are deafblind, whatever the cause and whenever the onset – congenital, early, late, or acquired during developmental years. It advocates with and for deafblind persons at all levels of government and the community to promote social, recreational, learning, educational, and employment opportunities for inclusion. It provides information to the general public, to organizations of and for deafblind persons, to caregivers, and to families and individuals who are deafblind in their preferred medium (Braille, large print, sign language, and various tactile communication systems).

The W. Ross Macdonald School, Deafblind Unit, and Resource Program
350 Brant Avenue, Brantford, ON N3T 3J9
tel: 519 759 0730   fax: 519 759 4741
The residential school program provides personal programs of instruction for school-aged children and youth. Specialist teachers and intervenors design and implement a twenty-four-hour, five-day a week program, in cooperation with the child's parents. The resource program provides support for infants, children, youth, and their families from the time of identification and support for children attending their local schools. The level of service support is determined on an individualized basis. The W. Ross Macdonald, in cooperation with the University of Western Ontario, provides a three-level teacher training course leading to certification as a Specialist Teacher of the Deafblind.

Czech Republic

Lorm: Society for the Deafblind
K vodojemu 29, 150 00 Praha 5,
tel: 420 2 55 17 61   fax: 420 2 55 17 61
A system attendance program for deafblind people, which aims at breaking and overcoming the negative psychological and social impact of deafblindness on afflicted individuals and their families. The program includes seeking and screening deafblind individuals; psychotherapy and sociability rehabilitation; communication development training; awakening, stimulating, and promoting self-help activities and self-confidence; tutorial, advisory, and information services for deafblind persons and surrounding people (family members, professionals, volunteers). Clients' individual needs are respected. Attendance is founded on group and individual work with deafblind people during psycho-rehabilitation stays, seminars, and meeting clubs. Group work is supplied by individual attendance at place of residence and at Lorm:'s advisory centre.

Lorm: Society for the Deafblind Advisory Centre
Radlicka 3. 150 00 Praha 5
tel: 420 2 57 09 54 18   fax: 420 2 55 17 61

Denmark

Aalborgskolen
Kollegievej 1, Postboks 7930 DK- 9210 Aalborg SØ
tel: 98 14 30 66   fax: 98 14 71 77
Aalborgskolen has a national deafblind department for congenitally deafblind children, who live at the school and receive education from start of school age and until eighteen years.

Information Centre for Acquired Deafblindness (Videnscentret for Døvblindblevne)
Generatorvij 2A, DK 2730 Herlev
tel: +45 44 85 60 30   fax: +45 44 85 60 99   email: dbcent@inet.uni-c.dk
home page: www.dbcent.dk
The aim of the centre is to gather, adapt, and develop knowledge on acquired deafblindness and, utilizing this knowledge base, to help to maintain the highest standards in local authority schemes to assist people who have suffered a serious impairment to their sight and hearing by the dissemination of information about acquired deafblindness. The centre aims to promote efficient and comprehensive access to professional knowledge and experience in the field.

Danish Resource Centre on Congenital Deafblindness (Videnscenter for Døvblindfødte)
Langagervej 4, DK 9220 Aalborg Ost
tel: 98 15 53 13   fax: 98 15 53 23   email: vcdbf@hum.auc.dk
home page: http://www.hum.auc.dk/vcdbf
The aim of the centre is to provide general and specific expertise on the special needs of congenitally deafblind children and adults in multidisciplinary and multisectorial cooperation, with the purpose of supporting and facilitating the development of advisory services and the local, regional, and national work. The task of the centre is to gather, coordinate, adapt, develop, and diffuse knowledge on congenital deafblindness.

Institutionen for Døvblinde
Sohngardsholmsvej 59, Postbox 142, 9100 Aalborg
tel: 98 15 53 13   fax: 98 14 73 44   e-mail: idb@vip.cybercity.dk

A national integrated living and school service for congenitally deafblind people aged eighteen to twenty-three, two housing-units, and a day centre for deafblind adults. The institution also has a national Special Supervisory Service for congenitally deafblind adults

Estonia

Estonian Federation of the Blind
Lai Str. 9, EE0001 Tallinn
tel: 372 6 411 972   fax: 372 6 411 831

Support Union of the Deafblind
Kalevipoja 4–39, EE0036 Tallinn
tel: 372 6 321 36 33

Finland

The Finnish Deafblind Association, Central Office
28 A Uudenmaankatu, FIN-00120 Helsinki
tel: 358 9 5495 350 texttel: 358 9 5495 3526   fax: 358 9 5495 3517
email: ehtinen@kuuros.sci.fi
The Finnish Deafblind Association is an interest and service organization founded in 1971. It advocates the following principles: 'A deafblind person has the right to be an equal member of society. He or she has the right to study and to work, to have hobbies and a family, and to cooperate with other people. A deafblind person has the right to lead an independent life.' From the Declaration of rights of deafblind people: 'The organization: The deafblind members of the organization have the highest authority in matters concerning the Association.' At the autumn meeting, the members elect a chairperson and nine members of the board.

Resource Centre for the Deafblind
Insin""rinkatu 10 , 33720 Tampere
tel: 358 3 3800 500   texttel: 358 3 3800 501   fax: 358 3 3800 502

Rehabilitation Centre for the Deafblind
Kukkum, entie 27, 40600 JYV   SKYL
tel: 358 14 446 110   textel: 358 14 446 1128   fax: 358 14 446 1140

Organizational Activities

1. Looking after interests of deafblind people in society and observing the development and implementation of legislation.
2. Informing cooperation partners, other organizations, and the public about deafblindness, education cooperation, with other organizations, and publishing information.
3. Providing and/or promoting local clubs for recreational activities, education for organizations, camps and other recreational activities, peer activities, and voluntary work
4. International activities: The association has a representative in the commission of the deafblind in the European Blind Union (EBU), in the European Deafblind Network (EDbN), and in the Nordic Staff Training Centre for Deafblind Services (NUD)
5. Providing services including:
   a) Resource and Expert Network: Ten regional counsellors, client work, cooperation with local authorities and service systems, education, courses for the deafblind, and volunteer work
   b) Resource Centre for the Deafblind, Tampere: Housing services, individually planned rehabilitation courses and adaptation training, facilities for work, hobby and rehabilitation activities, computer services and computer education for deafblind people, recreational and holiday activities
   c) Rehabilitation Centre for the Deafblind, Jyv skyl,,: Rehabilitation services for congenitally deafblind and hearing and visually impaired children, youth, and adults; adaptation training for hearing and visually impaired deafblind children and their families, educational guidance for children with Usher syndrome, and training for deafblind personnel
   d) Improving the access to information: (ADP-services, publishing newsletters and papers adapted for the deafblind,)

The Finnish Deafblind Association
Uudenmaankatu 28 A, 00120 Helsinki
tel: 358 9 5495 350   texttel: 358 9 5495 3526   fax: 358 9 5495 3517
The association is an interest and service organization for all deafblind people and work in the field of deafblindness throughout Finland.

The Service Foundation for the Deaf, Central Office
Ilkantie 4, P.O. Box 62, FIN-00400 Helsinki
tel: +358 9 580 31   texttel: +358 9 580 3651   fax: +358 9 580 3657
The Service Foundation for the Deaf provides accommodation services and

mental health services in sign language for the deaf and deafblind, together with various supporting services that are not available from the public sector. Activities, for example: service houses for the deaf and deafblind; service houses for the deaf and deafblind young people; work centre and service accommodation; development of social services and health services for the deaf and deafblind.

France

ANPSA Association de Patronage pour les Sourds-Aveugles   .
18 rue Etex, F-75018 Paris
tel: +33 1 46 27 48 10   fax: +33 1 46 27 80 92
Association of deafblind people, families, professionals, and institutions concerned with deafblindness. A good source of information concerning services for the deafblind in France

APSA 116 Av. de la Libération
7–86000 Poitiers,
tel: +33 5 49 62 67 89   fax: +33 5 49 62 67 90
Resource Centre for preschool deafblind children (CESSA Larnay) Boarding School for Deafblind Children, group homes for Congenitally Deafblind adults (Foyer La Varenne), Sheltered Workshop for Deafblind Adults. (CAT La Chume)

Establissement pour Sourds-Aveugles
37–39 rue Division Leclerc, 78460 Chevereuse
tel: +33 1 30 52 64 57
A boarding school for deafblind children.

Germany

Deutsches Taubblindenwerk gGmbH
Albert-Schweitzer-Hof 27, D 30559 Hanover
tel: 49 511 510 080,   fax: 49 511 510 08 57
email: 0511510080–1@btgate.de
The German Institute for the Deafblind, founded in 1967, is run by the German Federation of the Blind, the Federation of the Blind (Lower Saxony), and the German Welfare Umbrella Organization, and it is the largest organization of its kind in Germany. It aims to promote the needs of audio-visually handicapped and deafblind persons. The education, advancement, and care for audio-visually handicapped and deafblind persons include reducing isolation, promoting com-

munication, developing the skills of perception and mobility, daily living skills, creativity, and interaction with the environment. In addition to our intensive efforts to support the individual in meeting physical challenges and mental needs, special stress is placed on leisure-time activities and holiday events to overcome the problems of isolation and loneliness, create social relationships, and extend the skills of perception and mobility. The organization consists of three institutions, as follows.

Bildungszentrum für Taubblinde
Postfach 710460, 30544 Hanover
tel: 511 5100813   fax: 511 5100857
A private school approved by the government that provides both a residential program for school-aged children and youth and a resource program that provides support for infants, children, youth, and families from time of identification and adults who are adventitiously deafblind. A residential home for adults in Hanover with special workshops at the Blind Union of Lower Saxony. A residential home and workshop for deafblind young adults with additional handicaps in Fischbeck near Hameln

Blindeninstitutsstiftung
Ohmstrasse 7, 97076 Wuerzburg
tel: 0 931 2092 121   fax: 0 931 2092251
Provides a home-based early intervention program for infants from birth to eight years of age; a residential program for preschool and school aged children and youth from four to twenty-one years of age; and a residential program for adults including a sheltered workshop.

Oberlinhaus Potsdam Babelsberg (Rehabilitation Centre Innere Mission)
Rudolf Breitschied Strasse 24, 0–1591 Potsdam
tel: 33 763 5221   fax: 33 763 5230

Sonderheim für Taubblinde und Blinde Kinder, Jügendliche und Erwachsene
Dorfstrabe 16, 25767 Tensbuttel
tel: 0 48 35/999 0   fax: 0 48 35/999 30

Taubblindendienst e. V.
Fachverband im Diakon. Werk der EKD für Taubblinde und
    mehrfachbehinderte Blinde
Pillnitzer Strabe 71, 01454 Radeberg
tel: 0 35 28/4 39 70

Cecilienstift Halberstadt
Wohnheim für Taubblinde Menschen, Klusheim
38820 Halberstadt
tel: 0 39 41/44 28 13

Ghana

Centre for Deafblind Children
P.O. Box 33, Mampong-Akawpim
tel: 0872 220 34
Established in 1978, the Centre is a joint project between the Government of
Ghana and the Christoffel-Blindenmission (CBM) of Germany. CBM provides
the infrastructure, maintenance of physical facilities, and the supply of equipment and materials for the teaching/learning processes. The Ghanaian government provides staff and salaries. The Centre maintains links with Perkins
School for the Blind, Deafblind International, Sense International, and other
associations having an interest in deafblindness. The Centre provides educational and rehabilitative services to young deafblind students. Programs include
orientation and mobility training, vocational skills development, and the development of independent living skills.

Greece

Greek Association of Parents and Friends of Deafblind Children
Lighthouse of the Blind, Athinas 17 and Doiranis, Kallithea 17673
tel and fax: 1 6917774
The Association is the only association in Greece that is occupied with the
problems of deafblind persons. The main aims/activities are identification of
deafblind persons; education of deafblind children; rehabilitation; two-week
summer camp; and the creation of a 'home.' The Association works with the
state authorities for the creation of a school for deafblind children through the
Centre of Education and Rehabilitation of the Blind.

Hungary

Barczi Gusztav Training College for Teachers of the Handicapped
H-1443 Budapest 70, PF. 146
tel: 011 36 1 121 3526/40   fax: 011 1 122 6447

Iceland

Samskiptamidstod, heyrnarlausra og heynarskertra
Vesturhlio, 105 Reykjavik
tel: 562 7702   fax: 562 7714   email: valas@rhi.hi.is
The goal is to facilitate active integration into Icelandic society, run Sign Language courses and courses in untraditional communication for deafblind people and their families, and intervene as wishes indicate and need dictates. We do not have intervention services, but we do have interpreter services.

India

Helen Keller Institute for Deaf and Deafblind
Municipal Secondary School, South Wing Ground Floor, Near 'S' Bridge,
N.M. Joshi Marg Byculla (W), Mumbai 400011, India.
tel: 22 39 70 52   fax: 22 28 72 735
The Helen Keller Institute for Deaf and Deafblind has separate schools for the deaf (with sixty-two children) and for the deafblind (twenty-two children). The program for the deafblind offers individualized instruction from early intervention to adult rehabilitation, including infant and toddler to preschool (thrice weekly to every day), followed by monthly home visits for family orientation; all age groups are offered a graded functional curriculum catering to each individual. Curriculum content includes self-help skills, academics, pre-vocational skills, independent living skills, and job rehabilitation; co-curricular activities, such as swimming, camping, mobility, domestic science, mime, and dance, are also included. Hostel facilities for children residing outside Bombay are available.

Ireland

Anne Sullivan Foundation
40 Lower Drumcondra Road, Dublin 9
tel: 01 83 00 562   fax: 01 830 0562
Operates a residential centre for congenitally and early adventitiously deafblind persons (Anne Sullivan Centre, Brewery Road, Stillorgan, County Dublin) whose programs contain a substantial educational element on a life-long basis. The foundation also provides home support and outreach services.

Israel

Keren OR Inc, the Jerusalem Center for Multihandicapped Blind
Abba Hillel Silver 3, P.O. Box 23523, Ramot A, Jerusalem 91234
tel: 02 586 9626   fax: 02 586 9096
Keren Or provides a daily school curriculum for legally blind children ages one year to twenty-one years, with a wide range of additional handicaps, including deafness, physical disability, retardation, and communication disorders. The degree of handicap varies greatly from child to child. Paramedical programs are individualized, and emotional support is included. In addition, a residential home is provided from age five for children from all parts of the country.

Italy

Lega del Filo d'Oro
Via Montecerno, 1, 60027 Osimo (AN)
tel: 071/72451   fax: 071/717102   email: cdfilod@imar.net
web page: http://www.imar.net/filodoro
The Lega del Filo d'Oro is a national private association whose aim is rehabilitation, education, and assistance to deafblind and multi-sensorily impaired people. The Rehabilitation Centre of the Lega del Filo d'Oro offers services to people of all age groups. At the Diagnostic Centre a thorough psycho-pedagogic and medical assessment is made according to the multi-disciplinary method. The Documentation Centre allows a continuous updating of information and represents a point at a national level for materials on sensory impairment.

Japan

Japan Deaf-Blind Association
2-2-8 Nishiwaseda, Shinjyuku-ku, Tokyo 162
tel: +81 3 5272 1691   fax: +81 3 5272 1692
Established in 1991, the Japan Deaf-Blind Association now has identified about 400 deafblind people throughout the country. It undertakes several activities to establish the support to deafblind people. One important activity is the provision of support service providers to about 200 registered members with severe deafblindness, both adventitious and congenital, the maximum provision being 240 hours a year for each person. This is currently run on a 'model' project basis financed by subsidies from the central government in order to promote local initiatives to take over this service.

National Institute of Special Education, Department of Education for
the Multiply Handicapped
Address: 5-1-1 Nobi, Yokosuka 239
tel: +81 468 48 4121   fax: +81 468 49 5563   email: wchofuku@nise.go.jp
Directly affiliated to the Ministry of Education, the NISE carries out practical
research, in-service teacher training, and information dissemination concerning
special education. It also provides consultation services to families with children with disabilites upon referral. NISE is divided into different departments
according to categories of disability, including the Department of Education for
the Multiply Handicapped. There are seven staff in this department, and about
half of them have been engaged in the consultation service of children with congenital deafblindness upon referral.

Kodo-En
21-8-11, Ishidakami-cho, Sabae-shi, Fukui 916
tel: +81 778 62 1234   fax: +81 778 62 0890
email: kodoen@po.infosphere.or.jp
Kodo-En is a complex of residential homes and sheltered workshops for multiply disabled people with visual impairment, established and run by a private
organization. There is a residential home specifically for the deafblind with a
day centre where deafblind residents, some of whom are congenitally deafblind,
engage in productive work, recreation, and learning activities. Kodo-En recognizes the need for developing communication skills for deafblind residents, and
emphasis is placed on learning activities that promote communication. Currently, the program serves deafblind people.

Yokohama Christian School for the Blind
181 Takenomaru, Nakaku, Yokohama 231
tel: +81 45 641 2626   fax: +81 45 662 1710
This is a privately run school for the blind divided into two departments. One is
for vocational education for adventitiously visually impaired adults, teaching
acupuncture, moxibustion, and massage; the other is for multiply disabled children from age three to about twenty. There are about thirty children currently in
the Department for the Multiply Disabled among whom three are congenitally
deafblind. The school has had an enrolment of deafblind children, though small
in number, for more than twenty-five years, and the teachers have accumulated
the necessary skills and knowledge to work with these children. This feature is
difficult to find in public special schools in Japan, where teachers customarily
shift from one school to another in about three to ten years.

Kenya

Kabarnet School for Deafblind Children
P.O. Box 1340, Maralal
tel: 328 2107

Lithuania

Lithuanian Association of the Blind and Visually Handicapped
Labdariu 7/11, Vilnius
tel: 3702 619114 624866   fax: 3702 22 1464

Malaysia

St Nicholas Home
Locked Bag No. 3031, 4, Jalan Bagan Jermal Road, 10090 Penang
tel: 60 4 227 3294   fax: 60 4 229 0800   email: stnick@po.jaring.my
A residential program with six children. The children are given individual attention on self-help skills, basic writing, reading, counting, sign language, and
Braille. There are four teachers and two house mothers who attend to the recreational and physical needs of the children.

Netherlands

Centre Bartimeushage
P.O. Box 87, Oude Arnhemse Bovenweg 3, 3940 AB Doorn
tel: 343 526 500/526 501   fax: 343 526 798

Centre for Deafblind Children and Adults, Instituut voor Doven
Theerestraat 42, 5271 GD Sint Michielsgestel. The Netjerland
tel: 31 73 55 88 111   fax: 73 55 88 440
email: 100575.2522@compuserve.com
The Centre for Deafblind and Adults consists of the following units:
• A unit for parent guidance and family support for deafblind children ages
  birth to three years.
• A transition unit for children three to four years of age in cooperation with
  the school for the deafblind (Rafael).
• An outreach program for deafblind children who are served by other agencies, but have requested support from the Centre.
• A school and residential setting for children ages four to twenty. This com-

prehensive program provides instruction and education on the basis of an individualized educational program.
- A residential program for adults. This program provides job training, living accommodation, and a range of support facilities.
- A unit for multidisciplinary assessment, which provides medical, audiological (CI), visual, and psychological assessment and advice and rehabilitation services for all the deafblind students of the Centre, but it serves also as an outside clinic for all persons with deafblindness in the country.
- EUCO unit. Associated with the Centre, this unit provides information to agencies for the deafblind in the countries of the European Community.

New Zealand

Homai Vision Education Centre
Browns Road, Private Bag 801, Manurewa, Auckland
tel: 09 266 7109   fax: 09 267 4496
The Centre provides holistic transdisciplinary assessment of persons from birth to twenty-one who are congenitally and early adventitiously deafblind. Individual developmental and educational programs are developed to meet assessed needs.

Vision Hearing Impaired Association
c/o Royal NZ Foundation for the Blind, Auckland Regional Office Private Bag 99916, Newmarket, Auckland

Deafblind N.Z. Incorporated
P.O. Box 109–583, Newmarket, Auckland
tel: 09 355 6925
The society was registered in 1988 and is distinctive for being for people with the dual disability of deafblindness / vision and hearing impairment. It is organized and operated almost entirely by deafblind/VHI persons themselves to enhance the quality of life for persons with the unique dual sensory condition of 'Vision and Hearing Impairment.' One of the objectives of the society is To promote and forward the interests and well-being of persons aged eighteen years and over who are Deafblind / Vision and Hearing Impaired (VHI) and/or support those persons who are parents, guardians, spouses, or companions of Deafblind/VHI persons.

Norway

Norwegian Central Team for the Deafblind
P.O. Box 8042, Dep. N-0031 Oslo
tel: 47 22 24 81 80 textphone: 47 22 24 81 91   fax: 47 22 24 81 92   email: sentralteamet@sentralteamet.no   Internet: http://www.sentralteamet.no/
Our only task concerning congenitally deafblind persons is registration, while our focus group is made up of persons with acquired deafblindness, including persons with Ushers Syndrome. A special effort is made to identify elderly deafblind persons who were not previously registered.

Regionsenteret for døvblindfødte i Nord-Norge
Gimlev 64–68, Postboks 3323, N-9003 Tromsø.
email: regsendbf@online.no
The Regional Resource Centre for Persons with Congenital Deafblindness Northern Norway is situated in Tromsø. It offers services to congenitally deafblind persons of all ages. The Centre has an interdisciplinary staff of special educators, social workers, a physiotherapist, and a psychologist. A major part of the services includes assessment of mental, sensory, and communicative abilities and the implementation of individual intervention programs in the caretakers' own community. Consequently, much time is devoted to the supervision of caregivers and teachers in local communities in all parts of Northern Norway. In addition, the Resource Centre offers courses and seminars in Tromsø to professionals and non-professionals engaged in the services for congenitally deafblind and multihandicapped persons. Another major responsibility of the Resource Centre is connected to the management of its residential centre. At present seven congenitally deafblind adults have their own flats on a permanent basis, with day and night caretaking facilities. The residents are offered individual programs of teaching, work, medical treatment, physical training, and leisure-time activities.

Skadalen Resource Centre for Special Education of the Hearing Impaired
    and Deafblind
Postboks 13, Slemdal, N-0321 Oslo 3
tel: 22 14 52 90   fax: 22 14 76 51
The Centre provides highly specialized services for the congenitally deafblind in four main areas on the local, regional, and national levels.

1. The residential school for the congenitally deafblind (birth to twenty years) provides highly specialized personal programs of instruction.
2. The resource program provides assessment services focusing on identification of the congenitally deafblind on a national level and continual guidance and supervision to the networks around individual and groups of congenitally deafblind on a regional level. The Centre also provides supervision to consultants in other regions.
3. The staff development program provides continual courses to networks (staff and families) on a regional and a national basis.
4. The research program initiates, coordinates, and conducts development and research projects focusing on congenital deafblindness on a national level.

Solveigns Hus Hjemmet for Dove
P.O. Box 95, Sukke, N-3240 Andebu
tel: 47 3343 8700
The services provided by Solveigs Hus include residential settings and a resource centre. The residential homes provide housing and supported living for congenitally deafblind adults, to promote the individual's development of self-identity and quality of life. There is a continual search for motivating and developing daytime activities at different levels of complexity. It is our belief that, through social interaction and communication, these activities will serve as options that allow individuals to create their own quality of life. The resource centre provides services to congenitally deafblind persons of all ages in the southern part of Norway. In cooperation with local networks, the services include observation, assessment, and supervision. Specially designed courses are provided according to the network's individual needs.

Vestlandet Kompetansesenter Resource Centre for Special Education of
    Hearing Impaired and Deafblind
Jonas Liesvel 68, 5037 Solheimsviken
tel: 47 55 59 84 00   fax: 47 55 59 84 01

Philippines

Philippines National School for the Blind
Galvez Corner Figueroa, 1300 Pasay City
tel: 28 31 86 64

Poland

Polski Zwiazek Niewidomych Glowny
ul. Konwiktorska 9
tel: 22 31 33 83   fax: 22 63 55 793
The Association for the Welfare of Deafblind, often in cooperation with the Polish Association of the Blind, has created a rehabilitation and care centre for deafblind persons that includes residential provisions; developed a system of guide-interpreter services; organized two-week rehabilitation and training courses for varied groups of deafblind children and youth; prepared and distributed publications focusing on different issues, including didactic and training; providing rehabilitation equipment, including hearing and optical aids; and created and supported clubs for deafblind people and their families. In addition, the association provides information to the general population by publishing leaflets, organizing exhibitions of works of art created by the deafblind, and giving lectures.

Portugal

Casa Pia de Lisboa-CAACF
Rua d. Francisco Almeida 1, 1400 Lisboa
tel: 793 59 63   fax: 351 1 793 48 40
The College AACF of Casa Pia de Lisboa supports deafblind children and adults by promoting social and working integration leading to a good quality of life. The college also supports residences for deafblind people.

Romania

Department of Psychology, University Cluj-Napoca
Str. Kogainiceanu Nr. 1, 3400 Cluj-Napoca
tel: 95 11 61 01   fax: 95 11 19 05

Russia

Institute of Special Education, Russian Academy of Education, Laboratory for teaching children with compound impairments
8–2 Pogodinskaya St
119834 Russia, Moscow
tel.: 7 905 245 44 67; 7 095 246 44 67   fax: 7 095 230 20 62
email: root@ise.msk.ru

The Laboratory develops programs for teaching deafblind children of preschool and school ages, investigates the population of deafblind children, provides diagnostic assessment of deafblind people of different ages, consults parents and teachers who work with deafblind people, and develops training courses for specialists working with deafblind and multiply impaired children.

Home for Deafblind Children
20 Pogranichnaya St
141300 Russia' Sergiev Posad, Moscow Region
tel:/fax: 7 09654 2 52 08
A residential school accepting children from three to twenty-five years of age. The 120 residents are taught in groups of three to four students. Individual programs of teaching. Qualified teachers work with the children in and out of the classroom for sixteen of the twenty-four hours every day of the week.

Centre of Rehabilitation of the Blind
Department of Deafblind Rehabilitation
43 Panfilov St 143600 'volokolamsk, Moscow Region
tel: 2 33 05, 2 33 18
Rehabilitation course (2.5–5 months) for deafblind adults (eighteen to sixty years of age) from all over Russia: sources of communication; everyday routine skills; mobility; independent living. Specialized medical treatment and therapy. Social programs for students.

Singapore

Singapore School for the Visually Handicapped
51 Toa Payoh Rise, 1129 Singapore
tel: 250 3755, 250 5498   fax: 250 5348

Slovakia

Evanjelika pomocna skola internatna pre hluchoslepe deti
082 07 Cervenica 114, Slovakia
tel: 421 91 790215   fax: 421 91 790 215
Offers the only program for deafblind children in Slovakia. The residential school program provides the education and upbringing to children between three and eighteen years of age. Specialist teachers and educators design and implement a 24 hour, 7 day a week program. The school cooperates with parents and helps them to coordinate the work at home.

South Africa

Pioneer School for the Visually Handicapped
20 Adderley Street, 6850 Worcester
tel: 231 22313   fax: 231 23959   email: carrwoc@telkom.co.za
The Pioneer School provides individual programs according to the deafblind child's stage of development with particular emphasis on appropriate communication systems, developing social behaviour, practical skills for leading an independent life, developing self-awareness, and experiencing him/herself as a member of the community; and offering factual information and school subjects which provide general education.

Spain

CRE Antonio Vicente Mosquete, O.N.C.E. Programma de Sordociegos
Paseo de la Habana 208, 28036 Madrid
tel: +34 91 3453697, ext. 237   fax: +34 91 3507972
This program is aimed to cover the basic needs and deliver all possible services to the Spanish deafblind population. It offers education programs, sociocultural activities and support for adults and youth, interpreter services, and publishes *Tercer Sentido* among others.

Sweden

Ekeskolan
Box 9024, 700 09 Orebro
tel: 19 245 020   fax: 19 245 489

Resource Center Mo Gård
S-612 93 Finspång
tel: +46 122 23600   fax: +46 122 20117
For congenitally deafblind persons Mo Gård offers habilitation, independent living-services, group homes in Finspång; supervising, staff training, information, assessment, consultation for parents and staff on a local level. Stress is upon development work and networking.

Switzerland

Schweiz Stiftung für Taubblinde
Heim Tanne, Fuhrstrasse 15, 8135 Langau aA

tel: 00411 713 14 40   fax: 00411 713 14 35
Early advice service, school, sheltered workshops, residential facilities for deaf-blind children and adults

United Kingdom

Communication Works
32 High Street, High Wycombe, Bucks
tel: +44 1494 439222

Council for the Advancement of Communication with Deaf People
Pelaw House, School of Education, University of Durham, Durham DH1 1TA
tel: +44 191 374 3607   fax: +44 191 374 3605

Deafblind UK
Head Office: 100 Bridge Street, Peterborough PE1 1DY
tel: 0 1733 358100   fax: 0 1733 358356 text: +44 1733 358858
email: Jackie@deafblind.demon.co.uk
Deafblind UK is a charity whose aims are to further the interests and needs of
people who suffer from both hearing and sight impairments (deafblindness) and
also to generate public awareness of this condition. Deafblind UK caters for the
needs of deafblind people in all walks of life and provides many services.

Deafblind UK Scotland
Deafblind UK Scottish Office, Drena O'Malley, Development Manager
21 Alexandra Avenue, Lenzie G66 5BG
tel: 0141 777 6111   fax: 0141 775 3311
email: info@deafblindscotland.org.uk

Leigh Centre
41 The Archers Way, Glastonbury, Somerset BA6 9JB
tel: +44 1458 834986

Royal National Institute for the Blind
224 Great Portland Street, London W1N 6AA
tel: +44 171 388 1266   fax: +44 171 388 2034

Royal National Institute for Deaf People
19–23 Featherstone Street, London EC1Y 4AH
tel: +44 171 296 8184   fax: +44 171 296 8185 text: +44 171 296 8183

Sense – The National Deafblind and Rubella Association
11–13 Clifton Terrace, Finsbury Park, London N4 3SR
tel: +44 171 272 7774   minicom: +44 171 272 9648   fax: +44 171 272 6012
Founded as a parents' self-help group in 1955, Sense now serves people who were born deafblind or acquired deafblindness later in life. Families remain at Sense's core. Sense brings together the work of doctors, teachers, therapists, social workers, and other professionals, each looking at a different aspect of a deafblind person's life. Working in partnership, Sense offers integrated services to meet the range of needs of deafblind people and their families. Sense's specialist services include:

- Support for children, their parents and siblings
- Residential homes
- Education and training
- Holidays, leisure activities and respite care
- Intervenors who work one-to-one
- Communicator-guides and services for elderly people
- Support for people with Usher syndrome
- Sharing expertise throughout the United Kingdom as well as in other countries through Sense International

SCHOOL AND PRE-SCHOOL INSTITUTE SERVICES

Carnbooth School
80 Busby Road, Carmunnock, Glasgow G76 9EG
tel: +44 141 644 2773
Provides education for deafblind children from preschool to eighteen-plus.

Henshaw's School
Bogs Lane, Harrogate, North Yorkshire HG1 4ED
tel: +44 1423 886451

Northern Counties School for the Deaf
Great North Road, Newcastle-upon-Tyne NE2 3BB
tel: +44 191 281 5821

Whitefield School and Centre
Macdonald Road, Walthamstow, London E17 4AT
tel: 0 181 531 3426   email: WHITEFIELD_edu@classic.msn.com
The library has a special needs information service for subscribers. Members

may also subscribe to the bi-monthly current awareness bulletin, which reflects the needs of parents, educators, support services, health services, and administrators. The school provides education and support for deafblind children and children with sensory impairment and learning difficulties.

Royal School for the Blind
Church Road North, Wavertree, Liverpool L15 6TQ
tel: +44 151 733 1012

Royal School for Deaf Children
Victoria Road, Margate, Kent CT9 1NB
tel: +44 1843 227561

Royal West of England School for the Deaf
50 Topsham Road, Exeter EX2 4NF
tel: +44 1392 72692

Royal Schools for the Deaf (Manchester)
Stanley Road, Cheadlehulme, Cheadle, Cheshire SK8 6RF
tel: +44 161 437 5951/2/3

RNIB Condover Hall School
Condover, Shrewsbury, Shropshire SY5 7AH
tel: +44 174 372 2320

RNIB Rushton Hall School
Rushton, Nr Kettering, Northamtonshire NN14 1RR
tel: +44 1536 710506

Thorn Park School and Educational Services for the Hearing Impaired
Thorn Lane, Bingley Road, Bradford BD9 6RY
tel: +44 1274 497866/499746

The West of England School for Children with Little or No Sight
Countess Wear, Exeter, Devon
tel: +44 1392 454200

Education Service for Deafblind Children (South and West Wales): Resource
   and Assessment Centre: Ysgol Hendr
Bryncoch, Neath, West Glamorgan SA10 7TY
tel: +44 1639 631935

Sense – West of England Education Advisory Service
4 Church Road, Edgbaston, West Midlands B15 3TD
tel: +44 121 456 1564   fax: +44 121 452 1656

Sense – Ealing Family Centre
86 Cleveland Road, Ealing, London W13 0HE
tel: +44 181 991 0513   fax: +44 181 810 5925

Sense – Woodside Family Centre
Woodside Road, Kingswood, Bristol BS15 2DG
tel: 0 117 967 0008
Centre run by Sense for blind and deafblind children and their families.
Resource centre offering information and advice; toy library, sensory stimulation room, creche with many play resources and plenty of room.

Sense Scotland – Family Resource Centre
15 Newark Drive, Pollokshields, Glasgow G41 4QB
tel: +44 141 424 3222   fax: +44 141 424 1390   text: +44 141 424 1427
There are many schools in the United Kingdom, in addition to those given above, with specialist provision for deafblind children. For more information, please contact Education, Family and Advisory Services at Sense (see Organizations, above; tel: 0141 221 7577).

United States of America

American Association of the Deaf-Blind (AADB)
814 Thayer Ave, Ste 302, Silver Spring, MD 20910
email: aabb@erols.com
A national consumer advocacy organization for people who have a combined hearing and vision impairment. Membership is open to persons who are deafblind and individuals directly concerned with their well-being. The AADB provides technical assistance, consultants, and direct on-site assistance. Annual dues $15.00US.
Publishes *The Deaf-Blind American*

American Council of the Blind (Deaf-Blind Committee)
1155 15th Street, N.W., Suite 720 Washington, DC 20005
tel: 202 467 5081 or 800 424 8666   fax: 202 467 5085
Provides information, referral, scholarships, advocacy, consultation, and programming assistance.

American Foundation for the Blind
11 Penn Plaza, Suite 300, New York, NY 10001
tel: 800 232 5463, 212 502 7600   email: afbinfo@afb.org

American Printing House for the Blind
1839 Frankfort Ave., Louisville, KY 40206
tel: 502 895 2405 800 223 1839   fax: 502 895 1509   email: info@aph.ort
Produces materials in Braille, large print, and audiocassette; manufactures computer-access equipment and software.

Callier Azusa Scale
University of Texas at Dallas, Callier Center for Communication Disorders
1966 Inwood Road Dallas, Texas 75235
home page: http:/howw.utdallas.edu/dept/nd/text/cc/

CHARGE Syndrome Foundation, Inc.
2004 Parkade Blvd., Columbia, MO 65202–3121
tel: 800 442 7604   tel/fax: 573 499 4694   email: orphan@nord-rdb.com

DB-Link (The National Information Clearinghouse on Children Who
   Are Deafblind)
c/o Teaching Research Division, Western Oregon University,
345 North Monmouth Ave., Monmouth, OR 97361
tel: 800 438 9376   TTY/TDD 800 854 7013   fax: 503 838 8150
email: dblink@tr.wou.edu
Disseminates information as a public service. Keeps updated databases, including the names of consultants, information on early intervention, education medical, social independent living and health issues. Teaching Research publishes *Deaf-Blind Perspectives.*

Deaf-Blind Services, Rose Resnick Lighthouse for the Blind
214 Van Ness Ave., San Francisco, CA 94102
email: dpickering@lighthouse-sf.org
Services are available to all persons who have congenital or acquired visual and hearing impairments, including information and referral, advocacy, counselling and support groups, education and training, as well as adult retreat, service provider, and student education. Technical support is available to service providers and students to encourage better professional services.

Foundation Fighting Blindness
Executive Plaza 1, Suite 800, 11350 McCormick Rd, Hunt Valley,
MD 21031–1014
tel: 800 683 5555, 410 225 9400

Gallaudet University
800 Florida Ave., NE, Washington, DC 20002–3625
tel: 202 651 5551   fax: 202 651 5595   email: twjones@gallu.gallaudet.edu
Operates a deafblind program and supports individuals who are deafblind to
achieve educational success, disseminates information and publishes books,
pamphlets, and videos.

Hadley School for the Blind
700 Elm Street, Winnetka, IL 60093-0299
tel: 1 800 323 4238 or 847 446 8111   email: info@Hadley-School.org
Provides home studies in academic subjects, personal enrichment, rehabilitation, living without sight and hearing and supporting individuals who are deafblind.

Helen Keller National Center
111 Middle Neck Road, Sands Point, NY 11050
tel: 516 944 8900   fax: 516 944 7302   email: HKNCDIR@aol.com
A national program that provides diagnostic evaluation, short-term comprehensive rehabilitation and personal adjustment training, work experience, and
placement to youth and adults. The HKNC Technical Assistance Center assists
in transition from school to adult life, and supports groups who are promoting
integration. Publishes *HKNC-TAC News.*

REGIONAL REPRESENTATIVES

I. New England Region: Connecticut, Maine, Massachusetts, New Hampshire,
Rhode Island, Vermont.
HKNC, 313 Washington St. Suite 209, Newton, MA 02158; voice and TTY:
617 630 1580 and 617 630 1581   fax: 617 630 1579
email: HKNC1meb@aol.com

II. Mid-Atlantic Region: New York, New Jersey, Puerto Rico, Virgin Islands
HKNC, 111 Middle Neck Road, Sands Point, NY 11050
voice: 516 944 8900   TTY: 516 944 8637   fax: 516 883 9060
email: HKNCReg2BM@aol. com

538   John McInnes

III. East Central Region: Delaware, District of Columbia, Maryland, Pennsylvania, Virginia, West Virginia
HKNC, 6801 Kenilworth Avenue, Suite 100, Riverdale, MD 20737
voice: 301 699 6255, 6256   TTY: 301 699 8490   fax: 301 699 8564
email: HKNC.Region3@Juno.com

IV. Southeastern Region: Alabama, Florida, Georgia, Mississippi, Kentucky, North Carolina, Carolina, South Carolina, Tennessee
HKNC, 1005 Virginia Avenue, Suite 104, Atlanta, GA 30354
voice: 404 766 9625   TTY: 404 766 2820   fax: 404 766 3447
email: SB-HKNC@Juno.com

V. North Central Region: Illinois, Michigan, Indiana, Minnesota, Ohio, Wisconsin
HKNC, P.O. Box 6761, Rock Island, IL 61204-6761
voice and   TTY: 309 788 7990   TTY: 309 788 7089
fax: 309 788 7759   email: HKNC5@Juno.com

VI. South Central Region: Arkansas, Louisiana, New Mexico, Oklahoma, Texas
HCNC, 4455 LBJ Freeway, LB#3, Suite 814 Dallas, TX 75244-5998
voice and TTY: 972 490 9677, 9678, 9681, 9682   data line: 972 490 6054
fax: 972 490 6042   email: CCFUTBOL@aol.com

VII. Great Plains Region: Iowa, Kansas, Missouri, Nebraska
HKNC, 4330 Shawnee Mission Parkway, Suite 108 Shawnee Mission, KS 66205
voice and TTY: 913 677 4562   fax: 913 677 1544
email: HKNC7BJ@sprintmail.com

VIII. Rocky Mountain Region: Colorado, Montana, North Dakota, South Dakota, Utah, Wyoming
HKNC, 1880 South Pierce Street Suite #5, Lakewood, CO 80232
voice and TTY: 303 934 9037   fax: 303 934 2939
email: HKNCMO@tde.com

IX. Southwestern Region: Arizona, California, Guam, Samoa, and the Trust Territories Hawaii, Nevada
HKNC, 18345 Ventura Blvd Suite 505, Tarzana, California 91356
voice: 818 757 8921   TTY: 818 757 8922   fax: 818 757 8965
email: HKNCReg@aol.com

X. Northwestern Region: Alaska, Idaho, Oregon, Washington
HKNC, 2366 Eastlake Avenue East Suite 209, Seattle, Washington 98102-3366
voice: 206 324 9120 TTY: (D. Walt): 206 324 1133
email: NWHKNC@Juno.com

Older Adults Program
HKNC, 4455 LBJ Freeway, LB#3, Suite 814 Dallas, Texas 75244-5998
voice and TTY: 972 490 9677, 9678, 9681, 9682   fax: 972 490 6042
email: mbagley@earthlink.net

Howe Press
175 North Beacon Street, Watertown, MA 02172
May be contacted through the Perkins School for the Blind.

John Tracy Clinic
806 West Adams Boulevard, Los Angeles, CA 90007
tel: 213 748 5481   TTY/TTD: 213 747 2924   fax: 213 749 1651
email: jtclinic@aol.com
Provides a correspondence course for families of preschool children who are
deafblind. The course focuses on communication and skill development.

Mississippi State University Rehabilitation Research and Training Center
P.O. Drawer 6189, Mississippi State, MS 39762
tel: 601 325 2001   TTY/TDD: 601 325 8693   fax: 601 325 8989
email: rrtc@ra.msstate.edu
Conducts research projects, in-service training conferences. Publishes *Work-
sight.*

National Coalition on Deaf-Blindness (NCDB)
175 North Beacon Street, Watertown, MA 02172
tel: 617 972 7347   fax: 617 923 8076   email: davies@perkins,pvt.k12.ma.us

National Family Association for Deafblind (NFADB)
111 Middle Neck Road, Sans Point, NY 11050 1299
tel: 516 944 8900, 800 255 0411   fax: 516 944 7302
A national network of families of children, youth, and adults who are deafblind.
Focus on issues surrounding deafblindness by advocating, encouraging the
foundation and strengthening of family organizations in each state, and providing information and referrals. Publishes *NFADB Newsletter.*

National Federation of the Blind
1800 Johnson St Baltimore, MD 21230
tel: 410 659 9314   fax: 410 685 5653   email: epc@roudley.com.
Committee on the Concerns of the Deafblind evaluates and assists in establishing programs, public education, and scholarships.

National Technical Assistance Consortium (NTAC)
c/o Western Oregon University, 345 N. Monmouth, Monmouth, OR 97361
tel: 503 838 8807   email: ntac@wou.edu
NTAC provides technical assistance ato families and agencies serving children and young adults who are deafblind. NTAC combines the resources, expertise, and experience of two major organizations: Teaching Research and the Helen Keller National Center.

Office of Special Education Programs
U.S. Department of Education, 400 Maryland Ave. SW, MES Building, Washington, DC 20202-2570
tel: 202 205 5507   TTY/TDD: 202 205 9754   fax: 202 260 0416
email: charles-freeman@ed.gov

Administers the Individuals with Disabilities Education Act. Supports state and local educational authorities in implementing the special education mandates.

Overbrook School for the Blind
6333 Malvern Avenue, Philadelphia, PA 19151
tel: 215 877 0313   fax: 215 887 2466   email: denise@computerline.com
Serves children who are deafblind in a variety of programs. Staff use a variety of communication approaches and a functional curriculum is used stressing communication, vision related auditory training, daily living skills, vocational training, social skills, motor skills, recreational skills, O and M, and academics.

Parents of Deafblind Children Partnership
401 N. Pinon, Olathe, KS 66061
tel: 913 764 17231
Promotes networking of parents of deafblind children, sharing of information, and resources.

Perkins School for the Blind
175 North Beacon Street, Watertown, MA 02172
tel: 617 924 3434   fax: 617 926 2027
email: hiltonperkins@perkins.pvt.k12.ma.us

Provides day and residential educational services to students who are deafblind. The program offers both a functional and an academic curriculum, diagnostic/ transitional placements, extensive evaluation services, outreach, work experience, and transition planning.

SKI-HI Institute Outreach, Ski-Hi Institute
c/o Utah State University, 6500 Old Main Hills, Logan, UT 84322-6500
email: skihi@cc.usu.edu
A major focus is on family-centred early intervention for families with infants or preschoolers who are deafblind. Helps agencies to provide home intervention services for families who have children with disabilities by developing programs, materials, and curricula; training professionals; and developing direct service models.

Technical Assistance for Parent Programs (TAPP)
95 Berkeley St, Suite 104, Boston, MA 02116
tel: 617 482 2915   fax: 617 695 2939
Supports parent groups to work more effectively with professionals in educating deafblind children.

Texas School for the Blind and Visually Impaired
1100 W. 45th Street, Austin, TX
The Texas School for the Blind and Visually Impaired provides direct campus-based instruction for Texas students who are deafblind from six to twenty-one years of age based upon referrals from their local school districts. The program has a functional, community-based format, with emphasis on infused development of skills. Contacts for this program should be directed to Lauren Newton, Principal, newton_L@tsb1.tsbvi.educ   fax: 512 458 3395.

The TSBVI also provides training and support for school and community programs serving children who are deafblind from birth to age twenty-five and their families, through the Outreach Program. TSBVI Outreach offers local, regional, and statewide training specifically designed to target the needs of professionals and families with students who are deafblind as well as a quarterly newsletter, an accessible website at http://www.tsbvi.edu, and other resources and supports. Contacts for this program should be directed to Cyral Miller, Outreach Director, at miller_ca@tsb1.tsbvi.educ   fax: 512 206 9320.

Usher Syndrome Around the World (UAW)
P.O. Box 17318, Minneapolis, MN 55417
tel: 612 724 6982   email: kadbmn@aol.com

International Programs

Deafblind International
c/o Sense, 11–13 Clifton Terrace, Finsbury Park, London N4 3SR
tel: 0171 272 7774   fax: 0171 272 6012   email: rodney@sense.org.uk
Sponsors international conferences on issues concerning the support of educators, family members, and individuals who are deafblind. Promotes networking of families through Family Camps associated with the international conferences and the development of programs through the work of its individual members. Publishes *Deafblind Education.*

The EUCO Unit
c/o Instituut voor doven, Sint-Michielsgestel, NL. Theerestraat 42, 5271 GD Sint Michielsgestel
tel: 73 55 88 111   fax: 73 55 12 157
Provides staff training and development and information service for a European and international network.

Hilton/Perkins Program
175 North Beacon Street, Watertown MA 02172
tel: 617 972 7220   fax: 617 923 8076
email: 100575.2522@compuserve.com
Contact: Michael Collins, Director
Africa and the Caribbean: Aubrey Webson, Regional Coordinator
Latin America: Steve Perreault Graciela Ferioli, Regional Coordinators,
Eastern Europe: Dennis Lolli, Regional Coordinator,
Asia-Pacific: Kirk Hoerton, Marianne Riggio Regional Coordinators.
Internationally, the Hilton/Perkins Program assists in the development of educational services for deafblind and multi-handicapped blind children in developing countries. Hilton/Perkins staff work with more than eighty projects in fifty countries. Selected programs are supported in the Asia-Pacific Region, Africa, the Caribbean, Latin America, and Eastern Europe. Support includes assistance with program development, training, and technical assistance for staff and leadership training in the United States of America. Domestically, the program supports university training of teachers, training and technical assistance activities for schools and programs, development of parent organizations, and publications of literature for the field.

Nordic Staff Training Centre for Deafblind Services
Slotsgade 8, DK 9330 Dronninglund, Denmark
tel: 98 84 34 99   fax: 98 84 34 88

Sense International
11–13 Clifton Terrace, Finsbury Park, London N4 3SR
tel: +44 171 272 7774 minicom: +44 171 272 9648
fax: +44 171 272 6012   email: si@sense.org.uk
Sense International supports the development of services for deafblind and multiply disabled people throughout the world. We work with local partners in their own countries to support their ability to provide services themselves. Our main programs are in India, Eastern Europe, and Latin America, and we also offer an international staff development programme in the United Kingdom.

Deafblindness on the Internet

There many resources available on the internet. All over the world individuals and organizations (both national and international) are providing information so that the families of, and professionals working with, individuals who are challenged by this low-incidence disability will have access to resources and reference materials as well as the opportunity to establish networks among themselves to support each other. For example, Megue Nakazawa (email: nakazawa@*nise.go.jp*) of Japan is preparing a Deafblind Information Library for the home page of NISE. Anindya 'Bapin' Bhattacharyya provides an interesting and informative look at computers for the Deafblind at his web site, http://www.ualr.edu/~axbhatta/computer.html. Contributions like these to the area of deafblindness have made the internet a valuable source of up-to-date information.

Deaf-Blind Perspectives by Randy Klumph

Deaf-Blind Perspectives is a free journal-like publication, sponsored by the Teaching Research Division of Western Oregon University. This publication focuses on all pertinent issues important to people who are deafblind, and the people who serve them. *Deaf-Blind Perspectives* is dedicated to facilitating improved service delivery, limiting cross-purpose advocacy, and encouraging the sharing of ideas among all deafblind groups through accurate and contemporary information. *Deaf-Blind Perspectives* spans the entire age range from birth to senior citizen and includes discussions about those who are deafblind and cognitively able and those who are deafblind and cognitively disabled. Articles encompass early intervention, transition, communication techniques, syndrome characteristics, parental concerns, community living options, socialization, and so on. Controversy and discussion are welcome, and sometimes articles may represent opposing views on topics. The publication is a forum for ideas and discussion. Two important contributors are

- DB-LINK – The National Information Clearinghouse On Children And Youth Who Are DeafBlind (http://www.tr.wou.edu/dblink)
- NTAC – The National Technical Assistance Consortium for Children and Young Adults Who Are Deaf-Blind (http://www.tr.wou.edu/ntac).

Deaf-Blind Perspectives is published three times each year and is available in standard print, large-print, Braille, and ASCII formats. The current issue of *Deaf-Blind Perspectives* can be viewed on line (http://www.tr.wou.edu/tr/dbp), and previous issues (in ASCII) are available via FTP.

To order a free subscription to *Deaf-Blind Perspectives*, please send the following information: Your Name, Street, City, State, Zip, Country (if other than U.S.) and email address. Please specify preferred format. Grade 2 Braille, Large Print, disk (ASCII), standard print, email (ASCII) Send to: Deaf-Blind Perspectives, 345 N Monmouth Ave., Monmouth, OR 97361, U.S.A. tel: 503 838 8885;   fax: 503 838 8150;   email: dbp@wou.edu.

DEAFBLND Listserve

A listserve is an email discussion group that easily allows a person to send an identical mail message to all the members of a list simply by sending one message to the list server address. List servers have been used on the internet for years to share ideas, discuss issues, and announce events.

The topic of this email discussion group is Deafblindness. The purpose of this list is to share information, enquiries, ideas and opinions on all matters pertaining to Deafblindness. This list is open to professionals, to persons who are deafblind, and to their families and friends. There are 300 subscribers and it averages thirty-five messages per day. An archive of all messages is available for review at http://www.tr.wou.edu/archives.

To subscribe to the Deafblnd Listserve send the following command as an email message (note that 'deafblnd' is the correct spelling).
SUBSCRIBE DEAFBLND firstname lastname
Leave subject line blank if possible, and do not include a signature; send the email message to
LISTSERV@TR.WOU.EDU
You will then receive an email message asking you to confirm your subscription request. Save that message until your subscription is confirmed.

After you have joined the list, you can send messages to all members at deafblnd@tr.wou.edu. A list of answers to frequently asked question on deafblindness can be obtained from http://www.eng.dmu.ac.uk/~hgs/deafblind/ deafblnd_faq.html You can get an ASCII copy from the DEAFBLND listserver by sending an email message to: listserv@tr.wou.edu containing the command GET DEAFBLND.FAQ.

Places to Start on the Internet

James Gallagher (James@55wilma.demon.co.uk), who himself is deafblind, has put together an award-winning web site that is an excellent starting place for both parents and professionals who wish to access up-to-date information. His home page can be accessed at http://www.s55wilma.demon.co.uk/index. html. It lists topics such as the following:
Other Deafblindness, Resources on the Net
Equipment for Deafblind People
Mailing Lists and Newsletters for Deafblind People on the Net
Blindness Resources on the Net
Deafness Resources on the Net
Other Disabilities Resources on the Net
Equipment and Suppliers for Blind and Deaf People
Newsgroups and Listservs for Blind, Deaf, and Deafblind People
Some of My Friends on the Net

Hugh Sasse, (hgs@dmu.ac.uk) is one of a number of individuals who have worked to establish valuable centres. Hugh's homepage, 'A Deafblindness Web Resource,' is a wonderful mine of information about deafblindness around the world and should be accessed by everyone who has an interest in the field. It can be accessed at: http://www.eng.dmu.ac.uk/~hgs/deafblind/. Another excellent gateway resource page is <http://www.msstate.edu/dept/rrtc/irr/helen. html>

Finally, if you want to know more about services you can get through electronic mail, send an empty message to DrBob@mailback.com. You will receive over thirty pages of valuable information on how to use email to access the net.

Glossary

achilles tendon   the tendon behind the heel

acquired deafblindness   theterm 'acquired' is preferred by the majority of individuals who become deafblind as youths or adults (types 1, 2, and 3; see Preface), rather than the term 'adventitious'

adapted American Sign Language (AASL)   American Sign Language (ASL) adapted for use by individuals who are deafblind

adaptive intelligence   the extent to which measured intelligence has been effectively used in the pursuit of everyday goals

adventitiously   acquired after birth, not inherited

affective domain   concurring feelings and their expression

anterior head position   the head is held in an abnormal forward position

APGAR score   an evaluation of an infant's physical condition usually made one minute after birth and then repeated five minutes after birth Five factors: heart rate, muscle tone, respiratory effort, colour, and reflex irritability are scored from a low of zero to a normal of 2, and the five scores are combined to give a total score of 0 to 10; a total score below 7 indicates distress

attachment theories   theories in which the relationship between access to the caregiver and the initiatives of the child is emphasized and considered crucial to all development

automatization   the mastery of a skill or function to the extent that cognitive resources and attention are less necessary, thus liberating energy to learn new and more advanced functions

balance   equilibrium

behaviouristic approach   a model of learning based on the reinforcement / stimulus-response connections

blind   visual loss of 20/200 or greater in the best eye with correction or a visual field of less than 20 degrees

body image   concept of one's body and body parts and their relationship to each other

central hearing loss   loss due to processing problems in the brain

cerebral palsy   a non-progressive damage to the developing brain, which may occur before, during, or after birth

cognitive domain   of, relating to, or involving cognition – the *cognitive* elements of perception; based on or capable of being reduced to empirical factual knowledge

congenital(ly)   born with

cortex   the outer layer of certain organs such as the brain, kidneys, or adrenal glands; the innermost region of some organs is called the medulla

cortical visual impairment   visual loss due to processing problems in the brain rather than the eye itself or the optic nerve

crook lying   lying on the back with the knees bent and feet flat on the floor

cytoarchitecture   the specific arrangement of cells in tissue, often used to refer to the structure and functional organization of the brain

cytology   the study of individual cells

Deafblind International (DBI)   an organization representing people who work with individuals who are deafblind; membership is open to individuals and organizations; publishers of *Deafblind Education*

Deafblind List   an email site on the internet where information concerning deafblindness is exchanged

declarative   intent to share attention on a common focus and therefore include joint attention

deictic gestures   movements geared at 'showing,' for example, pointing or gazing at

dementia   a general decline in all areas of mental ability, usually due to brain disease; it is progressive, the most obvious feature being decreasing intellectual ability

dialogic ways   talking together

dialogue   communication requires a 'dialogic' activity, which means that the two partners are active participants and organize their contributions in a dialogic way; not necessarily verbal

disinhibition   loss or reduction of an inhibition (as by the action of interfering stimuli or events)

distance senses   vision and hearing

dizygotic   derived from two ova

dyad   the two people involved in a dialogue

dyadic joint space   joint attention, by both partners, to a third element that has not already been loaded with emotion *emotional bonding* the process of establishing attachment of individuals to each other, fostered through shared pleasurable experiences

emotional readiness the point at which facets of the landscape can be assimilated into the lifesphere

epistemology the study or a theory of the nature and grounds of knowledge especially with reference to its limits and validity

extended family includes parents, children, and all other relations, such as grandparents, uncles, aunts, and cousins

fading changing gradually (as in amount of physical support and manipulation by a caregiver)

father play roughhouse play stressing balance, holding on, and so forth, usually with the child sitting on the adult's knee; promotes bonding and social interaction

flaccidity state of complete muscle relaxation and lacking tone

fm systems a frequency modulation system used to broadcast signals from a microphone to a receiver (a microphone worn by an intervenor to broadcast speech sounds to a receiver worn by a deafblind individual)

formative evaluation an ongoing evaluation of a individual or program designed to identify and act upon changes

four-point kneeling kneeling with straight arms and legs at right angles to the trunk, shoulders, and hips, resting on flat hands and knees

frames of activities the detailed structure of sequences of events that ensure that opportunities to work on specific objectives will occur

frustration/reward a motivational technique: frustrating the child is expected to motivate him/her to speak; the reward is outside the interaction (which is not seen as the main motivator)

gait manner of walking

geniculate bent abruptly at an angle like a bent knee

goals a statement identifying a desired, future outcome; in the context of the Personal Plan, usually at the end of a five-year period

grade one Braille letter-by-letter representation using a six-cell format; read using tactile input

grade two Braille representation of words using a short-form code and contractions of words or parts of words; for example, dot five M stands for mother

habilitation to prepare an individual to fit into society

haptic memory memory relating to or based on the sense of touch

hydrocephalus an abnormal accumulation of fluid in the cranial vault causing an enlarged head; May be congenital or adventitious and have sudden onset or be slowly progressive

hydrotherapy the use of water to treat disorders; mostly limited to exercises in special pools *hypoactivity*   little or no activity

hypotonia   decreased tone of skeletal muscles; floppiness

imperative   relating to gestures used in an instrumental way; for example, pointing to obtain desired objects/events; does not include joint attention

incidental learning   non-directed learning; learning resulting from unplanned exposure to information or actions

Individual Educational Plan (IEP)   plan describing how an individual will benefit from an educational program, including any modifications to be made to meet his or her educational needs

Individual Pupil Plan (IPP)   plan describing how an individual will benefit from a modified educational program

instrumentation   process through which functions are developed and organized in the brain; for instance, vision is instrumented through the activity of the child, which connects movements and visual information

intellective   having, relating to, or belonging to the intellect

interactional exchanges   directional or reciprocal action or influence between or among individuals

interaction sequence   the stages of physical action/reaction between the instructor and the deafblind individual that progress from hand-on-hand teaching techniques, through reduced degrees of physical and communative support, to support being provided on request

interactional patterns   recognizable repetition of mutual or reciprocal action or influence

intersubjectivity   involving two individuals; primary intersubjectivity emphasizes interpersonal togetherness and interaction during which the partners start sharing emotions and attention; it gradually progresses to secondary intersubjectivity as communicative acts are sustained in face-to-face interaction and attention is directed at a third element which is the topic of conversation

IQ   an expression of how well a person performed on a standardized intelligence test in comparison with others of the same age group

kinaesthetic   sensorily mediated by end organs located in muscles, tendons, and joints and stimulated by bodily movements and tensions; also sensory experience derived from these organs

landscape   the objective world with which we are not yet familiar or comfortable

large print   print of 18 points or larger, making it easier to read

laterally rotated hips   hips rotated outwards

learned helplessness   a state resulting from not having the opportunity to experience, and learn from, one's actions; to be prevented from intellectual or physical development through the actions of others and thus causing one to function at a level significantly lower than that which could be attained

Life of Quality a lifestyle in which one has the same control over and expectations of his/her world as his/her peers

lifesphere that part of ourselves and the world with which we are familiar and comfortable

locus of security the figurative centre of one's lifesphere maintained through one's strongest emotional bonds

lumbrical action bending at the knuckles and the joints at the base of the fingers and toes

maldevelopment non, delayed, incomplete, or damaged growth

midline the median line or median plane of the body

millisecond thousandth of a second

monozygotic derived from a single egg

multi-sensory deprivation (MSD) deprived of a necessary level of information from the distance senses of vision and hearing

neurochemical chemical processes and phenomena related to the nervous system

neurological relating to the scientific study of the nervous system, especially in respect to its structure, functions, and abnormalities

neurological maturation the process or reaching full development of the nervous system

non-functional movements movements that serve no useful purpose, such as flicking fingers in front of eyes or head banging

non-verbal being other than verbal; involving minimal use of language; or ranking low in verbal skill; unable to use verbal language to communicate effectively compared with non-handicapped peers

nuclear family a family group that consists only of father, mother, and children

objectives specific success indicators, written in behavioural terms, that will be used to measure progress at the end of the time for which the objectives were written (term, six months, one year)

objects of reference objects that are used to refer to an activity as a way of informing a child, or of support an exchange (e.g., a towel, indicating it is time to have a bath)

on-line assessment evaluation of the child's responses during interaction with him/her to establish the level of functioning, the next level to be attained, and/or the new response desired; evaluation may be conscious or automatic

orientation and mobility   the ability to locate one's position in relationship to the environment and the ability to move about the environment safely

panencephalitis   an inflammation of the entire brain marked by progressive deterioration of mental and motor skills

pelvic rotation   situation where one pelvic bone lies farther forward than the other

perception   the learned ability to register consciously and give meaning to sensory stimulus

peripheral joints   fingers and toes

plantar-flexed feet   feet pointing downwards

positioning   placement of the body parts

posture   position of the body

prenatal viral insult   a viral infection occurring, existing, before birth

primary intersubjectivity   observed during the first six months of life during interactions between children and partners when no objects are integrated in the interaction (e.g., exchange of vocalizations)

pronation   act of turning the palms downward

prone lying   lying, face down

proprioception   the reception of stimuli produced within

protracted shoulder girdle   rounded shoulders with the shoulder joints sitting forward of the body midline

proximal senses   next to or nearest the point of attachment or origin, a central point, especially: located towards the centre of the body

psychologic   relating to the mind, its activity, or its products as an object of study

psychomotor domain   of or relating to motor action directly proceeding from mental activity

reactive environment   an environment designed to allow the individual who is deafblind to have the same control as the person who is non-handicapped; not without rules, regulations, responsibilities, or tasks; each individual is treated with respect by others, listened to by others, and encouraged to communicate his/her ideas

reciprocal social togetherness   a theory that postulates that the result of the simultaneous presence of an anxiety-evoking stimulus and an anxiety-lessening situation will be that the stimulus produces less anxiety

reciprocity   the quality or state of being reciprocal: mutual dependence, action, or influence

regulation   the maintaining of an interaction by both partners, for example, tempo, rhythm, intensity, space, novelty, timing

rehabilitation   restoration of a former capacity; return to a condition of health or useful and constructive activity

residual vision   remaining vision after a pre- or post-natal visual insult resulting in visual impairment or legal blindness

resonance   a phenomenon related to sharing in which the deafblind child is joined in an action already in his/her repertoire; this action is then modified using start/stop signals originating in the child

retinoblastoma   a malignant tumour of the retina that develops during childhood, is derived from retinal germ cells, and is associated with a chromosomal abnormality

secondary intersubjectivity   interaction between child and partner based on sharing or joint attention directed at a third element, usually an object; communicative acts are sustained in face-to-face interaction and attention; starts during the second half of the year

sharing   the experience of mutual attention with another

side lying   lying on the right or left side, with the lower leg bent for stability

signal   any object triggering a reaction; by contrast, a symbol signifies or represents a referent

Signing Exact English (SEE)   signing each word in the same order and form exactly as it is used in communication between two non-disabled individuals

silent page system   system in which a pager uses vibrations rather than sound to alert the person to whom a message is being delivered

somatosensory   relating to a sensory activity having its origin elsewhere than in the special sense organs (as eyes and ears) and conveying information about the state of the body proper and its immediate environment

spasticity   a state in which there is abnormal active pull or resistance of muscles to passive displacement of a limb, particularly in one direction of joint movement

spatial awareness   the ability to recognize and remember objects in space and their relationship to the body

spina bifida   developmental defect in which the vertebral arches of a part of the spinal column are missing and the spinal membranes and sometimes the cord protrude

strabismic   relating to inability of one eye to attain binocular vision with the other because of imbalance of the muscles of the eyeball – also called *squint*

success indicators   actions that will be observed, which indicate the attainment of a specific objective

summative evaluation   an evaluation that takes place at a specific time to identify an individual's level of functioning

supination   act of turning the palms upward

Tadoma   method of communication based on perceiving the voice of the speaker through touching the lips and neck

time-in   a social disapproval technique appropriate to deafblind children, in contrast to the 'time-out' isolation technique

TTY   an electrical device that uses a telephone connection to transmit and receive messages

two-hand manual alphabet   a representation of the alphabet using two hands, primarily used in the United Kingdom, in contrast to the one-hand representation used in North America

whole-whole approach   stresses the presentation of all aspect of the activity and the involvement of the person who is deafblind in a meaningful way throughout the activity, as opposed to breaking the activity into subroutines and teaching each such routine in isolation